Fundamentals of Medical Science for Medical Record Personnel

Contributors

Timothy E. Aldrich
Juanita S. Pursel

Fundamentals of Medical Science for Medical Record Personnel

Florence C. Amato
Florida International University
North Miami, Florida

AN ASPEN PUBLICATION®
Aspen Systems Corporation
Rockville, Maryland
Royal Tunbridge Wells
1985

Library of Congress Cataloging in Publication Data

Amato, Florence C.
Fundamentals of medical science for medical record personnel.

Includes bibliographies and index.
1. Medicine. 2. Medical sciences. 3. Medical record personnel.
I. Title. [DNLM: 1. Anatomy. 2. Diseases. 3. Pathology.
4. Physiology. QZ 140 A488f]
R129.A43 1985 610 84-24561
ISBN: 0-89443-567-1

Publisher: John R. Marozsan
Associate Publisher: Jack W. Knowles, Jr.
Editor-in-Chief: Michael Brown
Executive Managing Editor: Margot G. Raphael
Managing Editor: M. Eileen Higgins
Editorial Services: Jane Coyle
Printing and Manufacturing: Debbie Collins

Library of Congress Catalog Card Number: 84-24561
ISBN: 0-89443-567-1

Printed in the United States of America

2 3 4 5

To my husband,
Paul

Table of Contents

Preface

My career in medical record administration has encompassed many years both in the field and as an educator. Each area of endeavor has convinced me that medical record personnel need to have a better understanding of the fundamentals of disease processes. The current emphasis on medical record coding that has been brought about by the prospective payment system serves to emphasize the medical expertise that is so necessary to us as professionals.

This book is written at the request of the students with whom I have had the pleasure of working over the past 15 years. It is offered to them and their colleagues. It is designed to serve them in their expanding administrative roles by presenting diseases of the major diagnostic categories listed under the Diagnosis Related Grouping System. It is hoped that the book will aid employees who seek more knowledge in order to produce quality data and optimal hospital reimbursement. Most of all, however, it is offered to those who have a thirst for knowledge about the fundamentals of medical science as applied to medical records.

Acknowledgments

It has taken me four years to write this book. During that time, my husband, Paul A. Amato, was of immeasurable assistance because of his understanding and moral support. I am also grateful to Margaret Wade, M.D., who inspired me to do the writing—although at times I was not always so grateful for this task.

Special thanks go to members of Florida International University faculty—Lillian Lodge Kopenhaver, Ed.D., Communication Department; Timothy Aldrich, M.P.H., Ph.D., Department of Health Services Administration; and Juanita S. Pursel, R.R.A., M.S.W., Department of Medical Record Administration—for their comments and opinions. I also express my appreciation to Aspen Systems and their reviewers for their valuable suggestions. And to you readers, I am especially grateful that you have given me this opportunity to add my efforts to the advancement of the medical record profession.

Introduction

> Title VI of Public Law 98-21 added section 1886(d) to the Social Security Act (the Act) establishing a prospective payment system for Medicare payment of inpatient hospital services. Medicare payment is made at a predetermined, specific rate for each discharge. All discharges are classified according to a list of diagnosis-related groups (DRGs). (*Federal Register,* Rules and Regulations, Vol. 49, No. 1, Tuesday, January 3, 1984)

The purpose of this book is not to have the students and medical record personnel acquire a physician's depth of theoretical knowledge about medicine, but rather to have them gain the basic knowledge that is required for identifying documentation of clinical data found in the patient's medical record. It has been designed to be understood by those who are not physicians, but whose responsibility to code diagnoses impacts the financial stability of health care institutions.

The book is divided into two parts. Part I is an overview of body functions. Chapters 1 through 4 provide a brief description of cells, metabolism, tissues, and tissue adaptation.

Part II is the heart of the book. It comprises eleven chapters: a separate chapter for each body system—integumentary, musculoskeletal, nervous, endocrine, sense organs, cardiovascular, respiratory, digestive, genitourinary—and a chapter devoted to the female reproductive system. The format for each chapter is essentially the same. First the function and structures within the system are described, and then the diseases affecting that particular system are detailed, with concentration initially on the congenital or hereditary defects and then on the acquired diseases. Illustrations are given when relevant. Descriptions of diagnostic techniques and surgical procedures have been provided where applicable.

Because cancer is such a major concern of our health delivery system, as well as to the public at large, a special view of this complex of diseases is the subject of

Chapter 15. In a further effort to make this text suitable for the current needs of medical record personnel, Appendix A provides information on Diagnosis-Related Groups, including definitions and practical examples.

Part I

Overview of Body Functions

Chapter 1

The Cell: Basic Structure of Life

Juanita S. Pursel

Objectives

- Recognize and define specific terms related to the structure of the cell.
- List the types of cell and describe the function of each.
- Discuss the size and shape of cells in relation to their specific function.
- Describe the three basic components of the cell and discuss the function of each.
- List the subunits contained within the cell and discuss their various functions.
- Discuss and compare the two types of cell division.
- Explain the role of chromosomes and genes in cell division.

INTRODUCTION

Fundamental to understanding disease is the concept of the function of normal cells. The diagnosis of a disease often depends on cytology, or the study of cells, their origin, structure, and function.

All cells are not alike; they differ in function according to structure. A group of like cells form tissue. An organ is a structure composed of various types of tissue; thus, an organ is composed of thousands of cells and performs more complex functions than any single cells or type of tissue alone. The heart, lungs, liver, pancreas, stomach, kidneys, and uterus are only a few of the many organs in the human body. A group of organs working together form a system.

A system is the largest organizational unit considered in studies of the body. It consists of a group of organs working together to perform a more complex function than any one organ performs. The systems are as follows: integumentary, musculoskeletal, nervous, endocrine, sense organs, cardiovascular, respiratory, digestive, genitourinary, and reproductive systems.

CELL STRUCTURE

Cells, the basic structure of life, differ in size and shape, depending on structure. Muscle cells contract and nerve cells send impulses. A skeletal muscle cell may be several centimeters long. The length of a nerve cell depends on its activity. Nerve cell processes extend for a meter or more. Blood cells are small enough to pass through capillaries. The sperm is the smallest cell and the ovum, approximately 200 micrometers, is the largest.

The shape of cells depends on their function. Red blood cells are disk-shaped in order to provide adequate surface for oxygen exchange. White blood cells are always changing shape as they move throughout the body and engulf parasitic invaders. Some cells resemble stones; some are flat and round, like a coin; and some are long and thin, like threads.

Although cells differ in size and shape, the basic cell components are (a) a surface membrane called *plasma membrane,* (b) a semifluid substance called *cytoplasm,* and (c) a structure located centrally in the cytoplasm called the *nucleus* (see Figure 1–1).

Cell (Plasma) Membrane

The cytoplasm and nucleus are enclosed by an outer living edge of plasma cells, forming a membrane that separates the environment within the cell, intracellular, from that on the outside, extracellular. The membrane is usually pliable, but it may be rigid. It is capable of growth and repair.

Figure 1–1 Cell

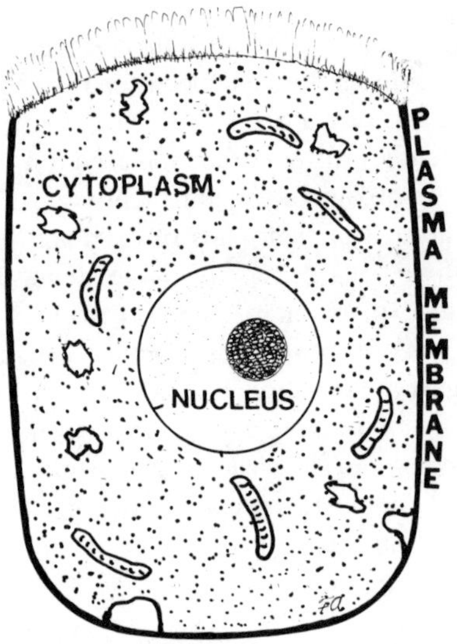

The plasma membrane is trilaminar (three-layered)—two protein layers separated by a lipid (fat) layer, which allows fluids, such as water and inorganic salt, to pass across the membrane. The outer and inner protein layers act as catalysts (slowing down or speeding up reactions) for specific metabolic or chemical reactions and regulate what passes in or out of the cell.

Regulation is brought about by the lipid layer sandwiched between the inner and outer protein layers. Only those substances that are soluble in lipid or in which lipid is soluble are able to pass through pores in the membrane. Therefore, the cell membrane is said to be semipermeable, allowing some substances to pass through and restricting others.

Although the cell membrane regulates the passage of some substances in and out of the cell through pores in the membrane, other materials cross the cell membrane through direct transportation. In some cells, the plasma membrane may surround solid particles and take them into vacuoles (a minute space or cavity in the tissues containing air or fluid). This process, called *phagocytosis,* is performed by white blood cells. Some large molecules dissolved in fluid are stored by the cell membrane in vacuoles. This is known as *pinocytosis*. These two functions are shown in Figure 1–2.

However, no matter by what means materials cross the cell membrane, it has selective permeability that can determine which materials enter or leave the cell.

In some cells the membrane has small fingerlike projections, called microvilli, on its surfaces. These projections increase the cell's area of absorption. Microvilli

Figure 1–2 Cell

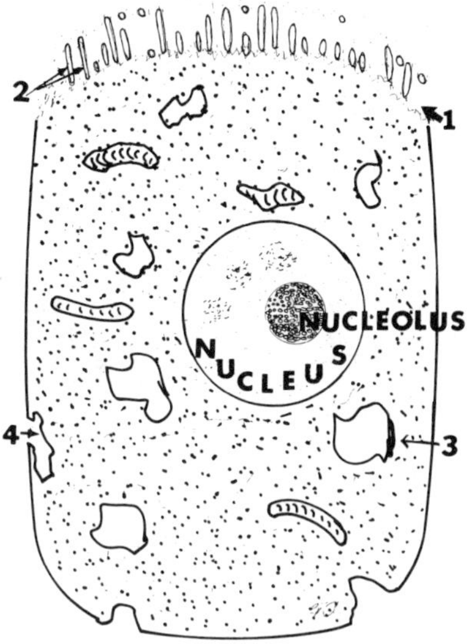

1. MICROVILLI 2. MICROTUBULES
3. VACUOLES 4. PINOCYTOSIS

contain a center of protein tubules (microtubules) that function in transporting materials along their surfaces. For example, in the trachea, cilia move material along the trachea's surface; on the tail of a sperm cell, an elongated cilium, the flagellum, transports sperm to unite with the ova.

Cytoplasm

The cytoplasm, the intracellular matrix surrounding the nucleus, contains subunits called inclusions and organelles.

Cytoplasmic Inclusions

Inclusions are nonliving materials, such as lipid (fat), carbohydrates (sugars), pigment, protein, and secretory droplets. They are stored in the cell to be used as sources of energy by the cell in its life processes.

Organelles

Organelles are membrane-bound organized living units that perform tasks of metabolism, reproduction, and growth for the cell (Figure 1–3). They are com-

Figure 1–3 Organelles

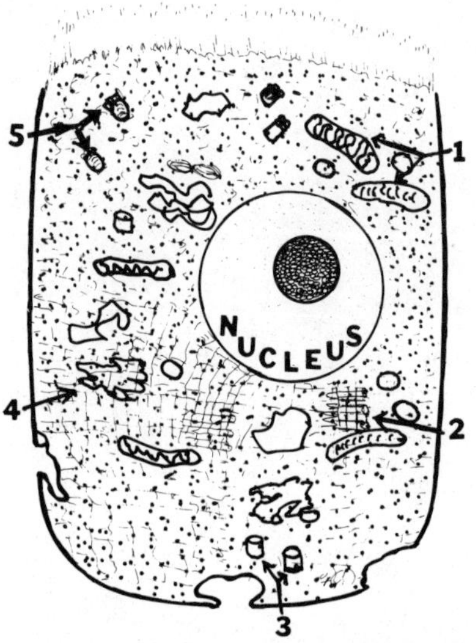

1. MITOCHONDRIA 2. ERGASTOPLASM
3. LYSOSOMES 4. GOLGI COMPLEX
5. CENTROSOMES

---

posed of membranes and enzymes, which are released by the regulation of the nucleus. Organelles occur in almost all types of cells, including (a) mitochondria, (b) ergastoplasm, (c) lysosomes, (d) Golgi complex, and (e) centrioles.

Mitochondria. Mitochondrial organelles are described by *Dorland's Medical Dictionary* as "small spherical to rod-shaped components . . . found in the cytoplasm of cells." They function by supporting the metabolism of the cells. Rich in enzymes, they attract high-energy phosphate compounds. Mitochondria are found in cells in which high metabolic activity is required, such as in the kidney tubules and the skeletal muscles. Exercise of the skeletal muscles increases the number of mitochondria present and disuse of muscles decreases their number and size.

Ergastoplasm. Ergastoplasm, or granular endoplasmic reticulum, is a complex network of delicate membranes roughened by small particles of ribosomes; the function of ribosomes is to synthesize new cell protein. Ribonucleic messenger (RNA), a nucleic acid, transmits information from the nucleus to the protein-forming system of the cell. Ribosomes function in accordance with the coded information carried by ribonucleic messengers from the nucleus.

Agranular endoplasmic reticulum has a smooth surface because of the absence of ribosomes. It is found in smooth muscle cells.

Both forms of endoplasmic reticulum are found in the liver.

Lysosomes. Lysosomes, microscopically dense bodies scattered throughout the cytoplasm, are membranous sacs containing approximately 20 potent hydrolytic enzymes. A hydrolytic enzyme is one that catalyzes the splitting of a compound into fragments by the addition of water. Such enzymes are capable of splitting polypeptide, lipid, and carbohydrate bonds. The enzymes found in lysosomes function primarily in digestion of proteins, nucleic acids, mucopolysaccharides, and glycogen.

Golgi Complex. The Golgi complex, continuous with ergastoplasm and adjacent to the nucleus, is composed of membranous plates that function by condensing and packaging proteins or mucus from the ergastoplasm for export from the cell. In the pancreas, the Golgi complex packages enzymes (protein) into droplets, which flow into the pancreatic duct. In the lining of the intestinal and respiratory tracts, the Golgi complex synthesizes secretions, thereby protecting the internal surfaces of the organs.

Centrioles. Centrioles are essential to cell division. Before cell division, the centrosome (a specialized area of cytoplasm containing centrioles) divides into two centrioles. During cell division, the centrioles are involved in the movement of chromosomes. A chromosome is the structure in the nucleus of the cell that contains genetic material, proteins, and RNA.

Nucleus

The nucleus is a spheroid body within a cell. It is the structure and functional center that controls metabolic processes and reproduction; it also provides hereditary mechanisms used in cell reproduction.

The nucleus consists of a nucleolus and chromatin in nucleoplasm, surrounded by a nuclear membrane.

Nuclear Membrane

The nuclear membrane is similar to the plasma membrane, as it regulates interactions between the nucleus and the cytoplasm but disappears during cell division. On the outer layer of the membrane are ribosomes and pores, which provide communication between the nucleoplasm and the cytoplasm. The outer layer of the membrane contains RNA. The nuclear membrane is continuous with the other membrane wall, the endoplasmic reticulum. When the cell divides, the membrane disappears.

Nucleolus

The nucleolus, a vacuolelike body rich in RNA within the nucleus of the cell, assists in directing the synthesis of protein in the cytoplasm.

Chromatin

Chromatin, which is composed of deoxyribonucleic acid (DNA) and protein, is the material found in chromosomes. The nucleus has 46 chromosomes, including 22 pairs of autosomes and 2 sex chromosomes. The chromosomes comprise chains of double-helix genes made from DNA. The genetic information is communicated to the cytoplasm by RNA molecules. RNA acts both as a messenger for DNA and as a constructor by gathering amino acid to make protein molecules.

Genes (DNA), subunits of chromosomes, control the metabolic activity and structural components of the cell, as well as the production of enzymes and hormones. They also direct the development and characteristics of each human being.

CELL DIVISION

There are two types of cell division: mitosis and meiosis.

Mitosis

Mitosis is the method of cell division whereby the cell grows by division, producing tissues and organs. The cell in the normal functioning state, interphase, passes through a continuous four-phase process: (1) prophase, (2) metaphase, (3) anaphase, and (4) telophase (Figure 1–4).

Prophase

In this first stage of mitosis, the chromatin network (DNA) becomes increasingly coiled as chromosomes become identifiable. The chromosomes may be described as two parallel pairs of coiled strands (chromatids) attached at the center (centromere). The cell nucleus begins to lose its identity as the nuclear membrane disappears. The centrioles migrate to opposite sides of the cell. A spindle of thin fibrils or astral rays forms to connect the two centrioles.

Metaphase

In the second phase of mitosis, two chromatids (coiled filaments) emerge from the chromosome as it divides. The chromatids migrate to the center of the cell,

Figure 1–4 Mitosis

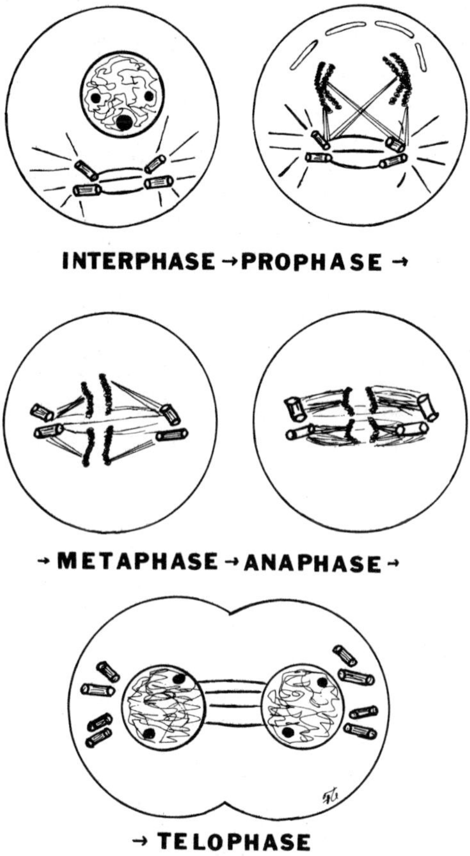

perpendicular to the spindles at the equatorial plate; here at their center (centromere), they are attached to the thin fibrils (astral rays) connecting the centrioles. The nucleus is no longer present.

Anaphase

During the third phase, the thin fibrils (astral rays) appear to pull the two pairs of chromatids apart as the centromere divides to form chromosomes for two cells. The importance of this phase is that one chromatid from each of the 46 chromosomes must be present in each daughter cell. The nucleus is still absent.

Telophase

In this last phase of mitosis, the chromosomes reach the location of the centrioles and begin to uncoil. As they uncoil, the thin fibrils (astral rays) disappear. A nuclear membrane surrounds each group of chromosomes and a nucleolus appears in the nucleus. Indentations from the cell membrane (plasmalemma) become visible at the equatorial plate as the cytoplasm divides, forming two cells each enclosed by a separate cell membrane.

Meiosis

Meiosis occurs in spermatozoa and ova, sex cells. The process is similar to that of mitosis but differs in that it consists of two successive cellular divisions with only a single replication of the chromosomes (Figure 1–5). Meiosis reduces the number of chromosomes in the daughter cells to 23, one-half the normal number. The egg and sperm each have 23 chromosomes. Therefore, when the egg is fertilized by the sperm, the 46 chromosomes are restored.

Figure 1–5 Meiosis

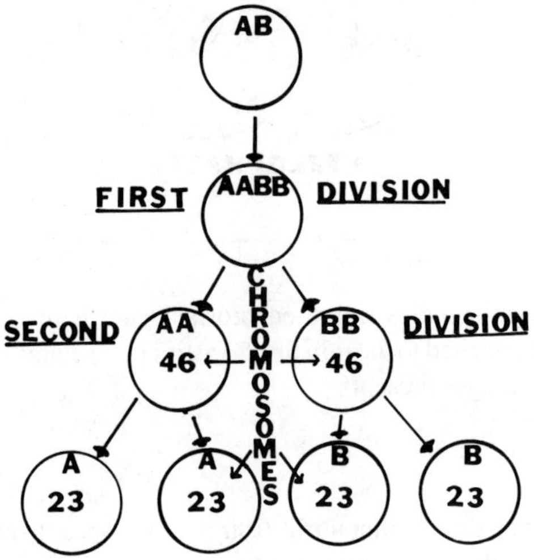

SUMMARY

This chapter has presented information about the structure and function of the cell. Components of the cell were explained. The role of the nucleus in reproduction was given. A group of like cells form tissues. The following chapter will discuss metabolism.

REFERENCE

Jacobs, Stanley, Francone, Clarice A., and Lassow, Walter J. *Structure and Function in Man,* 5th ed. Philadelphia: W. B. Saunders Co., 1982, chap. 3.

Chapter 2

Metabolism

Timothy E. Aldrich

Objectives

- Recognize and define specific terms concerning the process of metabolism.
- Describe, in general, the process of systemic metabolism.
- List and describe the three means by which substances are moved in and out of a cell.
- Describe, in general, the process of cellular metabolism.
- Discuss the three major metabolic processes.
- Discuss the interrelationship of tissues, organs, and cellular activities.
- Discuss the similarities and differences of cell types.
- Describe the relative time factor in cellular activities.

SYSTEMIC METABOLISM

As food and liquids are ingested or gases inhaled, the processes of metabolism are in place to function. Foodstuffs are digested (i.e., reduced to basic chemical composition) into a form that can be absorbed through the bowel. This process is called *catabolism*, the tearing down of substances. Both fluids and digested foodstuffs provide nourishment by way of the bloodstream's distribution throughout the body. Generally, these nutrients are used in *anabolism,* the building up of body tissue. Necessary gases (e.g., oxygen, nitrogen) are likewise diffused across the lung tissues and circulated to all cells by the blood. The tissue level processes involved are elaborated in Part II.

Anabolism and catabolism are in fact aspects of the single continuum, metabolism. Both are necessary, and both lead to waste or inert residues that must be excreted. Excretion, like absorption, involves more than one system. Waste gases are expired through the lungs. Fluids and solid waste are evacuated by the urinary and digestive systems, respectively. Thus the organismic perspective of metabolism is complete: Nourishment enters the body; it is broken down, distributed, and used for sustenance; wastes are eliminated.

This description, however, is too superficial, because the details of how the body survives are not included. What happens when the nourishment reaches the cells?

Distribution

As indicated earlier, nutrients are transported to single cells through the circulatory system. Fluids compose the serum and the dissolved gases are transported by specialized molecules (hemoglobin). At the cell surface, these nutrients are absorbed and wastes are released by basic diffusion mechanisms. The cell membrane is semipermeable; that is, it is selectively permeable. This means that molecules are absorbed across the membrane depending on their size, molecular weight, and electrical charge. Selective permeability is a critical aspect of the cell's protection and represents a marvelously simple first line of defense for the body.

Movement of substances in and out of the cell is accomplished by three means: (1) osmosis, (2) active transport, and (3) specialized transport.

Osmosis

Osmosis is taken from the Greek word for push. Simply stated, many chemicals will be transported in and out of the cell by a balancing of the concentration gradient. That is, the cell will seek to have its internal and external environments be compatible or static. Thus as more nourishment is available outside the cell than inside the cell, osmosis balances the gradient. The property of the body that causes it to maintain its internal stability is *homeostasis*.

Active Transport

Active transport permits a cell to move a substance from a part of lower concentration to one of higher concentration. This goes against the gradient of balance and thus is different from osmosis. An example of active transport involves nerve cells in which certain charged molecules (e.g., sodium, potassium) must be kept in critical balance to facilitate the chemical firing that represents nerve impulses. Sodium and potassium ''pumps'' move these molecules back into the nerve cell after firing.

Specialized Transport

Another form of active transport is specialized transport. The mechanisms of specialized transport involve a combining, or piggy-backing, of a molecule into the cell by a carrier molecule.

CELLULAR METABOLISM

The rudiments of moving substances in and out of the cell have now been introduced. What happens, then, while these substances are within the cell? Three principal activities within the cell constitute metabolism. Each activity is integrated into the operation of the cell so that all processes are occurring simultaneously. The steps that are involved in the process and the sequences in which events transpire are not presented in detail here. Only this comment is offered: Just as the body has a physical structure, it also has a temporal one. Activities of the cell, the tissues, and the organism follow a specific chronobiologic schedule. This schedule is delineated and individualized to some extent, yet it represents the natural order and is a critical part of human life.

This overview focuses on the three major metabolic processes in isolation: (1) energy production, (2) synthesis of proteins, and (3) internal regulation.

Energy Production

Energy is necessary for the body as it drives the chemical reactions that sustain life. Where does energy come from? Energy arises from chemical reactions themselves. Some chemical reactions require energy to proceed (endergonic) and others produce energy as they proceed (exergonic). Maintenance of equilibrium in the body has been previously mentioned and is exemplified here in the form of balanced chemical reactions. Energy is never truly lost or created; it is simply transformed. The transformation of energy begins in the cytoplasm of the cell and moves to the mitochondria, the body's energy factories.

Carbohydrates, the substrate for energy production in the body, are compounds that contain carbon, hydrogen, and oxygen in a 1:2:1 ratio. They may be either monosaccharides (as glucose), disaccharides (maltose), or complex strings called polysaccharides (glycogen). Energy is produced from a series of reactions that begins with a breaking down of glycogen (glycolysis) to glucose. Glucose is further reduced to pyruvic acid, which in turn is converted into a complex molecule called acetylcoenzyme A (acetyl-CoA). The acetyl-CoA enters a metabolic cycle called the *Krebs cycle* (after Sir Hans Krebs, who described its existence in 1937). The process is also known as the *citric acid cycle,* a term derived from the first step, in which the acetyl group is lifted from the Co-A and combined with oxaloacetic acid to form citric acid. The total process itself is considered a cycle, as the oxaloacetic acid is constantly regenerated.

The energy production of the Krebs cycle is mediated by enzymatic action. *Enzymes* are elemental units of the cell that react with specific chemicals to produce a change in the chemical. This production of a change, without being part of the change, is termed *catalysis*. The enzymes and coenzymes that act in conjunction with specific enzymes that participate in the Krebs cycle are a diverse group of highly specialized molecules. Suffice it to say that these enzymes drive chemical changes that result in the production of energy carriers. Figure 2–1 shows the Krebs cycle.

It is not necessary for you to memorize the chemical structures of the various compounds that are formed or to recall their names. This information is included only to provide you with the concept of enzymes working in an ordered sequence (like an assembly line) to produce energy for the cells.

Energy thus fuels the cells' metabolism. All working of the cytoplasm and nucleus requires energy. Myriad other enzymes are involved in the many chemical reactions that maintain life. These enzymes rely on the energy carriers to drive reactions to completion or to receive the energy released. Yet the independent process of energy production is necessary, as the body uses up more energy than it produces. Thus the balance needed for life requires input or fuel; this is the nourishment that is taken into the body. This process also produces wastes (e.g., water, carbon dioxide), which must be eliminated.

Synthesis of Proteins

Proteins are used both as structural elements by the cell and as regulators in cell processes. They are, then, both the functional unit of metabolism and the product of metabolism. Proteins are complex groups of nitrogen-containing molecules called *amino acids*. Only 20 known amino acids are found in living systems. Each of these building blocks of life contains an amino (nitrogen) group, a carboxyl

Figure 2–1 The Krebs Cycle

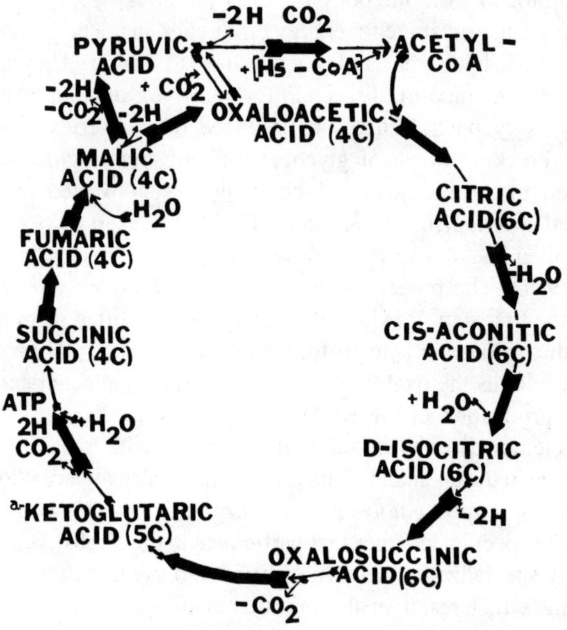

(carbon, oxygen, hydrogen) group, and a characteristic radical that differentiates it from the others. The amino acid groups float free in the cytoplasm; some are made in the cell, and others are obtained only through the food that is ingested.

In the cell, metabolic functions are controlled by the nuclear elements called chromosomes. The chromosomes contain the cell's genetic material, that is, the coded information inherited from preceding cellular generations. Through mechanisms that are largely unknown or too complex for elaboration here, the nucleus is stimulated to produce a particular protein. A section of a particular chromosome is then "opened" to be read by a messenger molecule. The messenger molecule makes a copy of the sequence of informational units (called *codons*) that call for a particular protein. It then exits from the nucleus into the cytoplasm, where it is transcribed (or read again) by an assembling unit, the ribosome. At each unit codon in the messenger's sequences, one amino acid is attached to a building string of other amino acids. The process of attaching amino acids involves the liberating of a water molecule to form a peptide bond (between the two amino acids). Thus the ribosomes "read" along the messenger molecule and attach the amino acids that are called for, to form a polypeptide chain (Figure 2–2).

The polypeptide chain is the basic unit of a protein molecule. Fibrinous protein (i.e., muscles) may be simply polypeptide chains. Single chains may coil about

Figure 2–2 Polypeptide Chain (6 of 20 Amino Acids)

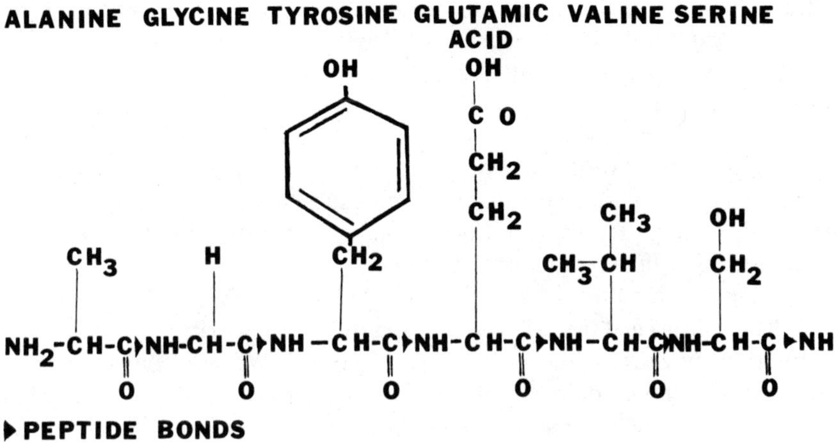

themselves or cross-bind to other polypeptide chains to form structural units. Peptide chains may fold into various shapes to form globular protein molecules. As mentioned previously, the functions of proteins are vast. They are the structure of all tissues and the products of cells; they represent the regulators of all higher functions (i.e., hormones, enzymes). Proteins may be either active in their original form or combined with other proteins or molecules (i.e., metal bearing), as in hemoglobin.

Other objects of cellular metabolism include polysaccharides (strings of sugars) and lipids. Sugar metabolism is mediated by several enzyme pathways (i.e., sequential process), somewhat as described for energy production. Likewise, lipid metabolism is a diverse proposition and is not elaborated here. It is important to recognize, however, that lipids are used both as structural elements of cells and as sources of energy. Lipids, as a group, are insoluble in water and are characterized by the structures in the cell membrane; they are polar molecules (i.e., oriented), so that one end is water soluble and the other is not. In the cell membrane, the insoluble ''heads'' of phospholipids are aligned in rows to contain the cell's watery interior.

Internal Regulation

The exact methods of internal regulation or systemic control are unknown. One aspect of regulation is recognition of when energy is needed and when certain proteins must be synthesized. How the nucleus detects these needs or receives the message is uncertain, but the information is transmitted. The manifestation of these stimuli on the body are seen as fatigue, hormonal signals, sentinel cell, and so forth.

On a cellular level, the process of internal control is primarily one of timing. As mentioned earlier, the body contains a chronologic structure that is a marvel of nature. Cells pass through definitive cycles of dormancy (rest), growth (synthesis), and division. A consideration of this cyclic existence is the maintenance of the cell's cytoplasm so that critical chemical levels are kept constant (e.g., water content). Disposal of wastes is another regulatory necessity. Wastes may be either gathered into circumscribed containers (vacuoles) for ejection from the cell, packaged for digestion (by the Golgi complex), or diffused out of the cell's membrane (as with excess water and gases).

Cell growth is a matter of careful regulation because the cell's volume increases from metabolism, and the cell membrane must be compensated to maintain the equilibrium pressure that maximizes cell activity. When sufficient mass is achieved and the cytoplasm volume will accommodate, then the division (mitosis–asexual reproduction) process must be orchestrated. With all these delicate processes needed to sustain life, one can easily see how fragile health is and how complex the proposition of illness can be. Loss of cellular regulation is among the most common afflictions. Significant molecules to be synthesized include those needed by the cell itself, those necessary for cellular or tissue organization (structured molecules), and those for excretion necessary in the body's function (enzymes or hormones). These processes of synthesis, energy production, and regulation are the same within each cell. Thus this brief look at the general form of these three mechanisms is adequate for grouping operations in all cells.

SUMMARY

The processes of cellular metabolism are dealt with only superficially in this limited coverage. The major considerations, such as cell division, are addressed in Chapter 1. These processes are under the control of the genetic material of the nucleus and are addressed earlier in this chapter. Several concepts that bear on later chapters need to be assimilated here. These concepts are an understanding that tissues and organs do not operate as autonomous units. Tissues and organs are aggregates of cells that act together in a highly refined manner, the primary activities being on a cellular level.

Each cell that makes up a tissue or organ is involved in the basic metabolism of life. There is energy to be produced and this uniformity in mechanisms for organisms composed of such diverse cell lines leads to two closing points. One should realize that what distinguishes one cell from another is the manner in which its nucleus conducts its operations. Given that all proteins are created by the same processes, the difference arises from which proteins are synthesized. Each cell line has its own set of characteristic products and its individual behavior. The other closing point is one of scale; reading about stepwise cellular activity can cause one to lose sight of how rapidly these processes occur. Cells operate on atomic and molecular levels; this aspect of the action is difficult to group, as is the rapidity of cellular events. Some cellular events occur as frequently as 3,600 per seond, thus defying conceptualization by our chronological perspective. That such order and fidelity exists within each of us is a marvel of nature and a tribute to our origin. This structure (both physical and chronological) represents the brief overview intended for this section.

REFERENCE

Anthony, Catherine Parker, and Thibodeau, Gary A. *Anatomy and Physiology,* 11th ed. St. Louis: C. V. Mosby Co., 1983, chap. 21.

Chapter 3

Tissues of the Body

Juanita S. Pursel

Objectives

- Identify the four major types of tissue by system.
- Explain the primary function of each type of tissue.
- Differentiate between the different types of epithelial tissue.
- Identify organs in the body that contain various types of epithelial tissue.
- List the types of specialized connective tissue.
- Explain the function of the various types of connective tissue.
- Identify areas of the body in which different kinds of connective tissue may be found.
- List and explain the function of various types of blood cells.
- Compare and contrast different types of muscle tissue.
- Identify organs and systems in which different types of muscle tissue may be found.
- Explain the function of nerve tissue.

INTRODUCTION

A brief overview of various types of tissues is presented here to provide a background for later discussion of diseases affecting these tissues. It is hoped that this overview also gives the reader a basis of comparison between the healthy and normally functioning body and the changes that occur owing to a disease process.

Tissues are groups of cells that, when combined, perform a common function. The tissues of the body are divided into four types: (1) epithelial, (2) connective, (3) muscular, and (4) nerve tissues. The characteristics and functions of each tissue type cause it to react to the advances of disease in specific and often predictable ways. They are part of the amazingly intricate means by which the body responds to ill effects.

EPITHELIAL TISSUE

Epithelial tissue performs four basic functions for the body—protection, absorption, secretion, and transportation of materials.

The cells of epithelial tissue, classified according to shape, arrangement of cell layers, and function, are (a) simple squamous, (b) simple cuboidal, (c) simple columnar, (d) stratified squamous, (e) stratified cuboidal, (f) stratified columnar, (g) pseudostratified, and (h) transitional. The various types of epithelial tissue are shown in Figure 3–1.

Simple Squamous

Tissue composed of simple squamous epithelium has a single layer of flattened platelike cells. Squamous epithelia are divided into endothelium, which lines the organs of the circulatory system, and mesothelium, which lines the body cavities. Both endothelium and mesothelium assist in the passage of substances through the body.

Simple Cuboidal

Epithelial tissue made of simple cuboidal epithelium has a single layer of cubical cells. Simple cuboidal epithelium, which lines the kidney tubules, the thyroid gland, and the surface of the ovary, aids in absorption and secretion.

Simple Columnar

Tissue composed of simple columnar epithelium has a single layer of tall, prismatic cells. The simple columnar epithelium that lines the stomach and small in-

Figure 3–1 Epithelial Tissue

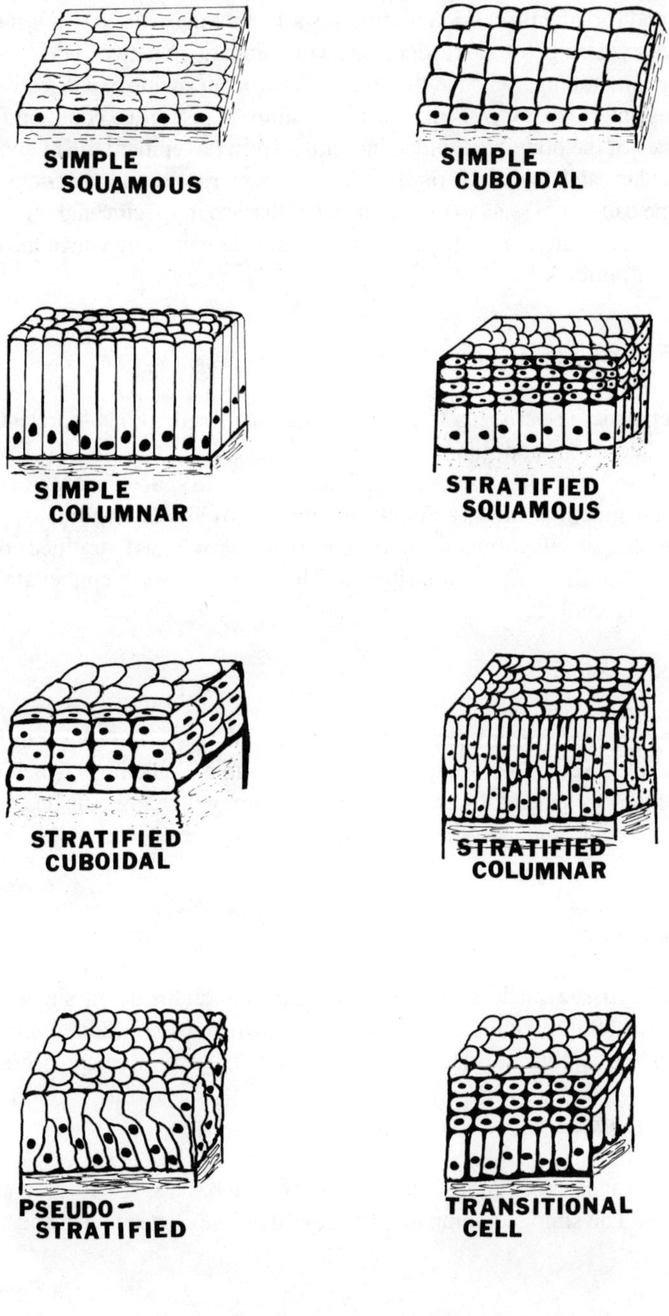

testines contains small microvilli (cylindrical processes on the surface of the cell), which increase the surface size of the cell for absorption and secretion. The simple columnar epithelium found in the uterus and uterine tubes is ciliated (fringed with hair), which provides for the movement of materials over the surface.

Stratified Squamous

Tissue with stratified squamous epithelial cells has flattened platelike cells arranged in several layers. These cells line the surfaces of the body that are subject to great wear, such as the outer skin (epidermis), the internal surfaces of the mouth, and the esophagus. The function of stratified squamous epithelium is to protect against invasion by microorganisms.

Stratified Cuboidal

Tissue containing stratified cuboidal epithelial cells contains several layers of such cells. These cells are found in the ducts of some glands, and their function is the transportation of glandular secretion.

Stratified Columnar

Tissue containing stratified columnar cells contains several layers of elongated pillarlike cells. Stratified columnar epithelium, which lines the pharynx, larynx, urethra, and salivary gland ducts, is responsible for the movement of material through the organs.

Pseudostratified

Epithelial tissue with pseudostratified cells is composed of one thick layer of cells but appears to have two or three layers because the nuclei are staggered in rows, resembling stratified epithelial cell tissue. Tissue with pseudostratified cells, found in the nasal passageway, trachea, bronchi, and male urethra, is responsible for transporting materials over its surface.

Transitional

Epithelial tissue with transitional-type cells is thought to represent a transitional form of tissue between stratified squamous and columnar epithelial cells. In the contracted stage, the epithelium appears to have many cell layers, but in the stretched condition, usually only two layers can be distinguished. Found in the excretory passages of the urinary system, transitional epithelium is changeable to accommodate pressure of urine.

CONNECTIVE TISSUE

Connective tissue, which is widely and diversely spread throughout the body, provides support by anchoring internal organs; it connects muscles to bone and bone to bone. Blood, a form of connective tissue, is transported throughout the body and protects the body against infection.

Connective tissue consists of cells and fibers in a gelatinous substance. The main types of connective tissue are (a) connective tissue proper, (b) cartilage, (c) bone, and (d) blood and lymph.

Connective Tissue Proper

The main types of general connective tissue, shown in Figure 3–2, are areolar, adipose, and dense fibrous.

Areolar tissue, also known as loose connective tissue, is soft and pliable and contains elastic and reticular fibers. It is found between organs and muscles; it surrounds the organs to give them support.

Adipose tissue is similar to areolar tissue; the difference is that the cells of adipose tissue contain fat. It is widely distributed throughout the body under the skin, giving insulation, support, food reserve, and protection.

Figure 3–2 Connective Tissue

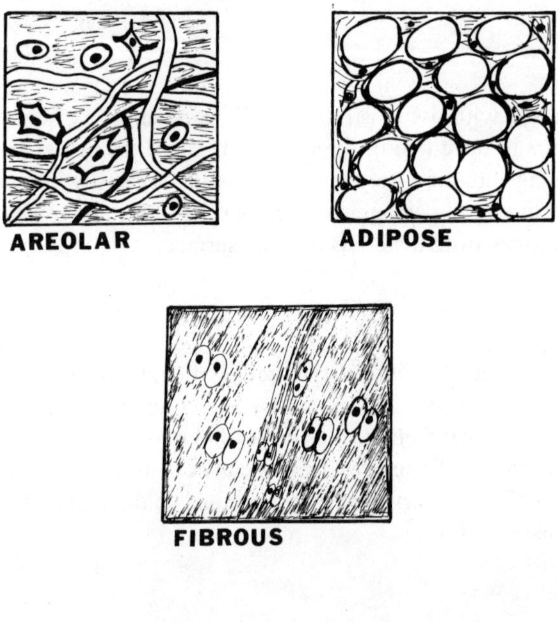

Dense fibrous tissue consists of collagenous bundles, with fibroblasts forming rows between the collagenous bundles. It is flexible but strong. Tendons, ligaments, aponeurosis, and deep fascia are composed of this type of tissue.

Cartilage

Cartilage is a specialized type of connective tissue consisting of cells called chondrocytes and extracellular fibers embedded in a gel-like matrix. It forms most of the temporary skeleton of the embryo, providing a model in which most of the bones develop. The most important types of cartilage are hyaline, elastic, and fibrocartilage (see Figure 3–3).

Hyaline cartilage, which is composed of chondrocytes and matric, contains many collagenic fibers. It is found in the tracheal rings, larynx, and sternal end of the ribs and on bone surfaces of joints. Its function is to give firm but flexible support to the organs.

Elastic cartilage differs from hyaline cartilage in that it is composed of elastic fibers, which gives flexibility to the structures formed by it. It is found in the epiglottis, external ear, and eustachian tubes.

Fibrocartilage contains collagenous fibers of cells, in single rows. It is found in the intervertebral disks and pubic symphysis joint.

Figure 3–3 Cartilage

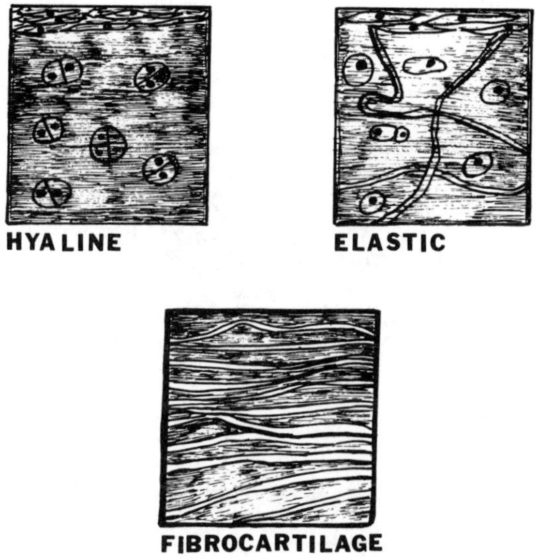

Bone

Bone, or osseous tissue, is the hard form of connective tissue that constitutes the majority of the skeleton. It consists of cells and matrix impregnated with a mineral component of 85 percent calcium phosphate and 10 percent calcium carbonate, which gives it rigidity. Compact bone forms the outer shell of bones; it varies in thickness. Spongy bone is found in the interior of many bones where the spaces are filled with bone marrow; it appears as a laced arrangement of interconnecting bone, with many spaces between the bone. Compact and spongy bone are shown in Figure 3–4.

Blood and Lymph

Blood and lymph are included under connective tissue because, as intracellular fluid, they travel throughout the body.

Blood

The intracellular fluid plasma is a free liquid containing blood cells. The blood cells circulated in the plasma are erythrocytes (red blood cells), leukocytes (white blood cells), and platelets (see Figure 3–5).

Erythrocyte formation takes place in the red bone marrow of adults and in the liver, spleen, and bone marrow of the fetus. *Erythrocytes* are biconcave disks about 7.7 micrometers in diameter that have no nuclei. They consist mainly of hemoglobin and stroma. Their function is to carry oxygen and carbon dioxide. They are also important in the maintenance of a normal acid–base balance. Because they are subject to much wear in circulation, the average life span is

Figure 3–4 Bone Tissue

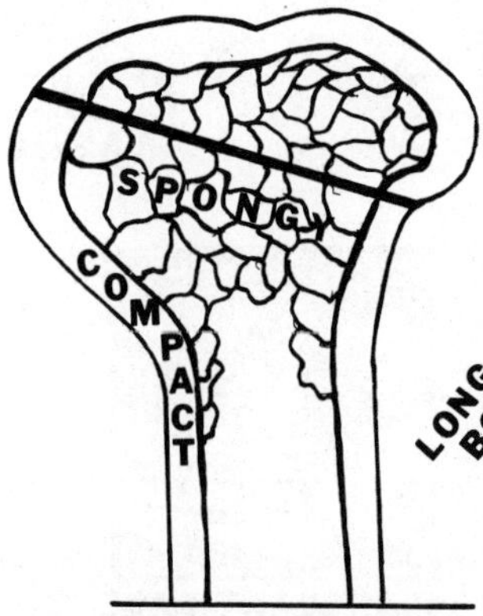

Figure 3–5 Blood

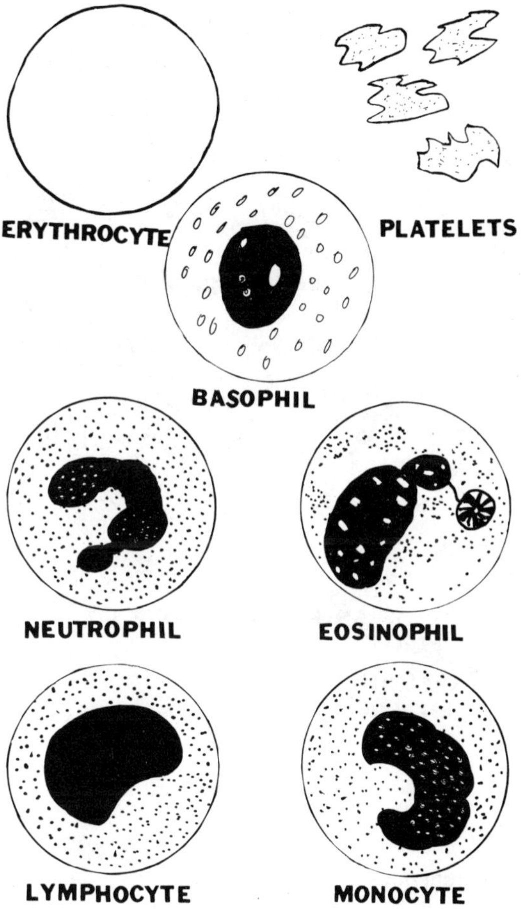

120 days. Erythrocytes are removed by cells in the bone marrow, spleen, and liver.

Leukocytes are colorless blood cells whose function is to protect the body against infection. There are two types of leukocytes: nongranular and granular. Nongranular leukocytes are lymphocytes and monocytes. Granular leukocytes are neutrophils, eosinophils, and basophils. Figure 3–6 shows the various types of leukocytes, grouped according to function, and the percentage of each found in normal blood.

Platelets are disk-shaped, nonnucleated blood elements having a fragile membrane. They play an important role in coagulation and the clotting of blood.

Figure 3–6 Leukocyte Count

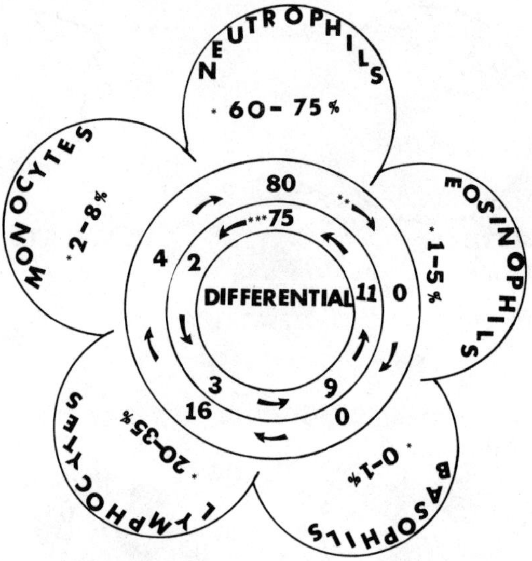

· NORMAL LIMITS

·· RIGHT SHIFT INDICATIVE OF PERNICIOUS ANEMIA

··· LEFT SHIFT, CHRONIC MYELOCYTIC LEUKEMIA

Lymph

Lymph is a transparent but slightly yellow liquid found in the lymphatic vessels and derived from tissue fluid. Lymph consists of a liquid material and cells, most of which are lymphocytes. It is collected from all parts of the body and is returned to the blood through the lymphatic system.

MUSCULAR TISSUE

Muscular tissue produces movement through involuntary and voluntary contractions. The three types of muscular tissue are smooth, striated, and cardiac (see Figure 3–7).

Smooth muscles are composed of elongated, spindle-shaped, nucleated cells arranged parallel to one another and to the long axis of the muscle. Smooth-muscle contraction is involuntary (autonomic control) and is produced chemically through

Figure 3–7 Muscle Tissue

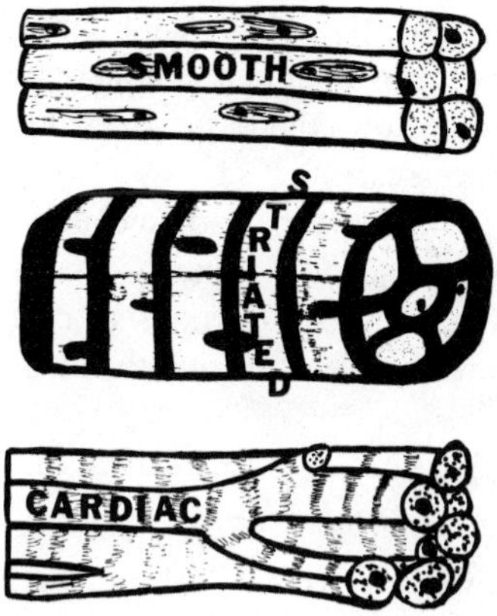

nerve endings or through hormones of the endocrine glands. Smooth muscles are found in the intestines, bladder, and blood vessels.

Striated muscles, which are covered with a thin layer of connective tissue, are arranged into bundles of fibers bound together with connective tissue to form specific muscles. Muscle fibers can be extremely long and contain several nuclei. The striations of skeletal muscles are due to actin and myosin filaments; these filaments interact chemically during contraction. Muscle movements are voluntary.

Almost all the heart is composed of *cardiac striated muscle.* The nuclei are located centrally in the cells. Sympathetic and parasympathetic (autonomic) nerves innervate the heart; the sympathetic nerves speed up the heart and the parasympathetic nerves slow down the heart. Thus the heart is able to contract accordingly.

NERVOUS TISSUE

A nerve consists of a connective tissue sheath enclosing bundles of nerve fibers; each bundle has its own sheath that conveys impulses between a part of the central nervous system and some other region of the body. A neuron is the cell unit of the nervous system. It contains a nucleus and surrounding cytoplasm. Categorized by their function, nerves are sensory, motor, or mixed. *Sensory nerves* (afferent) carry information from the outside world to the brain and spinal cord. *Motor nerves* (efferent) transmit impulses from the brain and spinal cord to the muscles. *Mixed nerves,* composed of both sensory and motor nerves, transmit impulses in both directions simultaneously.

SUMMARY

The intricacies of each tissue type are evident in the variety and complexity of the functions the tissues perform. A unique and incredible blending of the specific characteristics of each type allows the tissues to work together to perform even more elaborate bodily processes.

An organ is a group of tissues that perform a complex function for the body. It may contain as many as three or four types of tissue. The stomach, liver, and spleen are examples of organs. A system consists of a group of organs working together to perform a more complex function than a single organ.

REFERENCE

Jacobs, Stanley, Francone, Clarice A., and Lassow, Walter J. *Structure and Function in Man,* 5th ed. Philadelphia: W.B. Saunders Co., 1982, pp. 80–94.

Chapter 4

Cellular and Tissue Adaptation

Juanita S. Pursel

Objectives

- List and describe the methods by which tissue responds to changes in its environment.
- Describe the four common types of tissue adaptation.
- Explain how the five types of atrophic reaction respond to environmental changes.
- Contrast and compare the five types of atrophic reaction.
- Discuss metaplasia and describe the tissue reaction.
- Contrast hypertrophy and hyperplasia.
- Give examples of the four types of tissue adaptation.

INTRODUCTION

The response of the body systems to environmental changes, stress, injury, and aging can be reduced to the organs' smallest unit, the cell. In this chapter, the term *environment* pertains to any factor that is potentially injurious to the cell. The survival instinct of the cell to respond to a potentially harmful environmental change is manifested through abnormal alterations of cell structure and in tissue change, such as hypertrophy, atrophy, metaplasia, and hyperplasia. Sometimes such changes in tissue, when detected early, can be halted or reversed if the environmental factor bringing about the change in structure is removed. However, the structural changes in tissue that progress to cellular necrosis (death) cannot be halted or reversed.

HYPERTROPHY

Hypertrophy is the enlargement or overgrowth of an organ or a part owing to an increase in the size of the cells without an increase in the number of cells. The enlargement occurs because of increased combination of protein, nucleic acids, and lipid, as well as various intracellular organelles. The cells, in response to hormones or stress, compensate through overgrowth. Common types of hypertrophy are functional, physiological, compensatory, and complementary.

Functional hypertrophy of an organ or part is caused by its increased activity. It is widely known that today's athletes practice for hours to succeed in sports; this increased activity results in increased muscle size.

Hypertrophy experienced as a temporary increase in the size of an organ is produced by *physiological* change. An example of this is a new mother's breast enlargement occurs because of increased combination of protein, nucleic acids, and prolactin.

Hypertrophy is said to be *compensatory* when it results from an increased workload caused by some physical defect, such as the hypertrophy of the left ventricle owing to hypertension. Another example of overgrowth resulting from stress or pressure found in the cardiovascular system occurs when ventricles become enlarged because of the heart's effort to pump blood against a diseased valve in order to meet the body's requirements for blood. A kidney may become enlarged to compensate for the loss of the other kidney.

Lastly, hypertrophy is considered *complementary* when, for example, after a gastrectomy, the remaining part of the stomach increases in size to take the place of the portion of stomach excised.

ATROPHY

Atrophy, the opposite of hypertrophy, is the wasting away of the tissue or organ, with a diminution in cell size. Whereas hypertrophy is cellular adaptation to overwork, atrophy is the cells' response to a decrease in workload, use, blood supply, nutrition, or hormonal stimulation. Types of atrophy are functional, physiological, vascular, compensatory, and correlated.

Functional atrophy occurs from disuse of muscles, such as when a bedridden patient's leg muscles weaken and become atrophic (waste away) owing to lack of physical exercise. Microscopic examination of atrophic muscles reveals a decrease in the number of myofilaments. (Myofilaments are composed of myosin and actin, which together are responsible for muscle contractions.)

Physiological atrophy affects certain organs in all individuals as part of the normal aging process. Atrophy of the skin is revealed by the signs of aging in a person's face. Another example is found with endometrial atrophy occurring at menopause and accompanied by absence of menstrual flow and shrinkage of the uterus.

Vascular atrophy results from a progressive loss of substance in an organ or tissue when the blood supply to that organ or tissue falls below a critical level. A well-known example occurs in senile atrophy of the brain; brain cells become atrophic owing to the lack of circulation (blood supply).

An endocrine gland in particular, after excessive exogenous secretion by its paired organ, becomes atrophic to *compensate* for the oversecretion. Examples of this type of atrophy may be found in the suprarenal glands located over the kidneys.

Lastly, *correlated atrophy* may result from inflammation and disease, of which there are many types attacking the spinal and other muscles.

METAPLASIA

Metaplasia is the adaptive change of a specialized cell into another that is not normal for that particular tissue. Tissue lining the bronchi is columnar ciliated epithelium. The tissue cells in the bronchi of a smoker change into squamous epithelium because that type of epithelium is more adaptive to smoke. When a person quits smoking, the lining of the bronchus, over a period of time, reverts back to columnar ciliated epithelium.

HYPERPLASIA

Hyperplasia is the abnormal increase in the number of normal cells in regular arrangement of a tissue owing to an adaptive response. Such an increase may occur only in tissue that is capable of cell division.

Hyperplasia is possible when there is regeneration of an organ part after partial excision. It has been known to occur after the partial removal of the liver when the liver regenerates to return to its normal size. This differs from complementary hypertrophy, in which an organ becomes enlarged by stretching as it assumes the function of the part of the organ excised.

Hormones also play a part in hyperplasia when, under estrogen stimulation, the walls of the uterus become thickened in preparation for receiving the fertilized egg.

Neoplastic hyperplasia may occur in the uterus from prolonged estrogen hormonal stimulation, when the tissue undergoes malignant changes. This development has been documented in cases of women with endometrial carcinoma who have been on contraceptive hormonal therapy for an extended period.

SUMMARY

Hypertrophy, atrophy, metaplasia, and hyperplasia are basic concepts in the study of the fundamentals of medical science. They are occurring constantly in tissues as the body's systems respond to environmental changes. In some instances, when the injurious stimuli is removed, the tissue returns to its normal structure; in other cases it does not, resulting in neoplastic tissue and cellular changes.

REFERENCE

Price, Sylvia A., and Wilson, Lorraine McC. *Pathophysiology*, 2d ed. New York: McGraw-Hill Book Co., 1982, pp. 90–91.

Part II

Body Systems and Disease

Chapter 5

The Integumentary System

Objectives

- Name the structures of skin and their layers.
- Explain the function of skin.
- Differentiate between the functions of the various layers of skin.
- Compare albinism and leukoderma.
- Contrast a carbuncle and furuncle.
- Differentiate between organic and inorganic substances that cause dermatitis.
- Describe the three degrees of burns.
- Discuss the stages of decubitus ulcer.

FUNCTION AND STRUCTURE

The integumentary system consists of the skin and its accessory organs, including hair, glands, and nails.

SKIN

The skin is the largest organ of the human body and it varies in function. Its surface is as large as an average human body, approximately 18 to 21 square feet.

The skin functions by wrapping around the body, resisting and adapting to the ever-changing environment and to the demands placed on it by the body it covers. It protects the body from microorganisms, cold, and heat; protects the vital organs from injury; eliminates waste through perspiration; and assists with the manufacture of vitamin D. Skin plays a minor role in excretion and absorption but an important role in temperature regulation. The skin demonstrates in a diagrammatic way the manner by which tissues are joined to form organs.

The skin is relatively flat membrane containing two major layers: the epidermis and the dermis. Under the dermis lies another layer of tissue called connective tissue. Figure 5–1 shows the layers of skin.

Figure 5–1 Skin

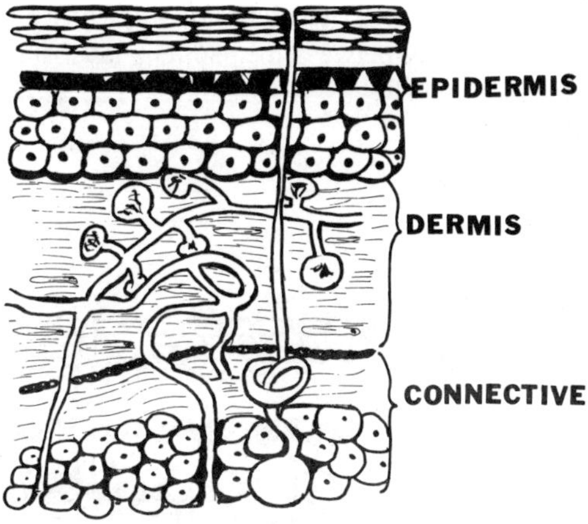

Epidermis

The epidermis, classified as stratified squamous epithelium, consists of four layers of tissue (stratum): corneum, lucidum, granulosum, and germinativum (see Figure 5–2). The epidermis has no blood vessels; it obtains oxygen and nourishment by diffusion of materials from the blood vessels of the underlying dermis.

Corneum

The surface cells, or corneum, are flat, scalelike, and dead; they consist of tough keratin, which forms a protective layer.

Lucidum and Granulosum

The next two layers of epithelial cells are very thin and are not present in all epidermis.

Germinativum

The first three layers of epidermis are continually replaced by new cells generated by the fourth layer. As the new cells from the germinativum move up, the old cells on the upper surface are shed. This layer also contains melanocytes, which are responsible for melanin, the skin's pigment.

Dermis

The dermis, the deeper and thicker of the two major layers of the skin, is composed of irregular, dense connective tissue. It has an outer papillary layer and an inner reticular layer. It contains a rich blood supply, with a plexus of vessels just below the epidermis. In the area between the papillary layer and the germinativum (the deepest layer of epidermis) lies a basement layer of epidermis that cements the epidermis to the dermis.

Figure 5–2 Epidermis

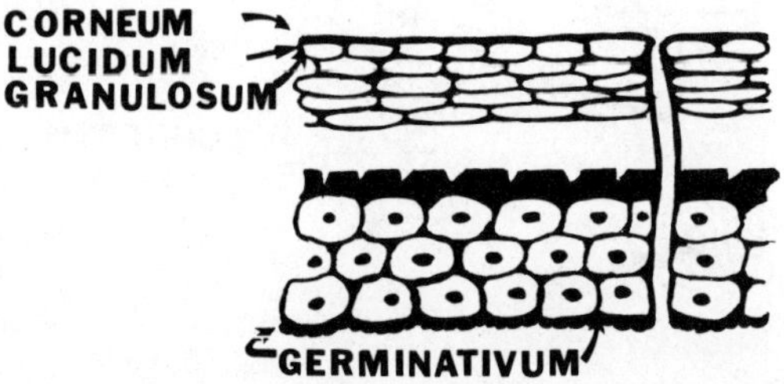

Papillary Layer

The papillary layer is named after papillae (elevations) that are arranged in ridges on its surface (Figure 5–3). The thin epidermis above the papillary layer conforms to this elevated surface; it also has ridges. These ridges, unique to each person, are known as fingerprints. The papillary layer is very vascular and supplies blood and nourishment to both the dermis and the germinativum.

Reticular Layer

The reticular layer is named after the reticulum (network) of collagen and elastic fibers that it contains. The collagen fibers resist tension and give toughness to the skin; the elastic fibers allow the skin to stretch and return to its original form. Therefore, the reticular layer functions mainly in giving the skin its toughness and elasticity. It also contains sweat and oil glands, hair follicles, sensory receptors, nerves, muscles, and blood vessels (Figure 5–4).

Subcutaneous Tissue

The subcutaneous tissue is the layer of loose (areolar) connective tissue under the dermis. It is attached to the dermis by bundles of collagenous fibers extending from the dermis. Connective tissue is variable in thickness and contains many fat cells. The function of subcutaneous tissue is to attach skin to the underlying structures; it covers organs to protect them and attaches skin to underlying muscle.

Figure 5–3 Papillary Layer

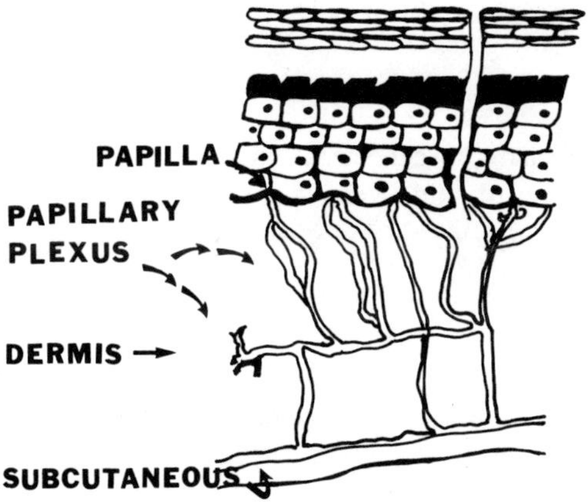

Figure 5–4 Reticular Layer

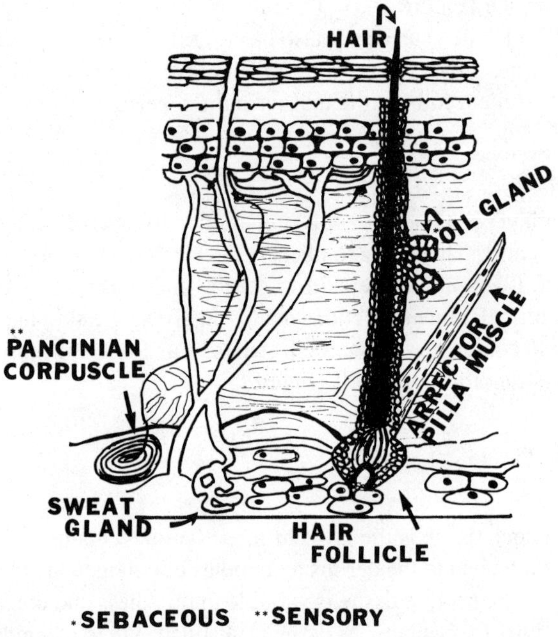

APPENDAGES

The appendages of the skin are nails, hair, and glands.

Nails

Fingernails and toenails have their roots in the nail beds of the mucosum formed from the coreum layer of skin. Nails themselves are horny, clear cells of epidermis.

Hair

Hair plays a role in protection, regulation of body temperature, and tactile (touch) perception.

Each hair has a shaft that projects above the epidermal surface of the skin and a root that extends downward into the dermis and subcutaneous layers. The root lies within a tubelike hair follicle, which is lined by cells from the epidermis and expanded at its lower end into a bulb. Sebaceous glands surround the hair follicle. Extending at an angle from the hair follicle to the papillary layer of the dermis is a narrow band of smooth muscle, the arrector pili muscle. When this muscle contracts, as in response to cold or fright, it elevates the hair follicle and the hair, causing goose pimples. This muscle in contraction also presses against the sebaceous glands, causing them to secrete sebum, an oily substance, into the hair follicle to lubricate the skin. The arrector pili muscle, sebaceous glands, and hair are shown in Figure 5–4.

Glands

The skin glands include the sebaceous, sweat, and ceruminous glands.

Sebaceous glands accompany hair everywhere. They secrete sebum (oil) through ducts (pores) to keep the hair supple and the skin soft. Sebaceous glands are stimulated by hormones during adolescence to increase secretion of sebum. Accumulation of sebum in pores on the skin sometimes causes pimples; an accumulation that turns black is called a blackhead.

Sweat glands contain a network of capillaries that assist in the maintenance of body temperature during hot weather and physical exercise. Evaporation of perspiration on the skin has a cooling effect. Another function of sweat glands is the secretion of salt, protein, and urea as waste products.

Ceruminous glands, found in the outer ear, secrete a waxlike substance called cerumen.

SKIN DISEASES

Diseases of the integumentary system generally are primarily or secondarily acquired. However, a few skin diseases are congenital or hereditary.

Primary lesions are categorized as follows:

- macule—freckles, moles, tattoos, port-wine marks, rashes from rubella and rubeola
- papule—warts, psoriasis, syphilis, drug eruptions, pigmented moles, acne
- vesicle—blister, insect bite, herpes simplex, herpes zoster, drug eruptions
- pustule—acne, furuncles, carbuncles, any pus-containing lesion

- wheal—an elevation caused by local edema, including stings, insect bites, and sensitivity to environmental conditions, such as cold, heat, and sunlight
- telangiectasia—dilation of superficial blood vessels resulting from systemic diseases

Secondary lesions, such as scales, scabs, erosions, and ulcers, evolve either from a primary lesion, owing to healing, lack of healing, or scratching, or from a systemic disease.

CONGENITAL AND HEREDITARY DISEASES

Albinism

Albinism is a hereditary condition, present at birth, in which melanocytes (cells) do not form melanin (pigmentation). It is characterized by white hair, pale skin, and pink eyes, often accompanied by nystagmus and refraction errors.

People with this disorder, albinos, are vulnerable to rays, sunburn easily, and are predisposed to skin cancer. Albinos should avoid sunlight and apply a 5% aminobenzoic acid-alcohol solution to the skin for protection. They should wear sunglasses to protect their eyes.

Pilonidal Cyst

A cyst is any closed cavity (sac) lined by epithelium containing liquid or semisolid material. A pilonidal cyst forms in the upper portion of the gluteal fold during embryonic development. It may be recognized at birth as a dimple or depression in the sacrococcygeal area.

Symptoms may begin with a bruise on the sacral area that becomes inflamed, red, and swollen. This may result in a sinus or fistula.

Treatment generally consists of incision and drainage to relieve pain, swelling, and suppuration. Excision of the sinus tract and the suturing of the cyst walls to the edges of the wound (marsupialization) are necessary to prevent recurrence of the cyst. The wound may be closed surgically or allowed to heal normally by granulation.

Nevus Flammeus (Port-wine Stain)

A nevus flammeus is a flat, red or purplish hemangioma that is present at birth; it is most often found on the infant's face. Color shade of the nevus depends on whether the superficial or the dermal tissue is involved. The nevus is generally only on one side of the body. If the face is involved, the nevus can usually be hidden with an opaque cosmetic cream. Sometimes electrodesiccation or cryotherapy is used to improve appearance. Laser therapy is used experimentally and someday may be the preferred method of treatment.

ACQUIRED DEFECTS AND DISEASES

The acquired defects and diseases of the integumentary system may be either primary or secondary, with etiology of bacterial or viral infection, trauma, and allergy. Not all the lesions listed earlier are presented in this section.

Acne Vulgaris

Acne vulgaris is characterized by papules, pustules, and comedones (blackheads) on the face, neck, and trunk. Its cause is not clearly understood. However, because it generally begins at puberty, it is believed to be an interaction between hormones, sebum, and bacteria, in which there is an overproduction of sebum and an obstruction to its outflow from the pores.

Treatment includes cleansing the skin carefully to prevent formation of an abscess from a bacterial infection, which may result in scarring. Disfigurement may embarrass an adolescent, causing difficulty with self-concept and personal adjustment. Understanding and supportive help for the adolescent are advisable. Tretinoin (vitamin A acid) 0.05% cream or liquid or 0.01% gel is usually effective. Benzoyl peroxide 5% to 10% is another topical medication used in acne treatment. Exposure to sunlight should be avoided.

Urticaria and Angioneurotic Edema

Urticaria and angioneurotic edema are characterized by medium-sized to giant wheals. These conditions are associated primarily with food or drug allergies, insect bites, infection, stress, and digestive disturbances.

Symptoms of urticaria are single or multiple wheals, ranging from the size of a dime to that of a silver dollar, on the eyelids, lips, hands, feet, and other parts of the body, and severe itching. Symptoms of angioneurotic edema are severe itching and swelling of the subcutaneous tissue of the hands, feet, eyelids, lips, genitalia, and mucous membranes, which may produce respiratory distress. The patient may also complain of nausea, vomiting, diarrhea, and headache.

The cause needs to be identified, since there is possibility of fatality owing to epiglottis angioedema. Emergency treatment includes administration of epinephrine 1:1000 (0.3 ml s.c.) and diphenhydramine (Benadryl).

Furuncle and Carbuncle

A *furuncle* (boil) is a skin infection of the corium and subcutaneous layers, characterized by one core or point of infection.

A *carbuncle* is a cluster of boils with multiple draining pustules, caused by staphylococcus microorganisms that enter through the hair follicles.

Although a furuncle and carbuncle may occur anywhere on the body, they have been known to occur most often in the nasal cavity owing to the large number of hair follicles rooted in the corium of the nose.

Multiple lesions with pus may require culture of the drainage for identification of the bacteria; this is followed by a sensitivity test for specific antibiotic therapy.

Paronychia

Paronychia is an infection around the fingernails or toenails. It may be either acute or chronic. Generally, a microorganism, *Pseudomonas* or *Proteus*, enters the epidermis through a break from a hangnail or cut. Sometimes nails become chronically infected owing to irritation from soap or water.

Symptoms are redness and swelling round the nail, which is painful to the touch. Treatment consists of applying hot soaks. An acute infection involving the tendon sheath may require incision and drainage of the pus pocket and removal of the nail. Antibiotics may be necessary.

Dermatophytosis (Ringworm)

Dermatophytosis is a fungal infection caused by members of the dermatophyte family, generally *Microsporum, Trichophyton*, and *Epidermophyton*. Such infections are categorized according to the area of the body that is affected. Only the most common are given here; all are caused by *Trichophyton*.

Tinea Pedis

Perhaps the best known type of dermatophytosis is tinea pedis (athlete's foot). It begins with infection between the third and fourth interdigital spaces and spreads to the plantar surface of the arch. The lesions may appear as scaling, weeping vesicles. The toenails may also become involved.

Treatment with griseofulvin has proved most effective. A mixture of 3% salicylic acid and 6% benzoic acid in 70% alcohol solution is also recommended. Good foot hygiene is necessary, with special attention given to drying the interdigital spaces after bathing and to applying powder. Light footwear is advisable in hot weather.

Tinea Capitis

Ringworm of the scalp may become epidemic in schools. The lesions are small and scaly. Initially, they occur in small patches but may spread over the entire scalp.

Application of 1% miconazole or 1% clotrimazole cream to the infected scalp prevents the infection from spreading to others. Oral microsize griseofulvin (125 to 250 mg PO b.i.d. with meals) may be used successfully with children until the infection subsides.

Parasitic Infections

Scabies and pediculosis are two types of parasitic infections.

Scabies

Scabies is an infection resulting from infestation with *Sarcoptes scabiei* (itch mite). The impregnated female mite invades the stratum corneum and deposits her eggs. The hatched larvae then attack the hair follicles. Scabies is transmitted through skin contact.

Symptoms are crooked, dark-lined lesions, from a millimeter to a centimeter long, that are generally found between the fingers; on the wrists, elbows, breasts, and lower buttocks; and in the axillary folds. The itch is intense, and secondary infection may result from scratching lesions.

Treatment advised is application of 1% gamma benzene hexachloride, 25% benzyl benzoate cream or lotion over the entire skin surface after bathing. For children under age two, a 5% to 10% sulfur ointment is generally used rather than gamma benzene hexachloride, which may be toxic.

Pediculosis Capitis

Epidemics of infestation by lice are well known to elementary and secondary school systems. The head louse lives directly on its host. It is transmitted by personal contact with shared clothing, hairbrushes, combs, and hats. Diagnosis is made through scalp inspection of children who tend to scratch their heads. On examination, small, round, gray-white ova (nits) are found on the hair shafts. Nits develop into mature lice in 3 to 14 days.

When an epidemic of pediculosis capitis is uncovered in a school, the school usually closes until the situation is under control. Treatment consists of applying 1% gamma benzene hexachloride, in shampoo, cream, or lotion form, once a day for two days. Application may be repeated in two weeks to destroy any mature lice. Combs, hats, and clothing should be boiled to prevent reinfestation.

Herpes Simplex

One of the most feared diseases of the 20th century is herpes simplex, a viral infection caused by herpes virus hominus (HVH) that attacks the skin and the nervous system. There are two types of HVH: Type 1, which occurs on facial areas, especially around the mouth, and Type 2, which occurs in the genital area. A pregnant woman with Type 2 HVH may transmit the infection to the fetus through the placenta or to the newborn by contact during birth.

Symptoms of Type 1 HVH are small, red papules that develop in the area around the mouth, followed by eruptions of small vesicles or fever blisters. These eruptions are accompanied by pain and severe itching.

Symptoms of Type 2 HVH in the male are small groups of vesicular lesions around the glans or prepuce that erupt into superficial ulcers; in the female, multiple superficial eruptions may develop on the surfaces of the cervix, vagina, or perineum. These eruptions are also accompanied by pain and severe itching.

Treatment is the same for both types and includes cleansing the area with soap and water, where possible, to reduce the risk of secondary infection, such as encephalitis, gingivostomatitis, and herpes simplex keratitis. Therapy for secondary infections may include antibiotics, blood transfusions, and intravenous solutions.

Herpes Zoster

Herpes zoster, an acute infection caused by varicella-zoster virus, is characterized by painful vesicular skin lesions following an underlying cranial or spinal nerve route.

Signs are generally unilateral skin lesions along a nerve route that, within two weeks, erupt, form crusts, and diminish. Symptoms may include gastrointestinal disturbances, fever, headache, malaise, and severe itching.

For mild attacks, treatment includes application of calamine lotion or other protectant to relieve itching and analgesics to relieve pain. Severe cases may be treated with topical corticosteroids.

Burns

Burns may be caused by exposure to such elements as fire, heat, chemicals, electricity, and sunshine and by other factors, such as friction or abrasion. Burns are classified according to the severity and degree of skin damage and the percentage of body surface involvement.

The skin damage of a first-degree burn involves erythema (redness), without loss of epidermis; a second-degree burn involves blistering of the epidermis, without injury to the dermis; third-degree burn involves the destruction of the epidermis and the dermis.

The percentage of body involvement with a second-degree burn over 29 percent of the body or a third-degree burn of more than 9 percent may be critical to the patient.

Treatment of a burn depends on the degree of the burn and the extent of body involvement. Generally, first-degree burns are treated at home with oil or ice applications.

Patients with second- or third-degree burns involving body areas as described earlier require careful monitoring in burn centers. During the first two days after severe burn, sodium and protein pass into the burned areas, resulting in edema and blister formation. Hypotension (low blood pressure), hypoproteinemia (low protein), hyponatremia (low sodium), and oliguria (diminished capacity to form and pass urine) are present. Depending on the severity of the burns and the patient's condition, parenteral fluids, antibiotics, and tetanus are given as ordered. Blood transfusion may be indicated. Extensive plastic surgery with repeated skin grafts may also be required for functional restoration.

Decubitus Ulcer

A decubitus ulcer is an inflammation of the skin over a bony prominence, such as shoulder blades, elbows, sacrum, hips, knees, ankles, and heels, usually owing to prolonged pressure. Such ulcers are most often seen in the aged who are confined to bed. They may be staged as follows:

1. Erythema (redness)
2. Blistering
3. Skin broken; possibly epithelium and dermis destroyed; drainage present
4. Deep ulcer present; possibly bone exposed

Preventive care includes keeping the patient dry, turning him or her frequently, straightening wrinkled sheets, and messaging bony prominences with lubricants frequently during the day.

Treatment of decubitus ulcer depends on the stage of the lesion. In addition to preventive care, a patient with decubitus ulcer may require a magnesium aluminum hydroxide gel, powder or ointment preparation; tincture of benzoin; and irrigation of the area with hydrogen peroxide. Debridement may be necessary.

REFERENCE

Freedberg, Irwin M. "Cutaneous Medicine." In *The Principles and Practice of Medicine*, 12th ed., edited by A. McGehee Harvey, 1473–1494. New York: Appleton-Century-Crofts, 1980.

Chapter 6

The Musculoskeletal System

Objectives

- Name the structures of the musculoskeletal system.
- State the functions and classifications of bone.
- Explain bone formation cycle and bone metabolism.
- Name and explain three congenital anomalies of the system.
- State some of the causes of osteomalacia, rickets, and scurvy.
- Contrast absorption and accretion and its relationship to Paget's disease.
- Contrast the following fractures: traumatic and pathologic, open and closed, complete and incomplete.
- Differentiate between the types of fractures: transverse, comminuted, compound, impacted, depressed, greenstick, Pott's, and Colles' fractures.
- Compare intracapsular, intertrochanteric, and subtrochanteric hip fractures.
- State the differences among sprain, strain, and dislocation.
- Explain the difference between amputation and disarticulation of a limb.
- Recognize types of diseases of the musculoskeletal system with symptoms.

FUNCTION AND STRUCTURE

The musculoskeletal system comprises the bones, muscles, tendons, joints, ligaments, and bursae.

BONES

Function

The bones provide the framework that (a) furnishes the foundation and support for the entire body, (b) assists the body in motion, (c) serves as a muscle attachment to bones by tendons, and (d) protects vital organs, such as the heart, lungs, and brain, from injury.

Bone Development

Bone originates from primitive connective tissue (mesenchyma). Some of the fetal bones are preceded by membrane and some by cartilage, so that two types of bone development (ossification) take place. From mesenchyma, bone passes through either a membranous or a cartilaginous (endochondral) type of bone development. Mesenchyma undergoing the membranous phase of bone development is gradually replaced by osteoid matrix, which calcifies to become bone. The bones of the cranial vault and the face undergo this process.

Mesenchyma undergoing cartilaginous type of bone development contains an embryonic hyaline cartilage model of bone, which is invaded by blood vessels; the cartilage cells are destroyed and replaced by bone. This bone is again replaced, so that by adulthood none of the bone is of cartilaginous origin. This process occurs in the long bones, spine, scapulae, ribs, sternum, and pelvis.

Osteogenic cells (osteoblasts) generate bone tissue in either membranous or cartilaginous bone formation. This process is shown in Figure 6–1.

Bone Metabolism

The following explanation of bone metabolism is a simple discussion of the bone cycle, that is, accretion, or building up bone, and resorption, or breaking down process necessary for bone growth. Accretion and resorption are occurring constantly to accomplish bone remodeling; this process accounts for the change in strength and size of bones corresponding to growth and for the different shapes of bones. Figure 6–2 shows the bone cycle of accretion and resorption.

Figure 6–1 Bone Formation

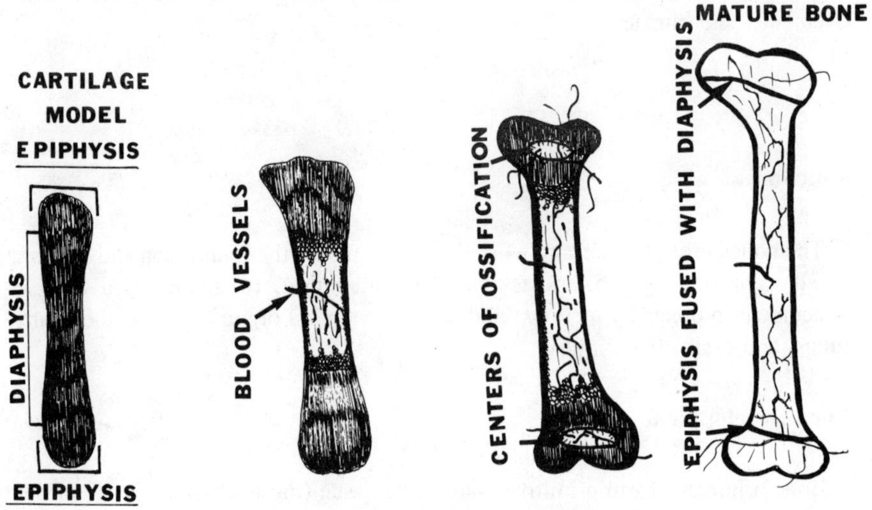

Figure 6–2 Bone Metabolism

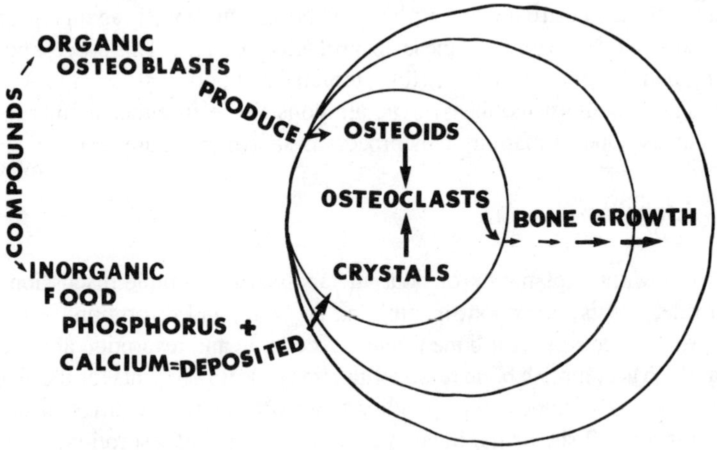

Accretion

Biochemically, compounds are divided into organic and inorganic. An organic compound contains carbon atoms, and an inorganic compound does not. Bones contain both organic and inorganic compounds. Chemically, bones go through both organic and inorganic phases during accretion.

Organic Phase of Bone Formation. Osteoblasts are continually producing osteoids, the organic matrix of bone. Within the organic matrix of bone, two substances, collagen and polysaccharide, are found. *Collagen* may be described as tiny ropes made of protein. *Polysaccharide* is a thick, gluelike substance made up of complex sugars and protein. Collagen is found in the complex matrix of polysaccharide. This completes the organic phase of bone formation.

Inorganic Phase of Bone Formation. Inorganic crystals containing phosphorus and calcium formed from the biochemical processing of food are deposited in the osteoid matrix to nourish the bone.

Accretion takes place through the production of osteoids and the depositing of inorganic crystals to build bone.

Resorption

Bone reconstruction takes place through bone phagocytes called osteoclasts, which reabsorb and digest bone tissue from the inside of the bone so that the bones gradually enlarge.

Structure and Classification

Bone consists of outer compact material, which is dense and hard, and inner cancellous material, which is spongy and porous. The amount of compact and cancellous material in each bone differs depending on the classification and specific function of the bone.

Bones are classified according to shape: short, long, flat, and irregular (see Figure 6–3). *Short bones,* found in the wrists and ankles, have a heavy shaft of inner spongy bone within a thin layer of outside compact bone.

Long bones, found in the upper and lower arms and legs, are composed of a shaft (diaphysis), capped on each end by an epiphysis. A fine line, or epiphyseal plate, separating the shaft and epiphysis on each end is the area in which cartilage is constantly being replaced by bone until growth is completed.

Flat bones—ribs, sternum, and skull—consist of spongy inner material between two coverings of compact bone; the outside coverings protect the internal organs. Ribs and sternum also provide a flat surface for attachment of muscles.

Irregular bones are those that do not fit the other three classifications. They are similar to the structure of the other bones, containing a layer of cancellous bone

Figure 6–3 Types of Bones

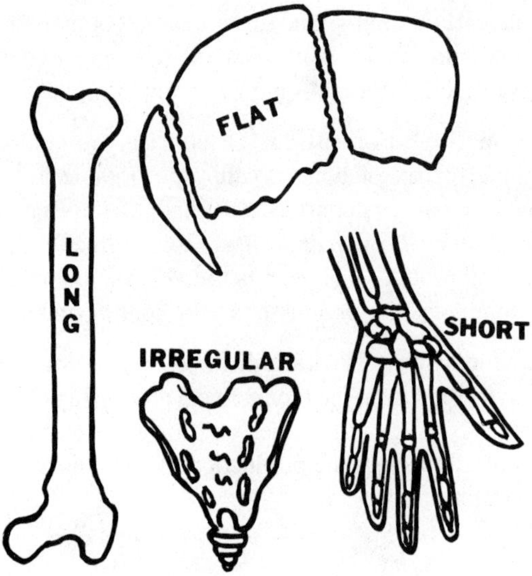

within and a layer of compact bone externally. Some of the parts of the body in which irregular bones are found are the vertebrae, sacrum, coccyx, and hyoid.

Layers of Bone Tissue

With the exception of long bones, all bones are completely covered by periosteum; the shafts of long bones are covered by periosteum and the ends that articulate with other bones are covered with cartilage cushions. Compact bone, the third hard, dense layer of bone under the periosteum, contains the haversian canals, which in turn contain blood vessels that function by carrying on internal respiration, that is, by bringing oxygen and nutrients to the bone and carrying away carbon dioxide as a waste product. The inner shaft, or medullary cavity, of long bone is filled with yellow bone marrow, which is composed mainly of fat cells. The center of the epiphysis, as well as the centers of most other bones, is made of cancellous or spongy bone that contains red bone marrow filled with blood cells in different stages of development. After full development, the sternum, ribs, pelvis, vertebrae, and epiphyses of long bones contain red bone marrow with cancellous tissue. As the child grows, the red marrow is replaced by yellow marrow. The layers of bone in the long bone and epiphysis are shown in Figure 6–4.

Figure 6–4 Long Bone

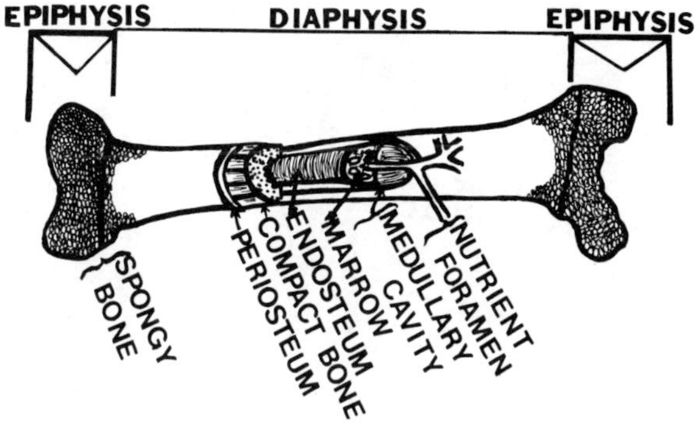

Bone Processes

The various types of processes, or projections, that extend from bones to attach bone to muscles and tendons, are as follows: round head, found in shoulder and hip sockets; tubercle, or site where the tendon or muscle is attached; the tuberosity, a rounded process that attaches muscles or tendon; condyle, a rounded process at the joint; fossa, a depression in a bone; foramen, an opening for the blood vessels and nerves; fissure, a deep, narrow opening; sulcus, a groove; and the sinus, an air-filled cavity within a bone. Figure 6–5 shows the various types of processes.

Skull Bones

The skull is supported by the vertebral column; it is composed of the face and the cranium. The face has 14 bones and the cranium has 8 bones (Figure 6–6). The facial bones include two of each of the following: nasal, superior maxillary, lachrimal, malar, palate, and inferior turbinated. The vomer and inferior maxillary account for the final two.

The eight cranial bones are the occipital, frontal, sphenoid, ethmoid, two parietal, and two temporal.

Vertebral Column

The 26 bones of the vertebral column (Figure 6–7) are divided into 7 cervical, 12 thoracic, 5 lumbar, the sacrum (five bones fused into one), and the coccyx (four bones fused into one). Between the bones are cartilaginous disks that function as cushions to buffer shock and provide flexion. The vertebra consists of the vertebral

Figure 6–5 Bone Processes

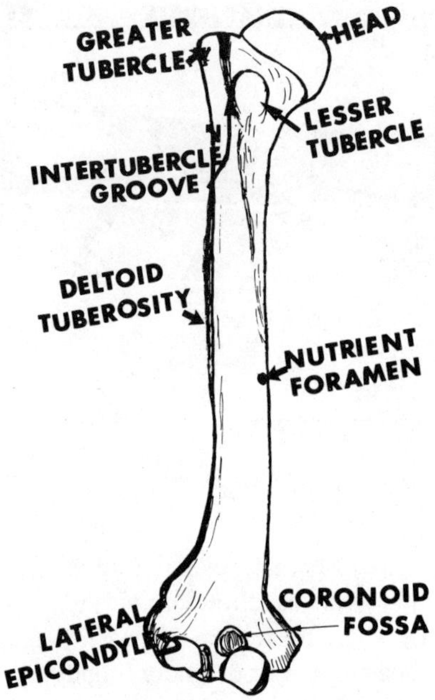

Figure 6–6 Skull Bones

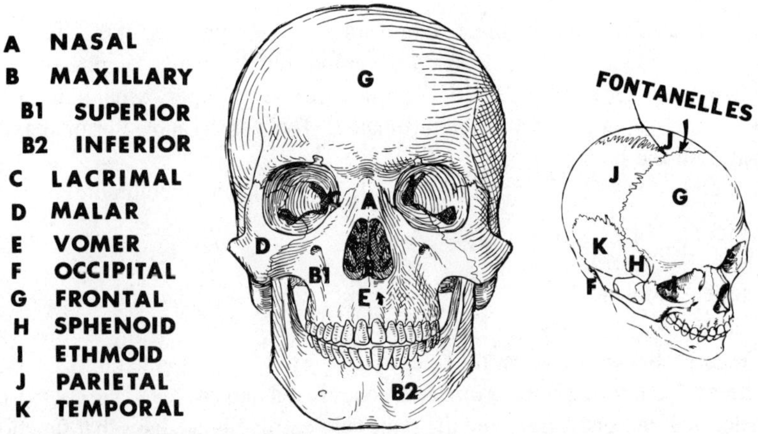

Figure 6–7 Vertebral Column

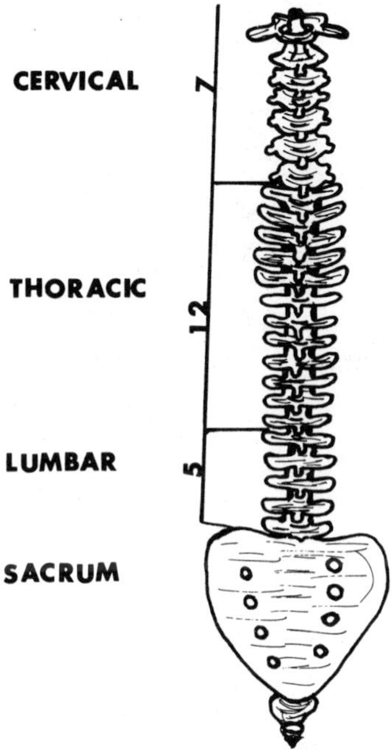

arch, spinous transverse and articular processes, and the laminae. The center of the vertebra is a hollow space through which the spinal cord passes.

Rib Cage

The clavicle, or collarbone, and the scapula bilaterally connect the breastbone to the shoulder in order to form the shoulder joint. The sternum, extending down the midline of the chest, articulates on the upper portion with the clavicle and ribs; on the lower part, the xiphoid process is attached to the abdominal muscles and the diaphragm. Of the 12 pairs of ribs, the first 7 are attached by costal cartilage anteriorly to the sternum and posteriorly with the vertebral column. Ribs 8, 9, and 10 join the 7th rib anteriorly, rather than the sternum and join the vertebra posteriorly. Ribs 11 and 12 are called floating ribs because they are unattached anteriorly. Figure 6–8 shows a posterior view of the rib cage.

Figure 6–8 Rib Cage

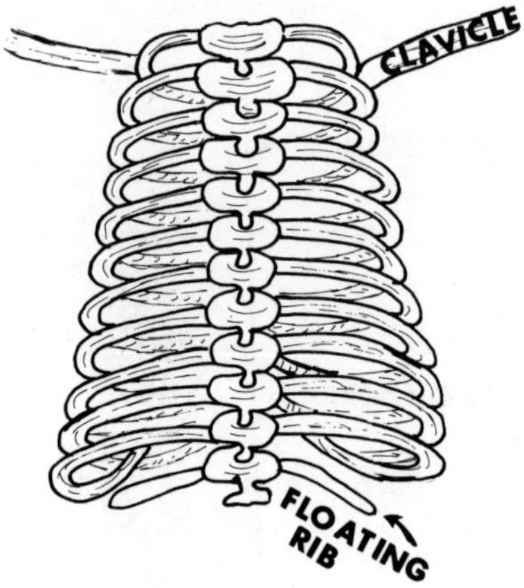

Arms, Hands, Legs, Feet

The humerus, ulna, radius, carpals, metacarpals, and phalanges make up the bones of the arms and hands; the femur, tibia, fibula, patella, tarsals, metatarsals, and phalanges are the bones of the legs and feet. The bones of the arms, hands, legs, and feet are shown in Figure 6–9.

MUSCLES

Function

The muscles provide a means of movement for the body. The point of attachment of the muscle is called *origin*; the junction where the muscle is joined to another bone is called *insertion*. When a muscle contracts, the bone to which it is attached remains firm and the bone to which the muscle is joined moves. For example, the brachial muscle has its origin on the anterior aspect of the humerus and its insertion in the coronoid process of the ulna. When the brachial muscle contracts, the forearm flexes (Figure 6–10). The foregoing is a simple explanation for a complex system.

Classification

The types of muscles are smooth, cardiac, and striated muscles (see Figure 6–11).

Figure 6–9 Bones of the Arms, Hands, and Legs

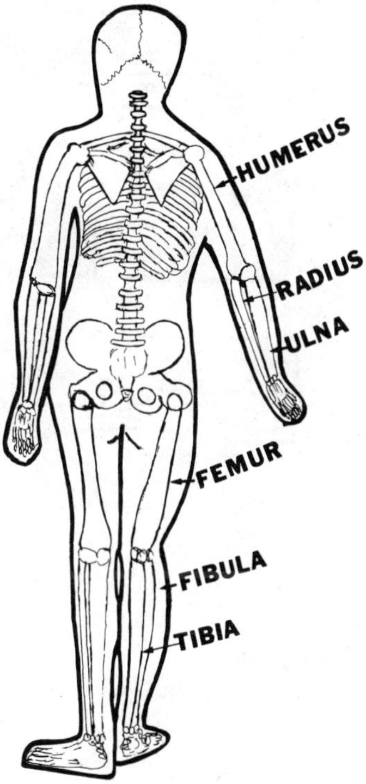

Figure 6–10 Brachial Muscle

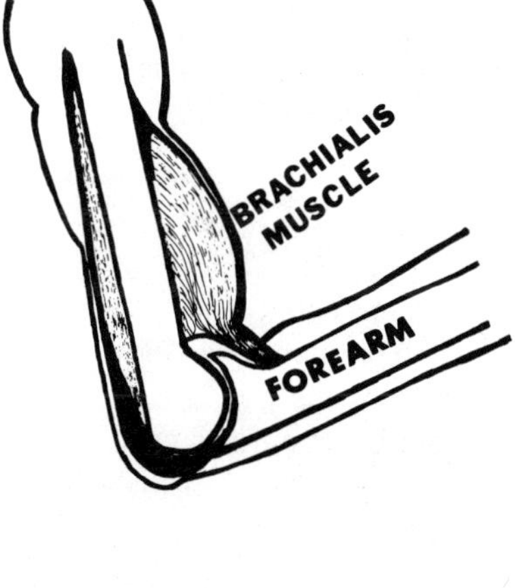

Figure 6–11 Muscles

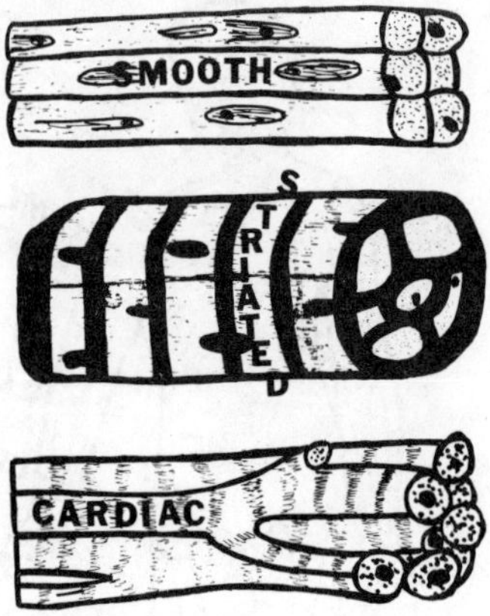

Smooth muscles, found in the digestive system, blood vessels, and secretory glands, move involuntarily. They react slowly to all stimuli and do not lose their tone if innervation is interrupted.

The *cardiac muscles,* involuntary like the smooth muscles, are found in the heart. These muscles are not paralyzed if they lose their neural stimuli.

Striated muscles are found throughout the musculoskeletal system. They do not react as quickly as other muscles of the body and are paralyzed by interruption of their innervation. In contrast to the smooth and cardiac muscles, the action of the striated muscles are voluntary and controlled by the individual. All skeletal muscles are striated.

TENDONS

Tendons are fibrous bands of connective cord. They are continuous with muscles and attach muscles to bone.

JOINTS

A joint is a place where bone connects with bone or with cartilage. It consists of the articular surfaces of two or more bones surrounded by a joint capsule and held in place by ligaments and muscles.

The articular ends of long bones are covered by compact subchondral bone and a thin layer of hyaline cartilage. The sparse cells within this cartilage lie in collagen fiber and protein polysaccharide matrix; they contain no blood vessels. The cartilage is nourished through diffusion of nutrients from synovial fluid.

The joint capsule is lined with synovial membrane and filled with a clear, light golden, viscid liquid called synovial fluid. The function of synovial fluid is (a) to nourish the joint with water and nutrients and (b) to lubricate the joint to allow only minimal friction on the movement over articular surfaces. Synovial fluid contains plasma dialysate and hyaluronate, which give it lubricating ability.

Some joints, like the vertebrae, have fibrocartilage disks between them, which permit limited movement and absorb shock.

Classification

The configuration of joints differs, depending on the type of joint and the function it serves. The three types of joints are (1) synarthrosis, (2) amphiarthrosis, and (3) diarthrosis (Figure 6–12).

Synarthrodial joints are immovable joints such as are found in the skull. *Amphiarthrodial joints* have slight movement, as, for example, the pubic symphysis; joints between the tibia and fibula with slight movement are bound by ligaments of fibrous connective tissue; joints between the hip bones (pubic symphysis) with slight movement are hyaline cartilage.

Diarthrodial joints are those that attach limbs with gliding, hinge, pivotal, or saddle movement. Joints between the carpal bones have gliding movements; the humerus and ulna have hinge movements; the hips have ball-and-socket movements; the radius and ulna have pivotal movement; and the carpal bone and the first metacarpal bone of the thumb have saddle movement.

Figure 6–12 Types of Joints

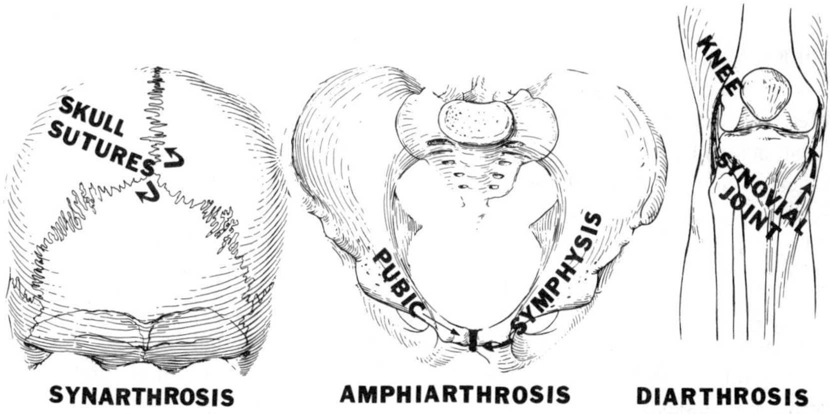

LIGAMENTS

Ligaments, fibrous bands of connective tissue, anchor the bones or cartilage around the joint capsule to give it strength. In the abdominal cavity, ligaments are double layers of peritoneum; they support the organs as they extend from one visceral organ to another.

BURSAE

Bursae, lined with synovial membrane and filled with synovial fluid, are sacs located in the spaces between tendons, ligaments, and bones. Their function is to lubricate the areas around the joint in order to eliminate friction and to facilitate movement over bony prominences around the joints. They are found in places in the tissues where friction would otherwise develop.

MUSCULOSKELETAL SYSTEM DISEASES

Patients with diseases and defects of the musculoskeletal system, when admitted to health care facilities, are generally assigned to the orthopedic service, a branch of surgery dedicated to restoring and preserving the musculoskeletal system's functions. Diseases and defects of the musculoskeletal system are divided into congenital defects and acquired diseases.

CONGENITAL DEFECTS

Congenital defects are physical anomalies present at birth that scientifically have been found to be due to (a) genetic, (b) intrauterine, or (c) both genetic and intrauterine etiology.

Genetic factors influencing congenital defects are chromosome and gene abnormalities. Variations in chromosome structure and number owing to abnormal cell division affect genes. In such cases, a newborn may have multiple congenital defects that are incompatible with living. A single gene abnormality from genetic mutation may be handed down to the newborn from parents or from other recent or distant ancestry. These defects are transmitted according to dominant, recessive, and sex-linked gene disorders.

The majority of congenital defects are due to intrauterine influences, such as drug and alcohol abuse, radiation effects, and disease contracted by the mother during pregnancy. The type and severity of congenital defects depend on the stage of development at the time the fetus was environmentally exposed.

Congenital defects may also result from a combination of genetic and intrauterine influences.

Preventive treatment consists in genetic counseling when there is a known familial chromosomal or genetic disorder. Early prenatal care for the mother and intrauterine pediatric care for the fetus may help to reduce congenital defects.

The Cranium

Craniosynostosis

Before birth, the bones of the vertex and sides of the skull are separated by a membrane into six areas. These six areas, called *fontanelles,* are found at the four angles of the parietal bones, as shown in Figure 6–6. The posterior fontanelle closes about two months after birth; the anterior fontanelle remains open until approximately age two.

Craniosynostosis, the premature closing of the sutures or fontanelles, results from a defect in ossification of bone in the skull or the conversion of cartilage into bone.

The severity of the defects depends on which suture is closed. The most common problem entails the premature closure of the sagittal suture with anteroposterior elongation of the cranium, allowing little room for growth. Because the brain doubles in weight during the first year of life, the fontanelles must be able to allow for brain growth through expansion. The premature closure of other sutures may affect personal appearance.

Radiology should rule out the possibility of microcephaly with the diagnosis of unfused sutures, in contrast to craniosynostosis, which will show fused sutures at birth.

Surgery, the only treatment, consists of removing a linear strip of bone along the fused suture. The edge of the bone is sutured with Silastic film to delay regrowth. Major skull reconstruction for premature closing of skull or facial sutures is now possible.

Hydrocephalus and Spina Bifida

Hydrocephalus and spina bifida require a team approach. These defects are discussed in Chapter 7.

Spine

Scoliosis

Scoliosis is the lateral curvature of the spine, with some degree of persistent rotation of a series of vertebrae from the normal spinal axis (see Figure 6–13). It is generally recognized in children through health examinations at school or in physical fitness classes when a child who is standing straight, with feet together,

Figure 6–13 Spinal Curvatures

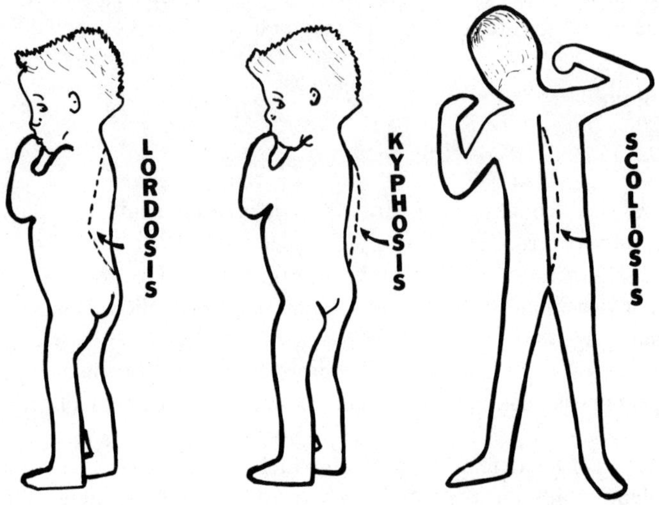

has one scapula lower than the other; or when a child who is bent over, with arms hanging loosely, has one side of the back elevated over the other; or when a teacher observes that a little girl's dress does not hang straight. Diagnosis is confirmed by x-ray.

Scoliosis is not a disease, but a condition or deformity. The etiology of scoliosis is not altogether known but may include congenital malformations of the spine and legs (unequal leg length), spastic paralysis, poliomyelitis, chest diseases, and incorrect posture. Two general types of scoliosis can be recognized: functional and structural.

Functional scoliosis can be differentiated from structural scoliosis in that the person is able to bend laterally on both sides. Functional scoliosis is spinal curvature owing to incorrect posture or one leg being longer than the other. Another cause of functional scoliosis may be sciatic pain from herniation of a lumbar intervertebral disk. This type of scoliosis is temporary; when the underlying problem is corrected, the spine is straightened.

Structural scoliosis presents a fixed curvature of the spine, with restrictions on bending in the direction opposite the curve. It may be caused by congenital malformation of the vertebrae, paralytic disorders, or unilateral chest condition.

Pathologic changes brought about by structural scoliosis include compression of the intervertebral disks on the concave side of the spinal curvature, thickening of the anterior longitudinal ligament, and turning of the spinous process toward the concave side.

The structures on the convex side remain normal; however, the intervertebral disks bulge, and the anterior longitudinal ligament becomes thin; the vertebral body turns toward the convex side of the spinal curvature.

The greatest damage is in the thoracic area, in which there is an anterior prominence of the thorax on the concave side of the spinal curvature. The chest wall rotates posteriorly on the convex side of the spinal curvature, and there is posterior prominence of the rib cage with decreased lung volume on the convex side.

As the condition worsens, the spine may collapse, allowing the rib cage to rest on the pelvis and compress the abdominal and thoracic viscera. Because of all these changes in the thoracic cavity, cardiopulmonary failure may occur.

Treatment of scoliosis depends on the degree of impairment and the patient's age at the time of first treatment. Initial treatment of scoliosis in a child may begin with traction, a brace, or a Risser cast. If scoliosis does not respond, spinal fusion may be necessary. The posterior spinal fusion is done in two stages: (1) vertebral body wedge resection and (2) spinal fusion after insertion of Harrington rods into the spine, one on each side of the curvature, forcing the spine into a more normal position.

The spinal fusion may be performed through a window in the Risser cast; then, at the completion of surgery, the cast is replastered. The patient is in the Risser cast for approximately one year. Follow-up x-rays are taken through the cast.

Kyphosis

Kyphosis is the anteroposterior curvature of the spine, where the convexity is posterior to the thoracic and sacral vertebrae of the spine (see Figure 6–13). This results in pathologic changes in the vertebrae and the intervertebral disks.

Kyphosis is not a disease, but a deformity that may be caused by chronic arthritis, tuberculosis, or posture. It occurs in children, teenagers, and adults.

In children, kyphosis generally involves only one vertebra in the dorsal spine, which is eroded until gradually it becomes flat (see Figure 6–14). The child may experience back pain, fatigue, muscle spasm, and tenderness on palpation. Differential diagnosis includes ruling out tuberculosis, tumor, compression fracture, congenital causes, and eosinophilic granuloma. Biopsy may be necessary in addition to x-rays. Treatment includes bed rest, a brace, or plaster cast until x-ray shows the area to be healed.

In a teenager, kyphosis generally involves three or more successive vertebrae of the dorsal spine. There may be anterior wedging of the vertebral body seen laterally on x-ray, whereas posteriorly, the nuclear material protrudes through the plates that separate the bone from the nucleus pulposus. Differential diagnosis is the same for the adolescent as for the child; kyphosis owing to poor posture does not show vertebral wedging. Treatment includes limited activity, bed board, and

Figure 6–14 Intervertebral Disc

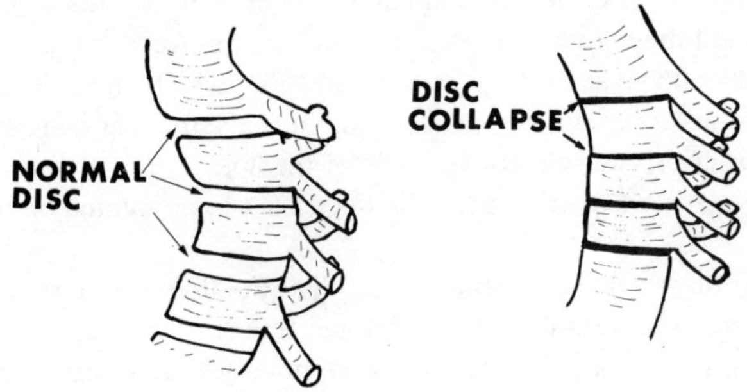

kyphosis exercises. In more advanced kyphosis, the patient may need to wear a brace for as long as a year or two or until the spine deformity has been somewhat corrected or the spinal lesion healed.

Kyphosis in the adult also involves the dorsal spine, where pathologic changes occur. The fibrocartilage capsule is composed of a center (nucleus pulposus) surrounded by a periphery of fibrous tissue. On each side of the fibrocartilage capsule is a plate of hyaline cartilage that separates the capsule from the vertebrae.

Pathologic changes occur when the nuclear material protrudes through the plate into the spongy portion of the bone of the vertebrae. As this condition progresses, the intervertebral disks become thin, collapse, and allow successive vertebrae to fuse. The hyaline cartilage plates may also degenerate, so that a bridge of bone gradually forms across the intervertebral space, resulting in ankylosis of the spine.

Differential diagnosis as to the primary cause of kyphosis in the adult patient is important; kyphosis may be secondary to spinal degeneration associated with aging, postmenopausal syndrome, senile osteoporosis, tuberculosis, drugs, and malignancy. Diagnostic laboratory tests include alkaline phosphatase, protein, serum calcium, and phosphorus. Biopsy may also be indicated.

Treatment includes maintenance of correct posture, with instructions for proper exercises, bed rest on bed board, spinal corset, or collar, depending on the progression of kyphosis. Treatment of the primary cause is important for improvement of adult kyphosis. Figure 6–13 illustrates kyphosis.

Arms and Legs

Congenital anomalies affecting the arms or legs often involve the absence of a limb. The words acheiria and apodia mean the absence of one or both hands and one or both feet, respectively. An arm or leg may be partially or entirely missing at birth.

Phocomelia is a developmental anomaly characterized by the absence of the arms or legs or both, so that the hands and feet are attached to the trunk. The condition, a side effect of the drug thalidomide taken during early pregnancy, is caused through interference with embryonic development.

Another cause of congenital malformations in the newborn may be due to the mother's contraction of an infectious disease, such as rubella (German measles).

Treatment may consist of surgical revision of the shortened arm for prosthetic fitting. In the case of a femur, extensive reconstruction may be necessary to make the stump suitable for prosthetic fitting and weight bearing.

Fingers and Toes

Polydactyly is a congenital anomaly of the hands or feet, where there are more than five fingers or toes. Supernumerary fingers or toes are generally removed shortly after birth. Congenital anomalies often occur together, so that a child born with polydactyly is likely to have syndactyly.

Syndactyly is the term used when two or more fingers or toes are joined together (webbed). This anomaly is more common in fingers than in toes. The webbed digits are separated surgically by dividing the soft tissue and sometimes the bone. This procedure may be performed when the child is between ages two and five. Advances in plastic surgery have brought excellent results. Generally, webbed fingers or toes do not interfere with function.

Feet

Talipes denotes deformities of the feet. The names of various types of talipes describe the position of the foot and ankle, such as varus (inversion), valgus (eversion), equinus (plantar flexion), and calcaneus (dorsiflexion). Figure 6–15 shows the types of talipes.

Figure 6–15 Talipes

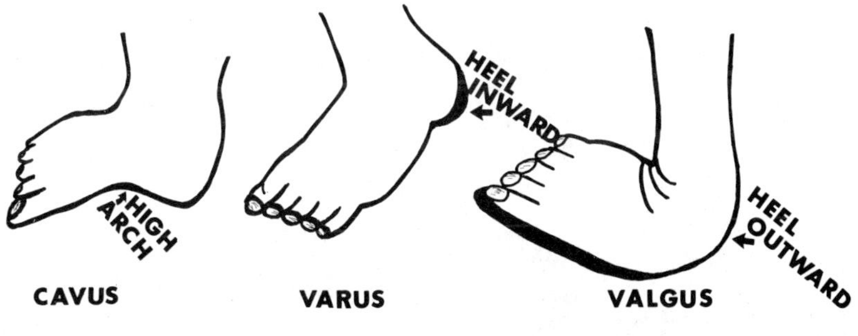

Talipes equinovarus (clubfoot) may be described as an elevated heel with the foot turned inward, toward the midline of the body. The degree of deformity ranges from mild to where the toes touch the medial side of the lower leg. Although generally thought of as being congenital, this defect may result from paralysis, poliomyelitis, muscular dystrophy, or trauma.

The earlier treatment begins, the better the results. Treatment of the newborn should start in the first weeks after birth, so that the deformity may be completely corrected without surgery. One method of treatment is the application of plaster casts to hold the feet in proper position. An alternate method is the Denis Browne splint (Figure 6–16). For infants that do not respond to casts or splints, the lengthening of the Achilles tendon to lessen the equinus (plantar flexion) deformity and the revision of the posterior capsule of the ankle joint to release tight contraction are performed, followed by the application of a cast. Depending on the severity of the deformity, many years of treatment and surgical reconstruction may be necessary for correction. Periodic follow-up examinations are required to detect any tendency toward recurrence.

Joints

A child may be born with a congenital hip dislocation (subluxation) or it may occur during infancy owing to the head of the femur not being properly aligned with the hip socket. This phenomenon usually occurs when the acetabulum, or hip socket, is abnormally lax and the ligamentum teres is elongated. If this condition is not detected and corrected, the child will walk with a defective gait and in later life will experience spinal problems and discomfort.

Figure 6–16 Correction of Clubfoot

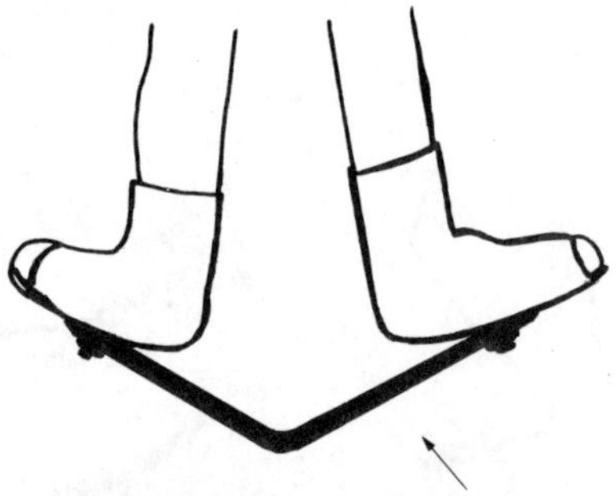

A simple procedure to test hip dislocation in an infant is Ortolani's sign, or click, which occurs when the flexed hips of the infant in supine position are slowly abducted. The clicking occurs when the hip slips into place. Another sign is limitation of abduction of the infant's flexed hips. This deformity is confirmed by radiologic changes and the child's gait.

Treatment varies with the patient's age, from splinting under age one, to open reduction with capsular arthroplasty up to age eight, and to replacement arthroplasty with Smith-Petersen metal cup prosthesis in older people.

Osteoarthritis of the hip, with degenerative joint changes in the femoral head and acetabulum of the hip, is a common complication in later years. Replacement arthroplasty with prosthetic device is an effective means of relieving pain and disability.

Early recognition of congenital joint dislocation in the infant with initiation of treatment almost always results in a normal joint. Treatment in the first years of life gives satisfactory results. Untreated hip dislocation results in defective gait and low back pain, which worsen with age.

ACQUIRED DEFECTS AND DISEASES

Acquired defects and diseases categorized under the musculoskeletal system are due to metabolic disturbances, infection, neoplasms, and trauma.

Metabolic Disturbances

It would be well to review the process of bone metabolism, explained earlier in this chapter, before proceeding to the diseases having a metabolic origin.

Rickets

Children with rickets are often seen on television programs about underdeveloped countries. Such children have deformities of the limbs, such as bowlegs and knock-knees.

In a child with rickets, calcium and phosphorus crystals are not deposited in the inorganic phase of bone metabolism; thus the bones become soft and do not gain rigidity. There are several reasons for this:

- dietary and environmental deficiency
- deficiency of vitamin D, normally produced by the sun in the skin
- problems with absorption of vitamin D from the intestines
- kidney problems, resulting in the loss of the mineral phosphorus.

The relationship of vitamin D to calcium and phosphorus is unknown.

Scurvy

In the 15th century, when European ships began making long sea voyages, scurvy became a well-recognized problem. Symptoms are bleeding gums, loss of teeth, and large bruises on the body. It was discovered in the 15th century that if sailors ate citrus fruits, symptoms subsided. Modern research has explained the phenomenon as the result of vitamin C deficiency. Vitamin C, referred to as ascorbic acid, is necessary for osteoid production. When osteoids are lacking in bone tissue, bone metabolism does not proceed in the normal fashion, so that deformed bones are produced. The role of osteoids in bone production is explained earlier.

Scurvy is found mainly in children in underdeveloped countries, where the diet is not balanced with citrus fruits. Symptoms found in infants aged 6 to 12 months are failure to gain weight, restlessness, anorexia, and irritability.

In the United States, scurvy is not prevalent because of a higher standard of living and public awareness concerning the necessity of vitamin intake. However, it may be found in children and adults due to malnourishment. Primarily, it is known as a disease affecting alcoholics due to improper diet.[1]

Adult symptoms are weakness, irritability, weight loss, arthralgia, and hemorrhages of the gums around the teeth. In severe cases, the gums are swollen and infection may occur.

Diagnostic testing for vitamin C deficiency includes determination of serum or white cell ascorbic acid levels. X-rays may show rarefaction of the long bones and swelling of the joints.

Treatment consists of large doses of vitamin C, which will bring about remarkable changes in symptomatology of weakness, irritability, and gum hemorrhages. Continual supplemental doses of vitamin C, in addition to dietary intake on a daily basis, are necessary over a long period.

Infection

The entire musculoskeletal system—bones, joints, and muscles—reacts to the invasion of microorganisms. An infection begins when the disease-producing organism enters the system (a) as a latent stage of a disease, (b) indirectly through the bloodstream, or (c) as the result of trauma, when the skin has been broken and the bone exposed, as, for example, in an automobile accident.

Osteitis

Osteitis is the general term used to describe inflammation of the bone owing to infection.

Paget's disease (osteitis deformans) is characterized by a bowlike deformity of the bone through increased bone mass. It attacks the bones in the legs, lower spine, pelvis, and skull. It is more prevalent in males than in females, attacking 3 percent of the male population over age 40 and 10 percent of the female population under age 70.[2] The disease has two stages; the first involves resorption and the second, accretion. It is during the accretion, or bone remodeling, stage that the bones are greatly malformed. In order to understand accretion and resorption, it would be advisable for the reader to review these concepts discussed earlier in the chapter.

Early signs of Paget's disease are difficult to detect. Initial discovery of the disease often occurs during routine physical examination, when serum alkaline phosphatase results are reported as elevated or x-ray examination reveals bone deformity.

Intervention requires no treatment for bone deformity, but rather drugs to decrease bone resorption and return bone metabolism to equilibrium.

Osteomyelitis

Acute Osteomyelitis. Acute osteomyelitis is a pyogenic, or pus-producing, infection that attacks the bone and bone marrow and spreads to joints. It is caused by *Staphylococcus aureus,* gram-positive and gram-negative bacteria, acid-fast bacilli, or fungi and may be secondary to another infection or introduced through bone trauma.

The patient experiences a rise in temperature, restlessness, irritability, and tenderness over the infected bone area. This results not only from a bone lesion, but also from a bloodstream infection with acute reaction.

Differential diagnosis must rule out acute rheumatic fever, polyarthritis, rheumatoid arthritis, and neoplasms. Early diagnosis is made with radionuclide scanning techniques and with technetium and gallium isotope scans. Because scans can give false positive results for osteomyelitis, it is important that such results be correlated with clinical findings to provide early antibiotic therapy.

In the acute stage, aspiration of the abscess and blood cultures may be necessary for identification of the organism before giving antibiotic therapy. In adults, antibiotics may be given in large doses, whereas in children, antibiotics should be given in continuous intravenous fluids.

Chronic Osteomyelitis. In the *chronic* stage, the disease becomes a low-grade infection manifested by drainage from one or more sinuses, recurrent episodes of pain, and increased swelling and inflammation. Drainage should be cultured for bacterial infection.

Over a long period, the bone becomes necrotic and breaks away from the healthy bone (sequestrum). A cellular debris or exudate collects at the site and develops into an abscess. The necrotic bone with abscess is surrounded by living bone, which forms an involucrum around the necrotic sequestrum. Through the cloaca (opening in the involucrum), pus drains out on the surface of the skin.

Treatment for chronic osteomyelitis may consist of aspiration of the abscess as well as culture of the drainage or aspirated material for antibiotic intervention. However, antibiotic therapy may be ineffective owing to tissue necrosis with the lack of circulation. In that case, sequestrectomy (surgical removal of the sequestrum) may be indicated. When more extensive treatment is indicated owing to the extent of bone involvement, saucerization of the bone area, with removal of scar tissue, sequestra, and granulation tissue and insertion of drains to allow for continuous irrigation of the area with antibiotic solution, may be necessary. A cast is generally applied. Limb amputation may be necessary when other methods of treatment fail.

Amputation. A limb is amputated (a) as a result of trauma from auto accidents or accidents involving industrial equipment; (b) when blood circulation in the limb cannot be restored, as in chronic osteomyelitis, diabetes, arteriosclerosis, Raynaud's and Buerger's diseases; or (c) when neoplasms or a congenital anomaly is present.

Types of amputation are disarticulation, open or closed amputation, and major or minor amputations. *Disarticulation* is an amputation through the joint. This method is preferred because an artificial limb can be easily fitted to the remaining limb. *Open or closed amputation* refers to whether or not the wound is closed with skin or left open for infection control. When the amputation is left open, a secondary closure is necessary. A *major amputation,* designed to produce a stump for an artificial limb, is performed on limbs proximal to the fingers and toes. A *minor amputation* is one performed on the fingers and toes, where as much function as possible is retained because the stump is not designed for an artificial limb. The decision of the type of amputation to perform depends on the site of the osteomyelitis and the severity of the chronic infection.

Arthritis

The American Rheumatism Association Nomenclature and Classification of Arthritis and Rheumatism lists 13 categories for arthritis and rheumatism. A major cause of disabilities in the United States, listed under the first category, Polyarthritis of Unknown Etiology, is rheumatoid arthritis. Another disabling disease, listed as the third category, is osteoarthritis, or degenerative joint disease.[3]

Rheumatoid Arthritis. When rheumatoid arthritis invades the joints, the inflammatory process attacks several joints, causing intense inflammation of the synovial membranes. The inflammation may subside entirely, without any damage to the joints, or pannus may develop, causing permanent damage. Pannus is an abnormal membrane of inflammatory exudate that blankets the synovial cells inside the joint, causing synovitis. This condition, over a period, causes the articular cartilage to erode so that the articular surface of the bone becomes exposed and replaced by fibrous tissue. The fibrous tissue forms an abnormal union between the two bone-eroded edges, resulting in the joint becoming consolidated and immobile. Immobility and consolidation of a joint is called *ankylosis*.

Rheumatoid arthritis attacks adults and children similarly. In children, it is known as juvenile rheumatoid arthritis and tends to strike the joints of the long bones, which stems the child's growth and development. Lymphadenopathy often precedes rheumatoid arthritis in children. Seventy-five percent of the children attacked by rheumatoid arthritis have experienced complete remission. Although children have a favorable prognosis for regaining joint function, debilitating arthritis owing to joint deformity may continue into adulthood.

Establishing a diagnosis during the early stages of rheumatoid arthritis is difficult because symptoms are similar to those of such diseases as acute rheumatic fever, gout, osteoarthritis, and tuberculosis.

Laboratory findings of a patient with rheumatoid arthritis show a positive agglutination test; cloudy synovial fluid from the infected joint contains between 3,000 and 50,000 white blood cells per cubic millimeter and has reduced viscosity. The Arthritis Foundation provides criteria to be used in diagnosing rheumatoid arthritis.[4]

Treatment is similar for adults and children, with the exception of hydroxychloroquine, which is not given to children, and includes bed rest, nutrition, salicylates, and anti-inflammatory drugs. Balanced diet for maintenance of normal weight is important in eliminating unnecessary weight on joints. Physical therapy is ordered to restore joint motion.

Severely deformed joints with ankylosis (Figure 6–17) that do not respond to drugs or physical therapy have been treated successfully with total joint replacement and the insertion of a prosthetic device. Surgery aims to improve mobility and relieve pain. The bones on each side of the prosthesis are resurfaced and anchored firmly to the prosthesis by cement, to avoid movement of the prosthesis and wear on the surrounding tissue.

Degenerative Joint Disease (Osteoarthritis). Osteoarthritis, also of unknown cause, has been attributed to mechanical stress, leading to cartilage cell damage and the release of proteolytic enzyme. This development is thought to bring about cartilage degeneration, subchondral bone thickness, and cyst formation. In contrast to rheumatoid arthritis, the changes occur in the articular cartilage at the ends of the bones, rather than in the synovial membrane (Figure 6–18). It is prevalent in men under age 45 and in women over age 45.

Symptoms include stiffness of short duration in a joint or two after inactivity, characterized by pain and mobility in the joint after exercise. There may be limited mobility in severe osteoarthritis with crepitus and enlargement of the joint with the presence of Heberden's nodes at the terminal interphalangeal joints.

Figure 6–17 Joint

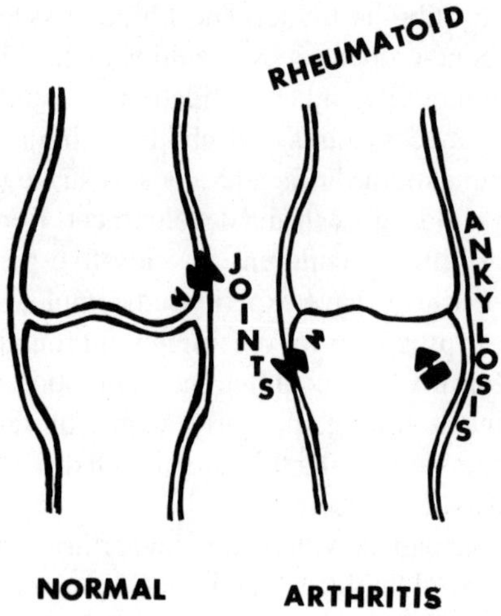

Figure 6–18 Osteoarthritis

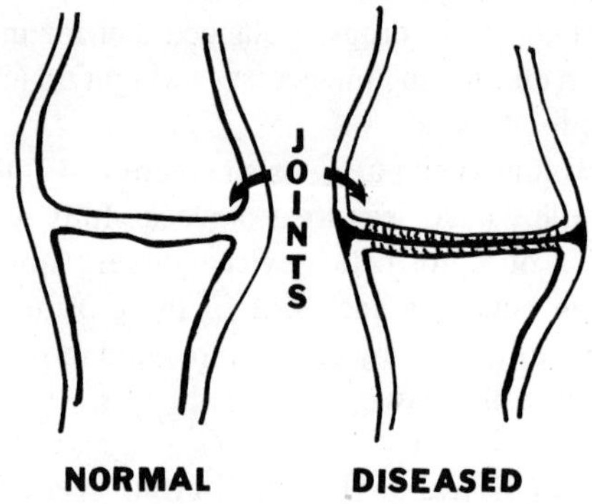

X-ray findings reveal subchondral bone thickness, cyst formation, and narrowing of joint space.

Keeping excess body weight to a minimum helps alleviate pressure on diseased joints. This is best accomplished by maintaining a well balanced diet and daily exercise within the individual's capacity. Injection of steroids (hydrocortisone) into joints sometimes gives temporary relief. Frequent injections are detrimental because they can lead to further damage by infection.

Several operations may be performed to relieve pain and to increase joint movement. A synovectomy may be indicated for thickened synovial membrane and a painful joint not relieved by other therapy. An osteotomy is performed to improve alignment and relieve pain.

The prognosis for less debilitation and joint damage is a more likely prospect for osteoarthritis than for rheumatoid arthritis. With proper and timely treatment, the joints in osteoarthritis can become less painful and disabling.

Trauma

Types of injuries that occur as a result of trauma are fractures, dislocations, sprains, and strains.

Traumatic Fracture

A fracture or broken bone, classified according to the nature of the injury, is either traumatic or pathologic. A traumatic fracture is the result of an injury. A fracture may be open or closed. An *open (compound) fracture* is one in which the skin is broken and the bone may protrude; a *closed (simple) fracture* is one in which no open wound is present.

Types of Fractures. A fracture may be complete or incomplete. A *complete fracture* is one in which the bone is broken completely across; an *incomplete fracture* is one in which part of the bone is broken and the other part is bent, such as a greenstick fracture that occurs in children before the bones are entirely ossified.

A fracture may be spiral with a twisted bone, transverse with the fracture at right angles to the axis of the bone, or comminuted with the bone splintered. Various types of fractures are shown in Figure 6–19.

Kinds of Fractures by Location. A fracture may be: (1) impacted with one fragment driven into another such as a hip fracture with the head of the femur driven into the acetabulum; (2) depressed with broken bones pushed inward, such as a skull fracture; (3) fracture-dislocation, which occurs when the bony structures of any joint are fractured and dislocated as well.

Treatment of Fractures. How a fracture is treated depends on many factors, such as the patient's condition, x-ray results, type of fracture (open or closed), and the location and displacement of the fracture.

A patient with multiple injuries, including fractures, may require immediate attention for other conditions, such as hemorrhage, respiratory failure, and shock.

A fracture may be evident through tissue swelling, tenderness to palpation, and deformity at the fracture site or, where a fracture is suspected, because a splint has been applied by a rescue squad.

Figure 6–19 Fractures

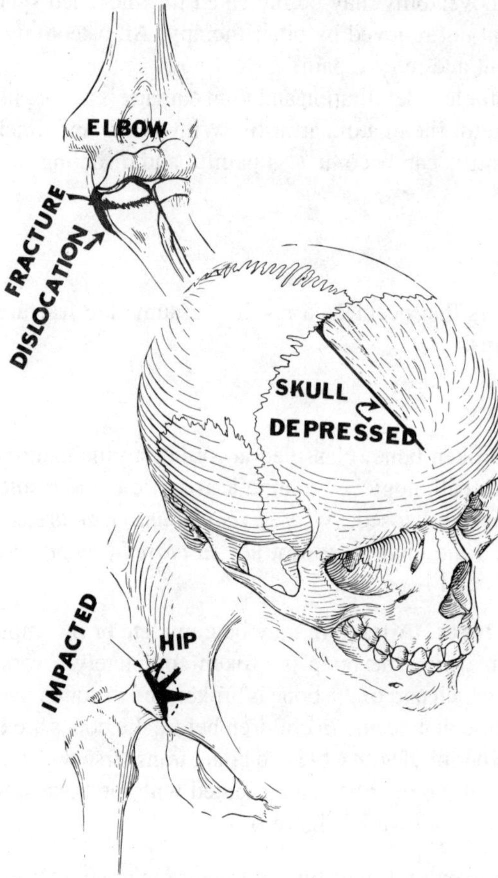

X-ray interpretation of the fracture, after the patient's general condition has been stabilized, is the determinant of the treatment necessary for the reduction of the fracture.

Fracture Reduction. Fractures with displacement may be reduced by closed reduction or open reduction. *Closed reduction* (without incision) of a fracture involves manipulation of the bone and external fixation with bandage, cast, or traction, for maintenance of fracture alignment and stability of the limb.

Open reduction, with incision into the fracture site, is performed for an open fracture and may be required for a closed fracture when closed reduction is unreliable or impracticable or has failed. Internal fixation is achieved with screws, rods, or metal plates. Many times after surgery external fixation with bandage, cast, or traction is also used to maintain fracture alignment.

Follow-up Care of Fractures. Periodically, follow-up x-rays need to be taken to ensure proper healing of the fracture. Three complications may occur: (1) delayed union, (2) nonunion, and (3) malunion. *Delayed union* occurs when the fracture has not healed within approximately 20 weeks. Common causes for delayed union are inaccurate reduction or immobilization, severe trauma, infection, fragment separation, and impairment of circulation in the limb. Treatment should be directed toward eliminating the reason for the delay. Ambulation, using a walking cast, may hasten healing.

Nonunion occurs when the process of bone repair ceases before producing a firm union between the fractured ends. Common causes for nonunion are essentially the same as for delayed union. Treatment consists of the use of orthopedic appliances to support, align, prevent, or correct deformities and to improve function. Surgical intervention may be necessary, with bone grafting. Generally, nonunited fractures require both internal and external fixation.

Malunion occurs when accurate reduction and mobilization cannot be obtained. It often can be prevented, but sometimes, when there are multiple injuries, prevention is impossible. Malunion results in shortening of the limb, deformity, and abnormal rotation owing to restriction of joint motion. If malunion is not corrected surgically, permanent disability may result.

Pathologic Fracture

A pathological fracture is a closed fracture that may occur in bones weakened by disease. The hip is a vulnerable site for this type of a fracture. However, hip fractures may also result from trauma. The three types of hip fractures are (1) intracapsular fracture, occurring in the part of the bone within the capsule; (2) intertrochanteric fracture, occurring between the trochanters; and (3) subtrochanteric fracture, occurring below the trochanters. These types of hip fractures are shown in Figure 6–20.

A symptom of pathological fracture of the hip is sudden pain on weight bearing. Fracture of the hip owing to trauma would include a history of an accident. In both cases, x-rays of the hip would reveal the location and type of fracture. Removal of a femoral head with insertion of a prosthesis is indicated (1) when the soft tissue attachments of a fractured head are destroyed; (2) to replace the head when necrosis or nonunion occurs after fracture reduction; and (3) to replace the head for mobilization of the joint in arthritic patients.

Treatment of Fractured Hip. The femur and acetabulum are generally referred to as the hip. Often with an intracapsular fracture, the head of the femur is

Figure 6–20 Types of Hip Fractures

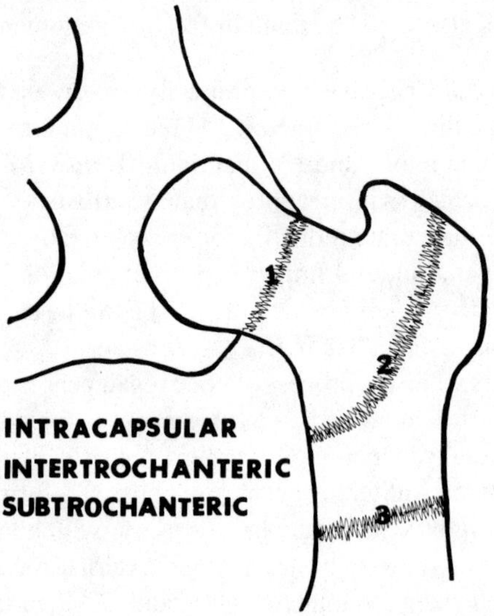

fractured and needs to be replaced. Fracture of the femoral neck and trochanter, without injury to the femoral head, may be reduced by inserting nails, pins, or rods across the fracture to bind the fragments together.

In surgery, when the head of the femur is removed, the neck is prepared for placement of the prosthesis, the prosthesis is fitted and driven into the medullary canal of the femur, and the incision is closed.

Dislocation

A bone such as a shoulder may be dislocated, or displaced, from the socket. This is the most common form of dislocation. Shoulder and spinal manipulation are often performed to replace dislocations of a joint.

Sprain

A sprain is a joint injury in which some of the fibers supporting the ligaments are ruptured. Sprains occur rather commonly among athletes. Symptoms are pain, grating, swelling, tenderness, and restricted motion.

Differential diagnosis includes ruling out minor fractures, strains, and bursitis. Treatment includes cold application immediately after injury, followed by rest, heat to relieve pain, and physical therapy.

Tendons and ligaments are often subjected to repeated trauma, which leads to irritation. Long-term debilitating effects after repeated trauma to the ligaments include osteochondritis dissecans and secondary changes in the radial head, with restricted movement.

Strain

Muscles are strained through injury, overexertion, and excessive exercise. In a strain, muscle pain is elicited by contraction and tenderness of the muscle. Treatment includes immobilization of the muscle by means of a plaster splint, adhesive plaster, or sling. Physical therapy, including heat and massage, is followed by gradual resumption of exercise.

Tenosynovitis

Tenosynovitis is an inflammatory process of the synovial lining of the tendon sheath caused by mechanical irritation, trauma, or rheumatoid arthritis. The most common causes are mechanical irritation and trauma.

Prolonged stress from gripping a device, such as hedge trimmer or a ball, can cause an abnormal growth of fibrous tissue to form within the lumen of the tendon sheath. The fibrous tissue gradually narrows the diameter of the sheath, increasing the friction between the tendon and the sheath.

Symptoms of pain and tenderness in the involved area are usually preceded by some type of traumatic episode.

Treatment includes immobilization of the injured area, with application of elastic bandages or adhesive strapping. Physical therapy is often recommended with heat application. Hydrocortisone is sometimes injected into the tendon sheath space to relieve pain.

Acute Suppurative Tenosynovitis

A puncture wound is often an entry point for tenosynovitis in the hands or feet owing to infection from *Staphylococcus* or *Streptococcus* organisms.

Symptoms are swelling and pain in the infected area. The infection may limit the extension of the fingers and toes when there is involvement of the digits. The patient may have fever and leukocytosis. Relief from pain is experienced when the pus pocket in the sheath ruptures and spreads to other areas.

Treatment consists of culture and sensitivity for antibiotic administration to control the infection. Aspiration or incision with insertion of drains may be necessary. When the infection is untreated, the tendon sheath may become permanently damaged, resulting in limited motion.

Calcific Tendinitis

An accumulation of calcium in the tendons of the shoulder, wrist, or hand secondary to previous trauma may cause tendinitis.

Symptoms are swelling and intense pain over the local area involved. Radiologic findings are positive for calcium deposits.

Preferred treatment is injection with hydrocortisone or local anesthetic.

NOTES

1. Philip D. Zieve, ''Bleeding Disorders.'' In *The Principles and Practice of Medicine,* 12th ed., ed. A. McGehee Harvey (New York: Appleton-Century-Crofts, 1980), 526.

2. Robert Berkow, ed., *The Merck Manual of Diagnosis and Therapy,* 14th ed. (Rahway, N.J.: Merck Sharp & Dohme Research Laboratories, 1982), 1242.

3. American Rheumatism Association, ''Primer on the Rheumatic Diseases,'' *Journal of the American Medical Association* 224 (April 30, 1973): 678–679.

4. Ibid., 799.

Chapter 7

The Neurologic System

Objectives

- Name the structures of the neurologic system.
- Contrast the functions of the central, peripheral, and autonomic nervous systems.
- Explain the difference between communicating and noncommunicating hydrocephalus.
- State the differences among cerebral, coronary, and pulmonary thromboses.
- Compare cerebral and coronary ischemia.
- Explain herniated intervertebral disk.
- Contrast the symptoms of Huntington's chorea and Friedreich's ataxia.
- Differentiate between spastic, ataxic, athetoid, and rigid cerebral palsy.
- Compare the symptoms of parkinsonian syndrome and Guillain-Barré syndrome; multiple sclerosis and muscular dystrophy.
- Differentiate between the types of epilepsy.

FUNCTION AND STRUCTURE

The nervous sytem, along with the endocrine system, correlates the adjustment and reaction of the human body to the internal and external environment. The nervous system communicates to all parts of the body through neurons by nerve-to-nerve impulses; the endocrine system communicates by secreting hormones into the blood through ductless glands, to be carried to all parts of the body. Nerve impulses and hormones work together to maintain homeostasis within the body, which is bombarded by internal and external environmental stimuli. This chapter is devoted exclusively to the nervous system.

The nervous system is divided into (a) the central nervous system, (b) the peripheral nervous system, and (c) the autonomic nervous system (see Figure 7–1).

Figure 7–1 The Nervous System

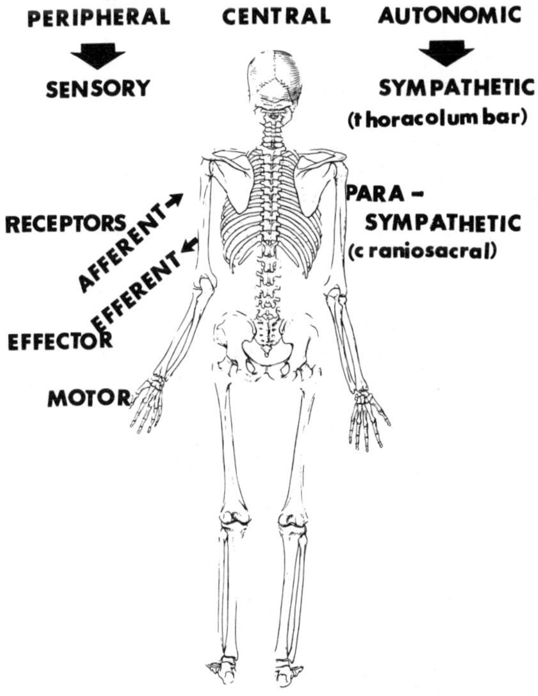

CENTRAL NERVOUS SYSTEM

The central nervous system (CNS) consists of the brain and the spinal cord.

Brain

The brain consists of the cerebrum, the brain stem, and the cerebellum (Figure 7–2).

Cerebrum

The cerebrum—right and left hemispheres—has a frontal, a parietal, a temporal, and an occipital lobe. The cerebrum functions by (a) initiating motor impulses to the muscles, (b) receiving sensory impulses from the periphery, and (c) thinking and reasoning for the individual. These functions are carried out in the cerebral cortex, a thin layer of gray matter that covers the hemispheres. Nerve cells in the cerebral cortex are grouped together by bundles of associated fibers to form nuclei, or centers. These centers function by giving off impulses in the performance of actions; impulses have been found to flow more easily through repetition and to form habits.

Figure 7–2 Parts of the Brain

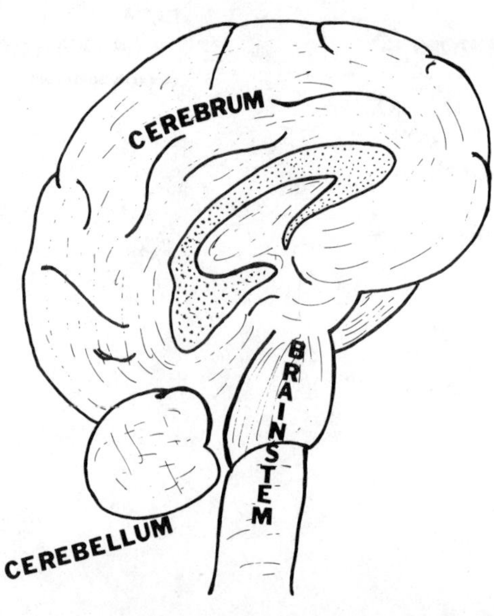

Brain Stem

The brain stem—midbrain, pons, and medulla oblongata—extending into the spinal cord, functions as a passageway and storehouse for (a) innumerable motor and sensory nerves and (b) the 12 cranial nerves extending to the eyes, ears, face, and mouth (Figure 7–3).

Cerebellum

The cerebellum function is coordinating and maintaining a state of balance in the body.

Spinal Cord

The spinal cord functions as a passageway for all nerves going to and coming from different parts of the body. Motor fibers from the brain end in nerve cells located in the gray matter of the spinal cord. From the nerve cells in the spinal cord, another group of nerve fibers carry motor messages to the muscles of the body. These nerve fibers are called *efferent nerves*. Nerve fibers from the upper

---

Figure 7–3 Cranial Nerves

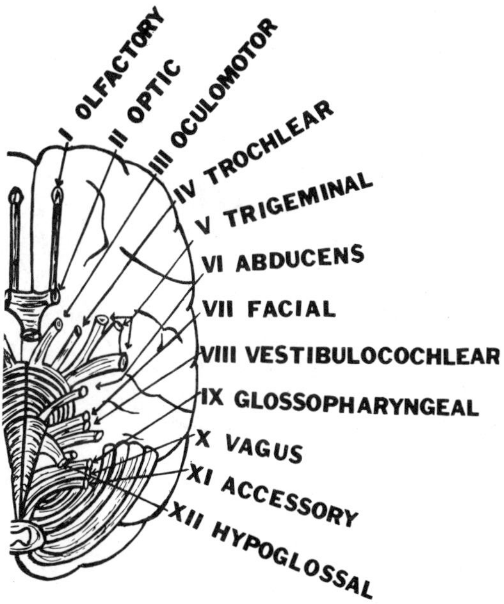

part of the body leave the spinal cord at the cervical region; nerve fibers from the lower part of the body leave the spinal cord at the lumbar region. Both groups exit through the anterior nerve roots to become peripheral motor nerves and fibers.

Sensory nerve fibers that carry messages to the CNS from the body *(afferent nerves)* enter the spinal cord through the posterior nerve root. Another group of nerve fibers go to centers in the brain where the messages are interpreted in terms of the outside environment. Figure 7–4 shows both the anterior and the posterior roots of the spinal nerves with synapse (the junction where an impulse is transmitted from one neuron to another).

CEREBROSPINAL FLUID

Cerebrospinal fluid (CSF) is so named because it bathes the brain and passes down the central canal and outside the spinal cord. It is produced by the choroid plexus and brain parenchyma; tracing its path, it is circulated through the openings in the roof of the fourth ventricle into the subarachnoid space and is absorbed into the venous system.

Changes in the carbon dioxide content of the CSF affect the respiratory center in the medulla oblongata, which helps to control breathing.

The volume of CSF in the adult brain is about 140 ml; approximately 23 ml are in the ventricles and about 117 ml are in the subarachnoid spaces of the brain and spinal cord.

Figure 7–4 Roots of Spinal Nerve

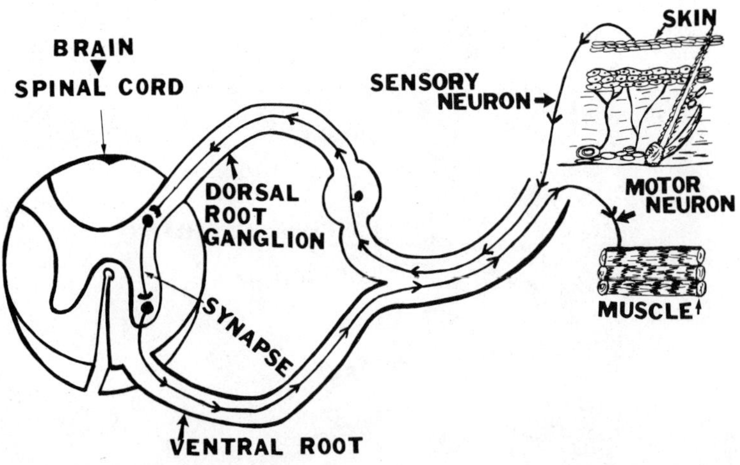

PERIPHERAL NERVOUS SYSTEM

The peripheral nervous system (PNS) includes all the nerves and ganglia outside the brain and spinal cord. A network of nerve fibers serves as a direct contact between the person and his or her environment for the purpose of survival. The function of the PNS begins with terminal nerve endings, known as *receptors,* which gather information and transmit it in the form of impulses by way of afferent, or sensory, nerves. The CNS interprets the information, and an efferent, or motor, nerve sends an impulse back to the part of the body that must take immediate action. The part of the body that responds with the desired activity is called the *effector*. Figure 7–4 shows the pathway of afferent and efferent messages.

AUTONOMIC NERVOUS SYSTEM

The impulses of the central and peripheral nervous systems are voluntary. The impulses of the autonomic nervous system (ANS) are involuntary. The ANS acts independently by carrying out functions without direct control of the body systems. The ANS is composed of (a) the sympathetic and (b) the parasympathetic nervous systems, which perform opposite functions. For example, the sympathetic nervous system is responsible for dilating the pupils of the eyes and the parasympathetic nervous system is responsible for constricting them.

NERVOUS SYSTEM TISSUE

The tissues of the nervous system are (a) neurons, or nerve cell, and (b) neuroglia, or interstitial tissue.

Neurons

Neurons consist of (a) the cell body including nucleus and cytoplasm, (b) an elongated projection called an axon, and (c) one or more projections called dendrites (Figure 7–5). The function of the axon is to transmit impulses away from the cell body. The function of the dendrites is to transmit impulses to the cell body. The axon of the cell of the CNS is surrounded by a myelin sheath. The axon of the peripheral nerve cell has an additional nucleated sheath called neurilemma (Schwann's membrane).

Interstitial Tissue

The interstitial tissue of the CNS contains (a) astroglia cells, (b) oligodendroglia, and (c) microglia cells.

Figure 7–5 A Neuron

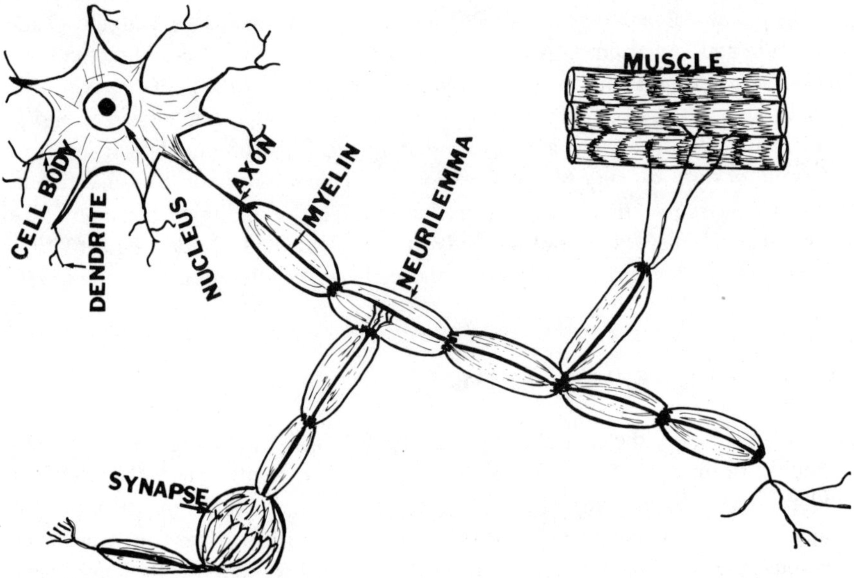

Astroglia Cells

Astroglia cells attached to the capillaries function by (a) carrying fluids, water, and electrolytes between capillaries and nerve cells and by (b) repairing the injured brain tissue. The common brain tumor gliosis has its origin in astroglia cells.

Oligodendroglia Cells

The function of oligodendroglia cells is unknown.

Microglia Cells

Microglia cells are small, nonneural cells of various forms. They are migratory cells and act like phagocytes to waste products of the nervous system.

NERVOUS SYSTEM DISEASES

Patients with diseases and defects of the nervous system, when admitted to health care facilities, are assigned to the neurologic service. Neurology is that branch of medicine dealing with diagnosis and treatment of nervous disorders. The diseases and defects of the neurologic system are divided into congenital defects and acquired diseases.

CONGENITAL DEFECTS

Hydrocephalus

Hydrocephalus is a congenital condition characterized by an abnormal accumulation of CSF within the cranial vault, with dilatation of the ventricles. It is generally accompanied by increased cranial pressure.

The two types of hydrocephalus are (a) communicating and (b) noncommunicating.

In *communicating hydrocephalus,* the CSF reaches the subarachnoid space but is not absorbed owing to other congenital anomalies, trauma, infection, or a brain tumor. In *noncommunicating hydrocephalus,* the CSF does not reach the subarachnoid space owing to a stricture or occlusion of the aqueduct of Sylvius.

A newborn with hydrocephalus may have enlargement of the head at birth, wide fontanelles, and downward displacement of the eyes within the orbital cavities. Or the infant's head may enlarge gradually, so that neurologic symptoms do not appear until early childhood or adulthood.

Signs and symptoms include progressive enlargement of the cranium, irritability, lethargy, vomiting, spasticity of the lower limbs, and abnormal reflex reactions. When the cranium becomes enormous, the patient also displays somnolence and seizures.

Diagnosis is confirmed by computerized axial tomography, encephalography, and arteriography.

Treatment consists of surgical correction to allow the normal flow of CSF. Such surgery involves the insertion of a catheter to siphon off excess fluid by ventricular bypass to either the right atrium of the heart or the peritoneal cavity. Recently, after in utero diagnosis, a shunt with bypass to the uterus was inserted successfully. The child, born by cesarean section, was without abnormal enlargement of the skull. After birth, the shunt was replaced with a bypass. The child's prognosis for leading a normal life is excellent.

Caring for a child with hydrocephalus entails proper handling for relief of strain on the neck and supportive nutrition. Maintenance of the shunt involves instructions to parents in the proper care of the shunt to avoid blockage and infection. Acetazolamide (Diamox) may be given to reduce CSF production. Spina bifida is often associated with hydrocephalus. Figure 7–6 shows a child with hydrocephalus.

Figure 7–6 Hydrocephalus Shunt Ventriculoatrial

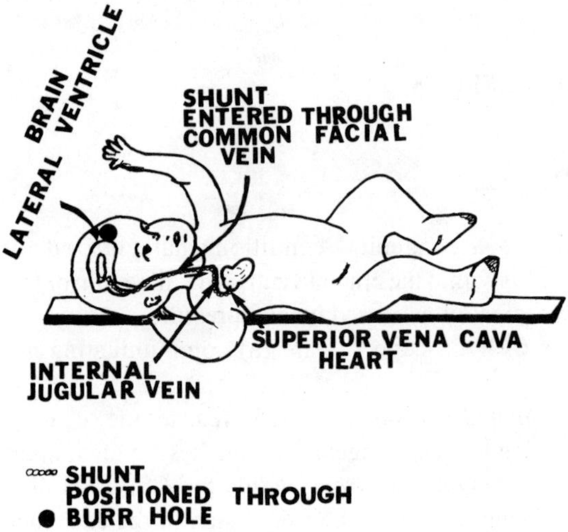

Source: Adapted from Youmans, J. *Neurological Surgery* (Philadelphia, Pa.: W.B. Saunders, 1973), p. 584.

Spina Bifida

Spina bifida is a general term used to define an opening in the bony encasement of the spinal cord through which the spinal cord and meninges may or may not protrude, called spina bifida cystica and spina bifida occulta, respectively.

Spina Bifida Occulta

Spinda bifida occulta is a defect in the laminar arch of the lumbosacral area without herniation of the spinal cord or meninges. It is characterized by a dimplelike skin depression. It is generally asymptomatic, but in some cases, the patient may experience urinary incontinence, weakness, and sensory loss in the lower lumbar area. In such cases, an intraspinal mass (dermoid or lipoma) may be demonstrated by myelography. Laminectomy for removal of the mass is indicated when there are progressive neurologic deficits.

Spina Bifida Cystica

Spina bifida cystica is a defect in the laminar arch of the lumbosacral area in which the protrusion through the spinal cord involves the meninges (meningocele), the spinal cord (myelocele), or both (myelomeningocele) (Figure 7–7).

Figure 7–7 Spina Bifida Cystica

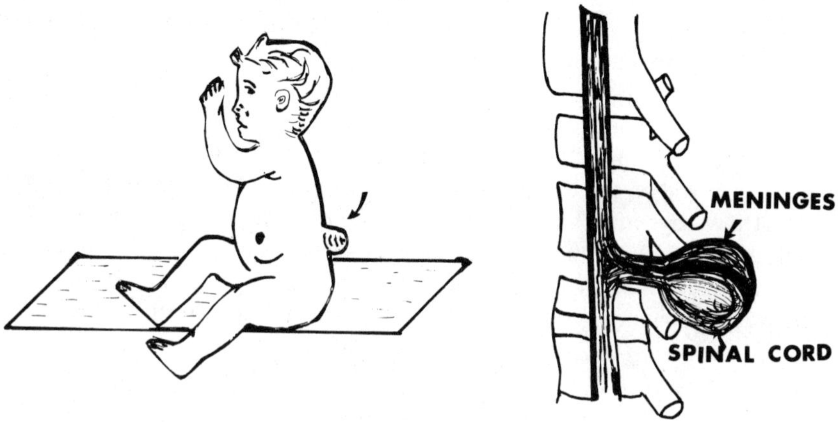

The suffix -cele, or sac, in *meningocele* indicates the saclike, thin membrane containing arachnoid and pia mater that protrudes through a defect in the skull or the lumbosacral region of the vertebral column. In *myelomeningocele,* the saclike protrusion contains spinal cord and its meninges. The sac is translucent and varies in sizes. The membrane may or may not be covered with skin. Before birth the sac is collapsed, but soon after birth, the thin-walled sac becomes distended with CSF. The sac has a high-risk factor of leaking or rupturing, which may lead to infection or meningitis.

Neurologic deficits may or may not be present with meningocele but are severe with myelomeningocele. They include paralysis of the lower extremities (paraplegia), with loss of bowel function and bladder control. The extent of paralysis depends on the level of the spinal cord defect. In myelomeningocele, there may be accompanying deformities, such as hydrocephaly, hip dislocation, and club feet.

Diagnosis is evident in cases of spina bifida cystica owing to the obvious cystic mass. However, radiology confirms the amount of bony defect.

Treatment of spina bifida cystica may require the teamwork of such specialists as the neurosurgeon, orthopedist, urologist, and physical therapist. Priority and type of treatment will depend on the location of the spinal defect, the amount of neurologic deficit present, the amount of skin covering the defect, and any accompanying congenital defect, such as hydrocephalus.

The goals of surgery should be the removal of the lesion and the prevention of infection and further neurologic deficits. Because of pressure from spinal fluid, the thin-walled membrane covering the herniated portion of the spinal cord may leak, requiring immediate surgery. Where there is no leakage but the skin coverage is deficient, surgery may be delayed until there is sufficient tissue growth to use the skin in surgically repairing the defect. Because meningocele and myelomeningocele are often accompanied by hydrocephalus, the insertion of a shunt may take priority over the removal of a spinal lesion to avoid evisceration of the spinal repair from increased CSF pressure.

The degree of neurologic deficit indicates the amount of rehabilitation required. Paralysis and deformity of the lower limbs may require surgery, casts, and braces. Control and prevention of urinary tract infection may also be necessary. Team treatment should be started during the first years of life. Mortality is high during the first few days after birth and remains so during the first year of life. With advances of science in the treatment of hydrocephalus, the early closure of the dural sac, prevention of urinary tract infection, and physical and occupational therapy, the prognosis of the severely handicapped has improved.

Encephalocele

An encephalocele is the protrusion of part of the brain through a defective opening in the skull. Similar congenital anomalies of the nervous system occur but are not mentioned here, since the infants born with these anomalies generally do not survive.

ACQUIRED DEFECTS AND DISORDERS

Acquired defects and disorders of the neurologic system may result from infection, circulatory dysfunction, trauma, neoplasms, and genetic causes.

Infection

Infections of the CNS may be caused by such pyogenic organisms as streptococcus or staphylococcus. The etiology may be *Mycobacterium tuberculosis,* syphilis, or fungi; aseptic infection may be due to viruses, such as herpes virus or poliomyelitis virus.

The foregoing infections present the same general symptoms: headache, fever, vomiting, and nuchal rigidity. The presence and variation of neurologic deficits depend on the location of the infection in the brain.

CSF analysis may reveal elevated levels of protein and leukocytosis. Electrocardiography, brain scan, and ventriculography are all aids in locating the area of the abscess. Culture and sensitivity testing of CSF is diagnostic in isolating the organism and helps determine the drug most likely to be successful in combatting the infection.

The patient is treated medically with antibiotics and supportively with an artificial airway and life-support measures. Dehydration and electrolyte imbalance are treated with intravenous fluids. Convulsions, seizures, and cerebral edema may occur. Although the prognosis is poor, antibiotics have greatly reduced the mortality. Survivors may have recurrent seizures, indicating brain damage.

Brain Abscess

A brain abscess is a localized collection of pus in a cranial cavity formed by disintegration of tissue. It may result from an infection in an adjacent area, such as the mastoids or sinuses, and spread through the meninges. This type of abscess may be found in the frontal lobe, the ipsilateral temporal lobe, or the cerebellar hemisphere.

An abscess may also originate from an infection in other areas of the body, especially the lungs, pleura, and heart. The infection is transmitted to the brain through the blood causing an abscess to form. This type of abscess may be distributed among the various areas of the brain.

A compound fracture of the skull after trauma may also result in a brain abscess through infection of the meninges.

A patient with a brain abscess who does not have the complication of meningitis has no signs or symptoms of infection, such as fever or leukocytosis. The lesion, diagnosed as an intracranial mass, is found on x-ray, electroencephalography, or brain scan and must be differentiated from a brain tumor, a hematoma, or some other type of lesion.

Treatment involves intravenous administration of antibiotics before surgical removal of the mass (craniotomy). The patient should be observed for cerebral edema, which would necessitate emergency surgery to prevent brain damage. Owing to the high incidence of seizures among such patients, prophylactic anticonvulsants may be prescribed.

Craniotomy

The brain and intracranial structures in the area of the lesion are exposed through an opening in the skull. A microscope may be utilized depending upon the location of the lesion. Incision is made in the scalp. The fibrous layer of tissue around the skull is incised with an electrocautery pencil and the skull is exposed. After bur holes are drilled, the skull is incised between the bur holes and the dura is lifted. The exposed brain lesion is excised, and the wound irrigated with antibiotics. The bone flap is reattached to the skull. Bur hole covers made of rubber or metal are fitted into the bur holes, which are covered with pericranium. The wound is closed with 4–0 synthetic sutures.

Poliomyelitis (Infantile Paralysis)

Poliomyelitis is a filterable viral infectious disease that attacks the nervous system, specifically the spinal cord and brain. It commonly attacks children aged 6 months to 15 years.

Symptoms are sore throat, nausea, vomiting, fever, diarrhea, constipation, aching muscles and joints. Muscles may also show weakness. There may or may not be paralysis, depending on the type of poliomyelitis.

Prognosis depends on the rapidity of diagnosis and treatment. After the infective stage, long-term rehabilitation begins.

The goals of the convalescent stage are to restore or obtain maximum muscle strength, to enable the patient to stand and walk, and to prevent deformity and malposition of the afflicted area. For paralytic defect, physical and occupational therapy may be needed for as long as two years. Leg or back braces may also be required for assistance in movement.

After the convalescent stage, the patient is reevaluated for residual defects. The purpose of the residual stage is to eliminate the need for braces by correcting residual deformities, improving muscle use, and stabilizing joints.

One method of correcting flexion contractures of the hips and knees uses cast application as a means of stretching the limb. The fascia, muscle, or tendon may also be released surgically. Muscle and tendon transfers are performed for any deformity or stiffness of the joint. Arthrodesis is performed to stabilize a joint. A triple arthrodesis of the talocalcaneal, talonavicular, and calcaneocuboid joints is performed to give the foot stability. Surgery is also done to equalize the length of the legs.

Poliomyelitis is no longer a problem in the United States, but it is in other countries. Travelers from the United States may be at risk if they have lost their immunity.

Poliovirus vaccines prepared to confer immunity are the Sabin and the Salk vaccines. The Sabin vaccine is an oral vaccine recommended for children under age 18 who have no specific contraindications. The Salk vaccine, given subcutaneously, is recommended for infants and children who are immunodeficient and for unvaccinated adults.

Syphilis

Tabes dorsalis is the name given to syphilis when, 5 to 10 years after the initial infection, it attacks the nervous system, causing degeneration of the spinal cord's dorsal column and the sensory nerve. The degeneration of the vertebral column brings about loss of sensation and reflexes, with accompanying failure of muscle coordination and irregularity of muscle action.

The most evident sign of tabes dorsalis is the gait displayed by the afflicted person, which shows lack of muscle coordination. Other symptoms are leg pain, loss of vibratory sense and reflexes, and analgesia. Pupils do not react to light but do accommodate.

Because the disease brings about demyelination of the posterior spinal roots, the prognosis is poor as the disease continues to progress.

Circulatory Diseases

In order to understand the circulatory diseases of the brain, it is necessary to review the circulatory system.

The cerebral arterial system is derived from a complex communicating system that forms what is known as the circle of Willis (Figure 7–8). In the anterior, the circle of Willis is formed by a branch of the internal carotid, the anterior cerebral arteries that are anastomosed with the anterior communicating artery. The circle of

---

Figure 7–8 Circle of Willis Arteries

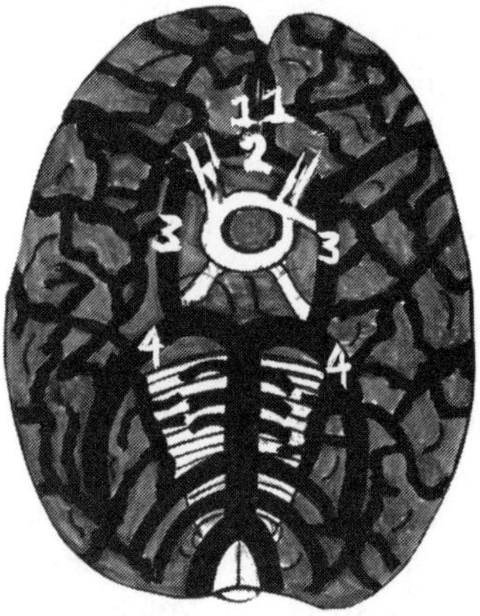

1. ANTERIOR CEREBRAL ARTERIES (2)
2. ANTERIOR COMMUNICATING
3. POSTERIOR COMMUNICATING (2)
4. POSTERIOR CEREBRAL ARTERIES (2)

Willis is formed in the posterior by branches of the basilar, the two posterior cerebrals; these are connected on each side with the internal carotid by the posterior communicating artery.

The cerebral hemispheres are supplied with blood from three trunks from the circle of Willis. This complex system of cerebral arterial communication makes it possible for blood circulation to continue, even though some vessels may be obstructed.

Review of the coronary artery diseases in Chapter 10 will assist the reader in understanding that artery diseases explained in that area apply to diseases of the arteries in any part of the body.

Cerebrovascular Accident (Stroke)

Cerebrovascular accident (CVA) is a disorder of the cerebral vessels that results from cerebral insufficiency owing to obstruction of the blood supply to the brain from arterial occlusion or hemorrhage.

Arterial Occlusion

The effects of occlusion of a vessel may range from slight to disastrous. The outcome depends on collateral circulation, that is, the ability and availability of collateral flow of blood from other near vessels.

It is difficult to differentiate between a thrombosis and an embolism. Generally, differentiation is made only at an autopsy. An *embolism* is an arteriosclerotic plaque or a blood clot that travels through arteries until it reaches an artery in the brain that is too small for it to pass through. The embolism lodges, and it is now called a thrombosis.

An embolism may cause an immediate and complete obstruction of the artery, or it may only partially block the lumen. In the latter case, the lumen may gradually close as debris from the blood collects around the partial obstruction. In either of these instances, the supply of blood to the brain is obstructed, resulting in cerebral insufficiency. The patient with stroke from cerebral insufficiency may experience vertigo, confusion, diplopia, weakness, slurred speech, and paresthesia in the extremities. The signs and symptoms depend on the location of the occlusion. Angiography can identify the involved artery.

Great care must be taken to differentiate the source of the symptoms because these same symptoms may also be indicative of other illnesses.

Treatment consists of identifying and treating the underlying cause; anticoagulation therapy or surgery may be indicated. An obstruction at the carotid bifurcation may require an endarterectomy. If the obstruction is intracranial, anticoagulation therapy may be indicated. Heparin is used for patients with daily attacks of ischemia; warfarin derivative is used when attacks occur less often.

Presently, 0.3 gm of aspirin once or twice a day is the drug of choice. Physical and occupational therapy may be required for rehabilitation of impaired limbs, as well as speech therapy for aphasia.

Cerebral Hemorrhage

Cerebral hemorrhage occurs when a blood vessel in the brain ruptures. The rupture may be associated with hypertension, arteriosclerosis, or an aneurysm. Cerebral hemorrhage from hypertension or an aneurysm is discussed here.

Hypertensive Hemorrhage. A hemorrhage from hypertension is a slowly seeping one, arising in small arteries. The hemorrhage may either progress until brain damage causes demise or cease spontaneously.

Symptoms may vary, depending on location, but generally include high blood pressure in an aged patient who complains of headache, diplopia, and vertigo. On examination there may be weakness or paralysis in the extremities, poor coordination, confusion, and collapse.

Laboratory tests consist of cerebrospinal fluid analysis, computerized axial tomography, or angiography to detect the size of the hemorrhage mass as well as the site of hemorrhage.

Treatment consists of immediate bed rest with sedation and antihypertensives to lower and maintain diastolic pressure in the range of 100 to 110 mm Hg. It should also include physical and occupational therapy for prevention of contractures and restoration of the use of limbs and speech therapy for regaining speech. Nursing goals should include prevention of decubiti, hypostatic pneumonia, and bladder infections.

Hemorrhage from Aneurysm. Most ruptured aneurysms are congenital and arise at the arteries forming the circle of Willis or near the basilar surface of the skull, from the internal carotid or middle cerebral arteries. In contrast with the seeping cerebral hemorrhage owing to hypertension, hemorrhage from a ruptured aneurysm is sudden and often strikes without warning. Ruptures frequently occur during strenuous physical activity, with the person experiencing an excruciating headache minutes before lapsing into unconsciousness.

Laboratory findings include the presence of blood in cerebrospinal fluid. Arteriography is essential for locating the aneurysm. Immediate surgical intervention requires accurate diagnosis and identification of the site of the lesion.

Surgery entails the exposition of the aneurysm for occlusion through a suboccipital or subfrontal craniectomy. Induced hypotension may be utilized to decrease the blood flow in the artery that feeds the aneurysm. The base of the aneurysm is clipped or ligated with end-to-end anastomosis. A microscope is used to facilitate the dissection of the delicate arteries at the base of the brain.

Prognosis is poor for the patient with a ruptured cerebral aneurysm, in that 50 percent of the patients expire between 24 and 48 hours after becoming symptomatic.[1]

Trauma

Cerebral Concussion

A cerebral concussion resulting from a blow to the head may be mild or severe. With mild cerebral concussion, loss of consciousness tends to come and go; with severe concussion, unconsciousness lasts for a long period, with transient loss of respiratory reflexes, vasomotor activity, and dilation of the pupils. Severe concussion may be accompanied by skull fracture.

Immediate treatment involves protection against shock, airway obstruction, and fluid (including blood) depletion. Oxygen may be administered to prevent arterial hypoxia. Subdural or intracerebral hematomas, accompanied by brain edema, may be present with signs of dilated pupils, pupillary fixation to light, and rigidity.

Anticonvulsant drugs, such as phenytoin, will protect the patient against seizures. Skull fractures that are aligned do not require surgery; depressed fractures may require emergency surgery owing to laceration of blood vessels. The convalescent period may be characterized by amnesia. Personality changes may occur.

Spinal Cord Injury

A fracture or dislocation of the spinal column causing compression of the spinal cord may result in permanent damage. Compression of the cervical cord may result in paralysis of the arms and legs or may be fatal owing to injury to the phrenic nerve, causing respiratory paralysis and death. Compression of the spinal cord above the first thoracic vertebra may cause paraplegia (motor or sensory loss of lower limbs) and below the first thoracic vertebra, quadriplegia (motor or sensory loss of both upper and lower limbs). An injury that transects the spinal cord, whether below or above the first thoracic vertebra, may cause permanent loss of motor and sensory functions below the level involved.

The injured patient experiences spinal shock characterized by placid paralysis and loss of skin sensation at the time of injury. After a few weeks, the involved muscles become spastic and some skin sensation may return. However, the loss of motor function is usually permanent.

Treatment of loss of bladder and bowel control and prevention of decubitis ulcers should be a great concern. Other therapy for a patient with a spinal cord injury depends on the type and severity of the injury. General treatment may involve physical, occupational, and psychological therapies.

Herniated Nucleus Pulposus (Intervertebral Disk)

The nucleus pulposus, consisting of pulpy elastic substance, is the central portion of each intervertebral disk. As a result of back injury, strain, or aging, the nucleus pulposus may slide through its fibrocartilage ring and cause herniation between the bodies of the adjoining vertebrae, commonly at the level of the last two lumbar interspaces. This results in irritation of the nerve root, causing pain in the lower back, buttocks, and leg along the sciatic nerve.

Radiologic examination reveals narrowing of the intervertebral space. Myelography may demonstrate the defect.

The goal of treatment is to relieve the pain so that the patient may resume normal functioning. Type of treatment depends on the extent and severity of the ruptured disk. Bed rest, leg or pelvic traction, and back manipulation are generally prescribed. If symptoms fail to improve with treatment and demonstrate progressive neurologic deficits, surgery may be required. Partial laminectomy consists of excising the herniated disk, along with any remaining disk material.

Brachial Plexus Injury

Perhaps the most common type of injury to the brachial plexus nerve is birth trauma, resulting from prolonged and difficult labor. The injury may range from slight to complete nerve rupture accompanied by soft-tissue injury to the humerus or clavicle. Depending on the severity of the injury, the newborn may have upper or lower arm paralysis, or the entire arm may be paralyzed.

Rehabilitation may begin the second week after birth and continue for months. This consists of exercises administered to the child by the parents. The prognosis for improvement or recovery depends on the extent and severity of the injury.[2]

Parkinson's Disease (Paralysis Agitans)

Parkinson's disease is characterized by involuntary shaking of the hands, a pill-rolling motion in the fingers, muscle rigidity, a masklike face, shuffling gait, and drooling.

The disease occurs between ages 50 and 60 and is of unknown cause. It can be detected in an early stage by the masklike facial expression and involuntary tremor, which worsens with time.

Drug therapy is generally not given until living impairment occurs. At that time, levodopa is usually given to lessen tremor and rigidity. Another drug that has about the same effect is amantadine hydrochloride. Because the disease progresses slowly, for an average of 10 years, the effect of long-term therapy with levodopa and amantadine is currently under research.[3]

Multiple Sclerosis

Multiple sclerosis (MS) attacks the myelin sheath of the nerve cells, producing sclerotic areas of demyelination and destroying the oligodendroglia cells.

Symptoms depend on the area of demyelination but generally include weakness, incoordination, inability to speak, diplopia, slight urinary retention or incontinence when the spinal cord is involved, and paresthesias in extremities, trunk, and face. Signs of impending hysteria, euphoria, and weeping are also common. On examination, the superficial reflexes are absent or diminished. Muscle weakness and a drunken gait may be observed.

There is no known intervention or cure; the patient should maintain a normal life style and avoid overexertion. Reduction of the spasticity often brings on excessive weakness. The National Multiple Sclerosis Society can provide valuable support for the patient with MS.

Guillain-Barré Syndrome

Guillain-Barré syndrome, or acute idiopathic polyneuritis, is a disorder of the peripheral motor nerves. The etiology is unknown but the syndrome may be caused by a breakdown in the individual's immune mechanism. Various mild forms of virus often precede the manifestation of the symptoms of this disease.

Initial symptoms are tingling and numbness in the toes and fingers, with muscle weakness and tenderness and progressive loss of tendon reflex. The patient may or may not have a low grade fever.

Because of the similarity of symptoms to peripheral polyneuropathies of sundry etiologies such as diabetic, alcoholic, toxic, carcinogenic, and others, careful diagnostic procedures should be followed.

Diagnostic confirmation of the disease is through CSF analysis, which reveals a low white cell count, high protein level, and normal pressure.

Intervention is of a crisis nature, requiring emergency medical treatment with constant monitoring and support of vital functions. The airway needs to be kept clear so that respiration can be assisted if necessary. Serum electrolytes need to be monitored. Physical therapy with heat application will relieve pain. Range-of-motion exercises must begin as soon as the crisis has subsided. Rehabilitation of residual defects may require months of physical therapy, braces, or corrective surgery.[4]

Tic Douloureux (Trigeminal Neuralgia)

Tic douloureux is a painful disorder of the fifth cranial (trigeminal) nerve. It is characterized by a brief, intense pain radiating down the trigeminal nerve in the superior mandibular or maxillary area. Cause is unknown.

The surgical intervention favored is that of removing pressures caused by arteries pressing on the nerve root.

Bell's Palsy

Bell's palsy, cause unknown, usually produces ischemia of the facial nerve in the area where it passes through the temporal bone.

Onset is marked by pain behind the ear, which is followed within a few hours by facial weakness, paralysis, a blank facial expression, and sometimes the inability to close the eye on the affected side.

Recovery depends on the extent of the nerve damage.

Epilepsy

Epilepsy may result from many of the diseases already discussed in this chapter, such as cerebrovascular accident, head trauma, and intracranial infections.

Generally, epilepsy is a convulsive disorder distinguished by sudden, passing symptoms of motor, sensory, or psychic deficiencies. Such symptoms are often associated with changes in consciousness. Seizures are classified as grand mal, petit mal, simple and complex partial seizures, and infantile spasms. Only the grand mal and petit mal seizures are discussed here.

Seizures may be controlled within three to five years with regular doses of phenobarbital or other anticonvulsant drugs. However, drug therapy may be necessary throughout life.

Grand Mal

A grand mal seizure, which may be preceded by an aura (odd motor or sensory sensation), usually begins with loss of consciousness and severe clonic convulsions. During the seizure, there may be loss of bladder and bowel control, tongue biting, and self-injury. Pupils may be dilated, deep reflexes absent, but Babinski reflex is present. After the seizure, the patient experiences a period of sleep and awakens in satisfactory condition.

Petit Mal

Petit mal seizures may consist of fleeting periods of unconsciousness that are not evident to the observer. They are characterized by vacant facial expression and cessation of motor activity.

Huntington's Chorea

Huntington's chorea, a hereditary disorder, has its onset between ages 30 and 45. The patient exhibits personality changes typified by mood swings, lack of interest in life, stubbornness, and inappropriate behavior. Sudden, jerky, irregular, involuntary movements begin first in the upper extremities and then progress to the legs. In the later stages, the patient loses the ability to walk and swallow, and speech becomes difficult.

The disease responds to perphenazine 20 mg per day and to haloperidol 0.5 to 12 mg per day. Nothing can be done to halt the mental decline that accompanies this disease. The prognosis is poor; the disease is usually fatal.

Muscular Dystrophy (Duchenne's)

Duchenne's muscular dystrophy is an inherited disease that affects boys exclusively. It usually begins between ages three and seven with progressive muscle degeneration and weakness, causing an unsteady gait, toe walking, lordosis, and frequent falling.

It is important to distinguish muscular dystrophy from muscular atrophy and polymyositis. This is accomplished through muscle biospy, electromyography, and measurement of serum creatine phosphokinase levels.

Intervention utilizes exercise, corrective surgery (if indicated), and a well-balanced diet to prevent exogenous obesity. Other than the foregoing, there is no recommended treatment.

By age 12, the child is extremely disabled and vulnerable to pulmonary infections and respiratory failure.[5]

Friedreich's Ataxia

Friedreich's ataxia, a hereditary disease usually transmitted through the autosomal recessive gene, commonly develops in children before age 15. It is characterized by weakness in the lower extremities, lack of coordination, and unsteady gait. The patient's condition progressively worsens, and she or he experiences nystagmus and a deficit in sensory modalities.[6] Prognosis is poor; the patient becomes disabled and may have an early death. No cure is known.

Cerebral Palsy

Cerebral palsy is a broad classification given to a number of nonprogressive voluntary motor deficits, including mental impairment. It is thought to result from either antenatal complications, such as prolonged labor, trauma at birth, and atelectasis, or from postnatal diseases and injuries, such as encephalitis, skull fracture, and circulatory disorders.

There are several types of cerebral palsy. Brain damage to the cerebral cortex results in *spastic cerebral palsy*. This is characterized by muscle movements with exaggerated responses, which results in the loss of precision control. Brain damage to the cerebellum results in *ataxic cerebral palsy,* which is characterized by lack of coordination with loss of balance. Brain damage to the basal ganglia results in *athetoid cerebral palsy*. This type of palsy is distinguished by involuntary slow, ceaseless movements that disappear during sleep. Widespread brain damage results in *rigid cerebral palsy,* which is a mixture of all the foregoing types of cerebral palsy.

Treatment goals for a patient with cerebral palsy should be realistic and based on the individual's potential. A child with normal mental capacity should have a comprehensive program that includes physical and occupational therapy, speech training, psychological and social adjustment, and education. The patient should be assisted in developing his or her maximum level of independence. There is a great need for educating the parents of a child with cerebral palsy.

Surgery may be performed on patients with spastic cerebral palsy. The procedure entails the partial division or excision of the motor nerves of spastic muscles to improve balance and increase the capability for muscle training. Other surgery includes tendon transfers, tenotomy, and lengthening of tendons to correct deformities and release contractures.[7]

NOTES

1. Thomas J. Preziosi, "Stroke Syndromes and Cerebrovascular Disorders." In *The Principles and Practice of Medicine,* 12th ed., ed. A. McGehee Harvey (New York: Appleton-Century-Crofts, 1980), 1278–1288.
2. H. Robert Brashear, Jr. and R. Beverly Raney, Sr., *Shands' Handbook of Orthopaedic Surgery,* 9th ed. (St. Louis: C.V. Mosby Co., 1978), 209.
3. Guy M. McKhann and Thomas J. Preziosi, "Parkinsonism and Other Disorders of Extrapyramidal Function," in *Principle and Practice of Medicine,* 1206–1213.
4. E.E. Specht, "Brachial Plexus Palsy in the Newborn: Incidence and Prognosis," *Clinical Orthopedics* 110 (1975): 32–34.
5. E.W. Johnson and J.H. Kennedy, "Comprehensive Management of Duchenne Muscular Dystrophy," *Archives of Physical Medicine* 52 (1971): 110–114.
6. *The Principles and Practice of Medicine,* 12th ed., 1217.
7. Brashear and Raney, *Orthopaedic Surgery,* 180–186.

Chapter 8

The Endocrine System

Objectives

- Name the endocrine glands and give their locations.
- Explain the functions of the anterior, middle, and posterior pituitary gland.
- Contrast symptoms of gigantism, acromegaly, and dwarfism.
- State the functions of the pancreas.
- Differentiate between the various types of diabetes.
- Explain the function of the thyroid gland in metabolism.
- Contrast hyperthyroidism and hypothyroidism.
- Explain the function of the parathyroid glands.
- Describe tetany and its cause.
- Explain recent concepts about the function of the thymus gland.
- Explain the functions of the adrenal glands.
- Differentiate between Cushing's disease and Cushing's syndrome.

FUNCTION AND STRUCTURE

The endocrine system, along with the nervous system, correlates the adjustment and reaction of the human body to the internal and external environments. The endocrine system communicates to all parts of the body by secreting hormones through ductless glands into the blood; the nervous system sends messages through the body through neurons from nerve-to-nerve impulses. Hormones and nerve impulses work together to maintain homeostasis within the body, which is bombarded by internal and external environmental stimuli.

The endocrine system, starting from the brain and going down through the body, is composed of the pituitary, thyroid, parathyroid, thymus, and adrenal glands, as well as the pancreas, testes, and ovaries. (The testes and ovaries are discussed in Chapters 13 and 14, Genitourinary System and Female Reproductive System, respectively). Figure 8–1 shows the location of these glands in the body.

Figure 8–1 Endocrine Glands

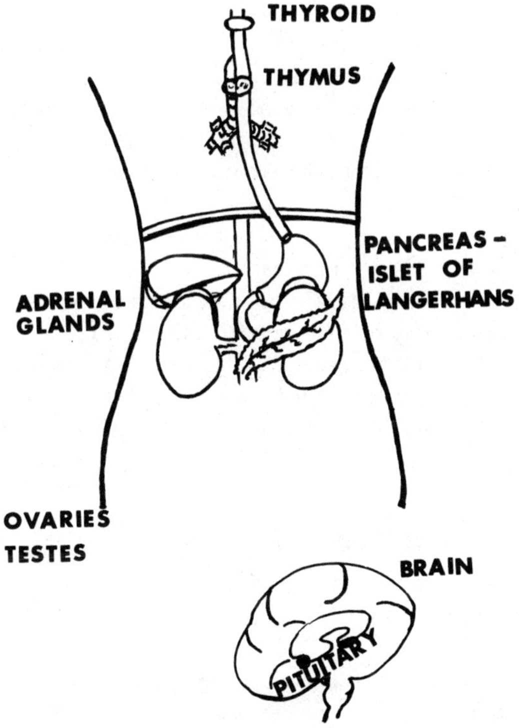

PITUITARY GLAND

The pituitary gland, a small structure about the size of a pea, is located in the saddle-shaped depression of the sphenoid bone, the sella turcica, in the brain. As an administrator, it directs the function of the other glands.

It is composed of the (a) anterior, (b) middle, and (c) posterior sections. The *anterior pituitary,* called *adenohypophysis,* secretes six hormones:

1. adrenocorticotropin (ACTH): affects the adrenal cortex
2. follicle-stimulating hormone (FSH): stimulates development of ovarian follicles and production of sperm and estrogen
3. luteinizing hormone (LH): regulates the reproduction cycle and stimulates the production of male hormones
4. growth hormone (GH): influences body growth
5. thyroid-stimulating hormone (TSH): stimulates the thyroid gland
6. prolactin: stimulates the secretion of milk

The function of the *middle portion* of the pituitary gland is vague. A substance called intermedin (melanocyte-stimulating hormone) is produced in this area. This substance is thought to be similar to corticotropin and may have some relationship to the amount of pigmentation in the human skin.

The *posterior pituitary,* called *neurohypophysis,* produces the hormones vasopressin, or antidiuretic hormone (ADH), and oxytocin. ADH conserves water in the body by acting on the kidneys to promote reabsorption of water through the tubules so that excessive urine is not secreted. It also stimulates the smooth muscles of the blood vessels to increase the blood pressure. Oxytocin functions by stimulating the lactating breast to release milk from the glandular cells into the ducts. Initially, the suckling infant is the stimulus for the release of oxytocin. The uterus is stimulated by oxytocin to contract at the time of childbirth.

One way to understand the diseases of the endocrine system is to realize that their symptoms are due to either an overproduction or underproduction of hormones.[1] Figure 8–2 shows the interrelationship of the pituitary hormones and their target organs.

PITUITARY DYSFUNCTIONAL DISEASES

Gigantism and Acromegaly

Gigantism, an overgrowth of all body tissues, occurs only during childhood and adolescence, when bone development is taking place. GH, or somatotropin, causes the bones of the child and adolescent to grow in length in the process of

Figure 8–2 Pituitary Hormones

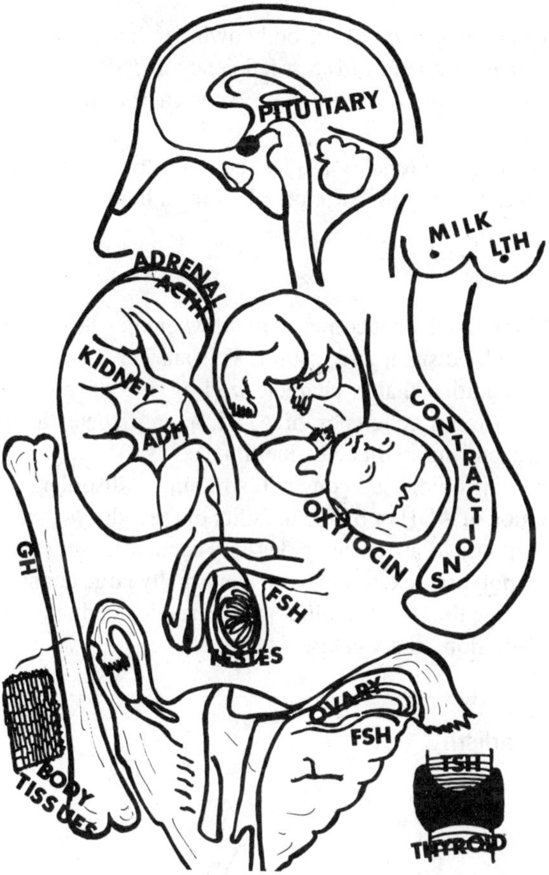

converting calcified cartilage into bone. However, excessive secretion of GH speeds up growth in the epiphyseal cartilage, and the person may become a giant. A tumor of the anterior pituitary may cause this oversecretion.

When excessive secretion of GH occurs after puberty, it is called *acromegaly*. This disease causes bone thickening and softness of tissue. It is characterized by abnormally large hands, feet, lower jaw, nose, and tongue sometimes to such an extent that the person looks disfigured. When acromegaly is caused by a pituitary tumor, the patient experiences headaches and visual problems.[2]

Treatment of pituitary tumor includes radiation and surgery. For patients without tumors, administration of bromocriptine mesylate has been known to restore plasma levels to normal.

Dwarfism

Dwarfism is an undergrowth of the body owing to insufficient secretion of GH (Figure 8–3). It may also result from a deficiency in TSH or ACTH or both, and heredity. Diagnosis needs to differentiate between various types and causes of dwarfism.

Deficiency in hormone production is less complex to treat than is oversecretion. GH may be replaced with a preparation taken from human pituitary glands.

Diabetes

When people are asked what comes to mind when they hear the word diabetes, most answer high blood sugar and insulin. This answer is not altogether correct.

Diabetes is a condition that is characterized by excessive excretion of urine, which may result from a deficiency of ADH, as in diabetes insipidus, or from hyperglycemia, occurring in diabetes mellitus.

Primary diabetes insipidus is a congenital or familial disorder, characterized by deficient production of ADH or by the inability of the kidneys to respond to ADH. Secondary, or acquired, diabetes insipidus may occur after surgery or an accident.

Symptoms are polyuria (excretion of an abnormally large quantity of urine) and polydipsia (excessive thirst). In adults, onset is sudden and may be accompanied by pyrexia, dehydration, and weakness.

Figure 8–3 Dwarfism

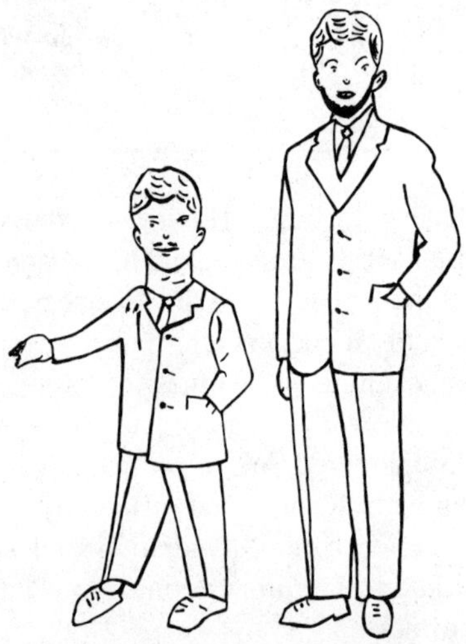

Urinalysis reveals low specific gravity of 1.001 to 1.005, which increases with water intake.

Prognosis is guarded, depending on the replacement of water loss owing to polyuria. The goal of therapy is to reduce polyuria. Either hormonal (ADH) or nonhormonal (chlorpropamide or clofibrate) treatment may be used. A thiazide diuretic may be given for salt depletion.

PANCREAS

The islets of Langerhans, which produce insulin, are found in the pancreas. Insulin regulates carbohydrate metabolism and glucagon in the blood.

PANCREATIC DISEASES

Diabetes Mellitus

Diabetes mellitus is a metabolic disorder in which the ability to oxidize carbohydrates is decreased owing to an insulin deficiency.

Symptoms include glycosuria (abnormal presence of glucose in the urine), polyuria, polydipsia, weakness, emaciation (excessive leanness), acidosis (acid–base imbalance), weight loss, and ketoacidosis.

Ketoacidosis, the accumulation of ketones in the body, may result from the inability of the body to metabolize carbohydrates. Symptoms are fruity breath odor, mental confusion, dyspnea, nausea, and vomiting. The characteristic breath odor is one of the key symptoms of diabetes mellitus.

Laboratory tests consist of fasting blood sugar, glucose tolerance, and urinalysis for ketones and glucose.

The goal of treatment is to maintain a balance among insulin and glucose utilization. Mild cases of diabetes may be controlled with diet alone. Severe cases require restricted diet and insulin injections. The kind of insulin prescribed and the dosage depends on the patient's condition. Regardless of the type or severity of the condition, each patient needs education in self-management, including diet instructions, how to test urine for sugar and interpret test results, how to recognize signs of shock or coma, and self-administration of insulin.[3]

Gestational Diabetes

Gestational diabetes, a metabolic disorder of insulin deficiency, occurs in pregnancy. It may be detrimental to the fetus if not controlled. Intrauterine fetal deaths prior to 35 weeks of pregnancy are attributed to uncontrolled diabetes.

Symptoms are the same as for diabetes mellitus. Treatment consists of diabetic diet and insulin to maintain blood glucose found in the nondiabetic. Generally, gestational diabetes is not present after delivery but may return in later life.

Juvenile Diabetes

Juvenile diabetes, a metabolic disorder occurring in children, is characterized by an inability to metabolize carbohydrates owing to insulin deficiency.

Symptoms are the same as for diabetes mellitus, with the addition of irritability. The child experiences a rapid onset with remission after treatment, generally within a three-month period. Remission may continue for years, only to have the condition return and progress quickly to total insulin dependency.

Clinical laboratory testing includes measurement of serum insulin and glucose levels.

Treatment depends on the severity of the disease. Active children who require diabetic diet and insulin are at risk for developing ketoacidosis, as explained in diabetes mellitus.

Patient and parent education should include review of diet regimen, physical activity, urine testing, insulin schedule (if prescribed), and the risk of ketoacidosis.

Hyperglycemia and Hypoglycemia

In *hyperglycemia,* the amount of sugar in the blood exceeds 110 mg of glucose per deciliter of blood. This condition occurs in diabetes mellitus. It may also occur after administration of intravenous fluids or after regular intake of foods or beverages containing excessive sugar.

In *hypoglycemia,* the blood contains less than the normal amount of sugar. This condition also occurs in diabetes mellitus with an overdosage of insulin, excessive exercise without reducing insulin dosage, inappropriate carbohydrate intake while taking insulin, or dietary deficiency.

Hypoglycemia may also result from excessive insulin secretion (hyperinsulinism) by the islet cells of the pancreas owing to a pancreatic tumor. Symptoms include weakness, convulsions, and loss of consciousness.

Immediate treatment for the diabetic with hypoglycemia is orange juice, with reinforcement of dietary instructions and insulin administration. Intervention for pancreatic tumor is surgical resection.

THYROID GLAND

The thyroid gland, which is attached to the trachea, consists of bilateral lobes connected in the middle by an isthmus. It is a sensitive gland, for during puberty, pregnancy, and stress, it increases in size and becomes more active.

The thyroid gland, stimulated by TSH from the pituitary gland, produces two iodine-containing hormones: thyroxine (T_4) and triiodothyronine (T_3). Both are bound to protein in blood when traveling through the body. In the liver, kidneys, and other organs, thyroxine is converted to triiodothyronine. The serum protein-bound iodine (PBI) test is an index for thyroid function.

The functions of the thyroid hormones are to regulate metabolic rate and the use of protein, fat, and carbohydrate in cells; to maintain GH secretion; to assist with central nervous system development; to stimulate the production of enzymes; and to assist in regulation of body temperature.

THYROID DISEASES

Hyperthyroidism and Hypothyroidism

Hyperthyroidism results from thyroid hormone overproduction. Just the opposite occurs with *hypothyroidism*.

Symptoms of hyperthyroidism are nervousness, lack of concentration, irritability, and, in extreme cases, bulging eyes. Patients with hyperthyroidism are thin because they are constantly burning up energy. They have an excessive appetite and rapid heart rate and experience insomnia.

Almost the opposite symptoms are found in hypothyroidism, with obesity, fatigue, drowsiness, and sensitivity to cold in warm weather.

The serum protein-bound iodine (PBI) test is an index for these conditions, as well as measurement of serum triiodothyronine (T_3) and thyroxine (T_4) levels.

The goal of therapy is to regulate the amount of thyroxine excreted. Treatment depends on the underlying cause of hyperthyroidism or hypothyroidism.[4]

Graves' Disease

Graves' disease is characterized by exophthalmos (abnormal protrusion of one or both eyeballs), a goiter (pronounced swelling in the neck), pretibial myxedema (edematous mucin deposits on anterior surface of the legs), restlessness, palpitation, atrial fibrillation, tachycardia, and warm, moist skin. Eye signs may include lid lag, lacrimation, irritation, and photophobia.

Diagnosis of Graves' disease depends on patient history and physical examination, combined with results from serum T_4 assay and T_3 resin uptake test.

Treatment is determined by the severity of the disease and the patient's age. Antithyroid drugs, propylthiouracil, and methimazole have been used with success. Radioactive iodine is used with patients who are past their childbearing years. Surgery is indicated for patients who cannot tolerate antithyroid drugs or radioactive iodine.[5]

Cretinism

A pregnant woman with hypothyroidism usually does not produce sufficient iodine during fetal development, which may result in infantile cretinism. In the newborn, cretinism is characterized by small, slanted eyes; the child may also be mentally retarded.

Cretinism can be avoided with early detection and treatment of hypothyroidism with iodine during pregnancy. If it is discovered at birth and is due to iodine deficiency, it can be treated with iodine.[6] If it is due to fetal hypoplasia of the thyroid gland, administration of iodine will be ineffective.

PARATHYROID GLANDS

The parathyroid glands are four tiny structures attached to the posterior portion of the thyroid gland.

PARATHYROID DISEASES

Hyperparathyroidism

The parathyroid glands secrete parathormone (PTH), which controls the metabolism of calcium and phosphate. Low blood calcium increases PTH secretion; hormone secretion raises blood calcium to its normal level by increasing bone resorption. Hyperparathyroidism is an increase of PTH after blood calcium levels are reached. Calcium continues to be utilized through bone resorption until the bones are almost depleted of calcium. This leads to softening and weakening of bones. Excessive calcium (hypercalcemia) in the blood is excreted by the kidneys in the form of stones. This condition is caused by a neoplasm. Treatment consists of calcium intake to halt calcium depletion in bone and surgical removal of the neoplasm. Figure 8–4 illustrates the concept of hyperparathyroidism.

Hypoparathyroidism

Elevated levels of blood calcium decrease the secretion of PTH. This is accomplished by stimulating the secretion of calcitonin by the thyroid gland; calcitonin lowers blood calcium by inhibiting bone resorption. Hypoparathyroidism occurs when there is a deficiency of PTH; when calcium is low and resorption and accretion are not balanced; and when hypocalcemia occurs. This concept is shown in Figure 8–5.

Figure 8–4 Hyperparathyroidism

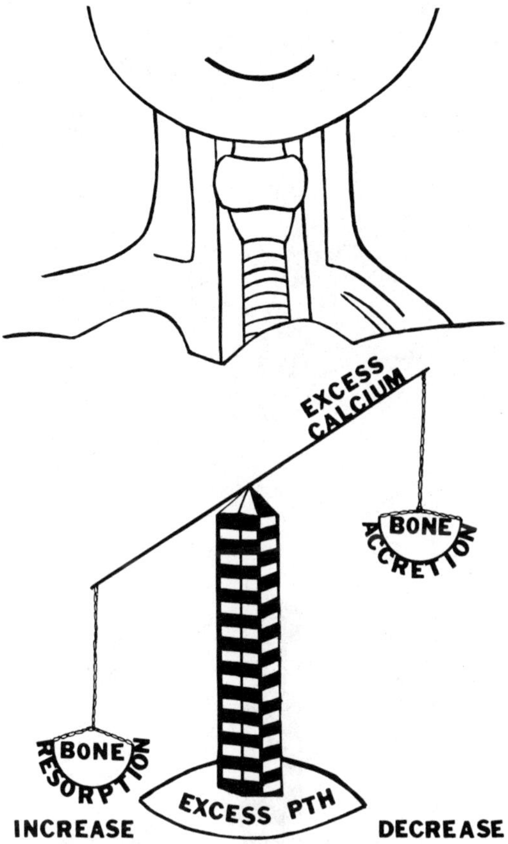

The acute stage of hypoparathyroidism, tetany, may occur after thyroid surgery, when part of the parathyroid is also removed. Tetany is characterized by muscle spasms and convulsions. Treatment is restoration of serum calcium level to normal through intravenous injection of calcium salts.[7]

THYMUS GLAND

The thymus is a gland-like structure located anterior to the lower trachea, inferior to the thyroid, and superior to the fourth costal cartilage in the mediastinal

Figure 8–5 Hypoparathyroidism

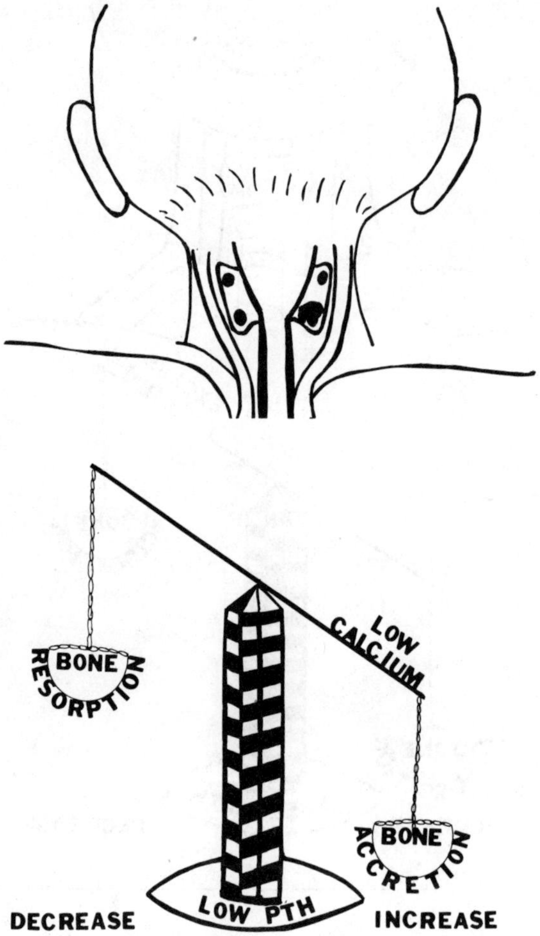

cavity. At birth and up to age 2, the thymus is large in comparison to the body. It continues to grow until puberty when atrophy begins. Not a great deal was known about the thymus until recently and not much is understood fully now. It was credited with forming antibodies to protect the body from disease. Now it is thought that the thymus also plays an active part in the lymphatic system.

The hormone thymosin has been isolated from thymus tissue. Normally present in sufficient quantities in the child, thymosin decreases with age. Thymosin is a group of peptides that play an active role in maturation and development of the T-cells. T-cells, or thymus-dependent lymphocytes, are thought to resist infectious diseases such as those attributed to some bacteria and viruses, cancer, and homograft.

Indications for immune deficiencies in a child younger than six months are infections with persistent lymphocyte counts below 2,000 cubic mm (lymphopenia). X-rays of the chest and abdomen are taken to verify the presence of the thymus and spleen.

Children lacking immunity are isolated within a sterile atmosphere (bubble); other treatment depends entirely upon the etiology of the immune disorder. Generally, these children do not live long.

Synthetic thymosin is being used in research for treatment of rheumatoid arthritis, which is thought to be caused by an immune disorder. Conclusive results have not been reached.

ADRENAL GLANDS

The adrenal glands are located on top of each kidney. Some consider them two glands contained in one because each has two main parts, the cortex and the medulla, which perform specific functions.

The *adrenal cortex* is made up of three layers of cells: the outer layer, glomerulosa, secretes hormones called mineralocorticoids; the middle layer, fasciculata, secretes glucocorticoids; and the inner layer, reticularis, secretes both glucocorticoids and sex hormones.

The principal mineralocorticoid, aldosterone, functions by maintaining homeostasis of blood sodium concentration. Aldosterone stimulates the renal tubule cells to recycle sodium ions from tubule urine back into the blood.

Glucocorticoids break down proteins to amino acids in all cells except the liver. The amino acids then move from the cells into the blood, where they are carried to the liver. In the liver, the amino acids, through a chemical reaction called gluconeogenesis, are converted into glucose. A high concentration of glucocorticoids in the blood results in a higher-than-normal blood glucose concentration, hyperglycemia. Glucocorticoids also mobilize fat from adipose cells and maintain normal blood pressure. Glucocorticoid secretion increases during stress.

The adrenal cortex secretes significant amounts of androgen in males and insignificant amounts of estrogen and androgen in females. Oversecretion of androgen in females produces masculine features and may cause a beard to grow.

The *adrenal medulla* secretes two hormones, epinephrine and norepinephrine, which serve to increase and prolong sympathetic nerve reaction to both smooth and cardiac muscles and glands. In response to stress or fright, secretion of epinephrine is increased.[8]

ADRENAL DISEASES

Addison's Disease (Adrenocortical Insufficiency)

Addison's disease results from insufficient secretion of glucocorticoids and mineralocorticoids. It may be caused by adrenal calcification, tuberculosis, or coccidioidomycosis.

Symptoms are weakness, malaise, myalgia, nausea, vomiting, diarrhea, irritability, and pigmentary changes.

Laboratory findings diagnostic of Addison's disease are an abnormal amount of lymphocytes in the blood, low serum sodium and chloride levels, and elevated serum potassium level and blood urea nitrogen.

Adrenal Virilism (Adrenogenital Syndromes)

Adrenogenital syndromes are a group of diseases in which genital abnormalities are caused by steroidogenesis (production of steroids by the adrenal cortex). The production of steroids by the adrenal cortex is begun by the action of ACTH. It follows a chemical roadway in the production of androgen secretion. Androgen is any substance that possesses masculinizing qualities such as testosterone and androsterone. Androsterone is found in males and females. There are four chemical pathways that lead from ACTH to androgen synthesis. A blockage in any one of these pathways causing a rise in ACTH will cause excessive androgen production by the adrenal cortex.

Adrenal virilism (in the mild form, rarely extreme) is the most common of these diseases relating to overproduction of androgen. It is the presence of male characteristics in the female owing to an adrenocortical tumor or hyperplasia. Rarely does it present itself as feminization of the male.

Symptoms include amenorrhea, hirsutism, acne, and a male voice. Preferred intervention is adrenalectomy and drug therapy to reduce androgen production.

Cushing's Syndrome

Cushing's syndrome, a metabolic disorder, may result from chronic and excessive production of cortisol by the adrenal cortex or may be secondary to a pituitary tumor. In addition to the foregoing, Cushing's syndrome may be iatrogenic, resulting from the administration of large doses of synthetic glucocorticoids as an anti-inflammatory agent for rheumatoid arthritis, asthma, lipoma, or some type of skin disorder.

Symptoms are decreased glucose tolerance, moon face, obesity with protuberant abdomen, weakness, headache, hypertension, hirsutism, and some degree of emotional change.

The diagnosis of glycosuria from a glucose tolerance test is diagnostic of Cushing's syndrome. Urinary 17-ketosteroids are (a) low or within normal limits owing to adenoma, (b) high or within normal limits owing to hyperplasia, or (c) high owing to carcinoma. Computerized tomography scanning, ultrasonography, angiography, and ^{131}I-19-iodocholesterol scanning demonstrate adrenal tumors or glandular hyperplasia.

Favored intervention is surgical removal of tumors or resection of the adrenal glands with hyperplasia.

Cushing's Disease

Cushing's disease, a metabolic disorder, is characterized by an abnormal increase of adrenocortical steroids. It is caused by the pituitary secretion of adrenocorticotropin.

Symptoms include an accumulation of fat on the chest, back, and face; hyperglycemia; increased gluconeogenesis; muscle weakness; and osteoporosis.

Hyperglycemia resulting from Cushing's disease does not respond to treatment; the patient may eventually develop diabetes mellitus. The adrenals may have to be totally or subtotally resected, after which drug preparations of adrenal steroids are administered.

NOTES

1. Sylvia A. Price and Lorraine McC. Wilson, *Pathophysiology* (New York: McGraw-Hill Book Co., 1982), 698–705.

2. Ibid., 739–740.

3. G.J. Cahill, Jr., "Diabetes Mellitus: A Brief Overview," *Johns Hopkins Medical Journal* 143 (1978):155–159.

4. Robert I. Gregerman, "The Thyroid Gland." In *The Principles and Practice of Medicine*, 12th ed., ed. A. McGehee Harvey et al. (New York: Appleton-Century-Crofts, 1980), 869–892.

5. Price and Wilson, *Pathophysiology*, 751–752.

6. Gregerman, "The Thyroid Gland," *Principles and Practice of Medicine*, 884.

7. Samuel A. Wells, Jr., "The Parathyroid Glands," *Textbook of Surgery*, 11th ed., ed. David C. Sabiston, Jr. (Philadelphia: W. B. Saunders Co., 1977), 725–738.

8. Turner Bledsoe, "Disorders of the Adrenal Gland," *Principles and Practice of Medicine*, 776–794.

Chapter 9

Sense Organs: Eyes and Ears

Objectives

- Name the structures and accessory organs of the eyes.
- Explain the functions of the eye structures.
- Describe the mechanism of sight.
- Describe the symptoms of cataracts, glaucoma, and detached retina.
- Name the external and internal structures of the ear.
- Explain the functions of the structures of the internal ear.
- Describe the mechanism of hearing.
- Describe the symptoms of otosclerosis and Meniere's syndrome.
- Recognize the conditions for which stapedectomy and stapedioplasty are performed.

FUNCTION AND STRUCTURE

The eyes and ears are sense organs of sight and hearing that, in embryonic development, are extensions from the brain. Throughout life, as sense organs, their receptors continue to send and receive messages that link a person with his or her exterior environment.

EYES

The eyes are perhaps the most treasured of a person's possessions. The structures of the eyes consist of the eyeballs, cavities and humors, crystalline lens, and muscles. The accessory structures of the eye are the eyebrows, eyelashes, eyelids, and lacrimal apparatus (Figure 9–1).

Eyeballs

The eyeballs lie in two bony orbits, where they are protected by surrounding bones. The three layers of eyeball tissue are (a) the sclera, or outer layers; (b) the choroid; and (c) the retina (Figure 9–2).

The *sclera* surrounds the entire eye. The opaque posterior surface has an opening for the optic nerve. The transparent convex anterior surface is called the *cornea*. On an average, it is 10 to 11 mm in diameter. The cornea is the principal refracting medium of the eye. It bends light rays to help focus them on the retina. This is accomplished by changing the curvature of the lens.

Figure 9–1 Eye

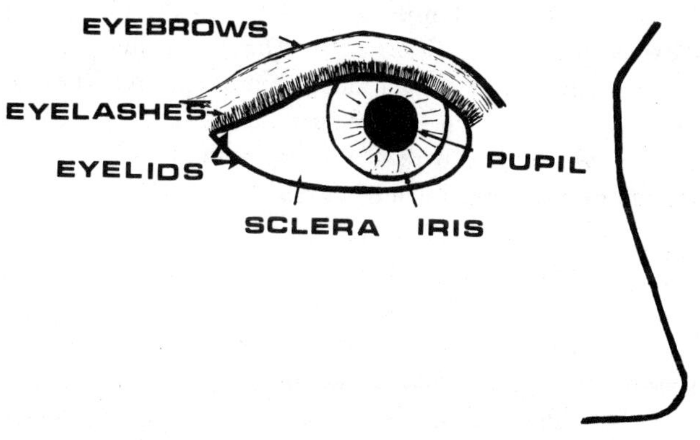

Figure 9–2 Layers of Tissue

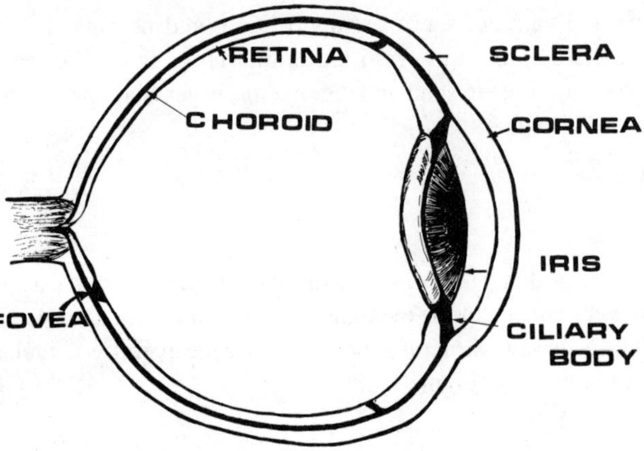

At the anterior part of the sclera, at its junction with the cornea, is a ring-shaped sinus (channel), called the canal of Schlemm.

The *choroid,* a membrane posteriorly lining the sclera, is darkly pigmented and highly vascular. The anterior of the choroid forms the ciliary body. The ciliary body is triangular, with its apex extending from the choroid on both ends. It encircles the iris. The iris, located anteriorly to the lens and posteriorly to the cornea, has a colored, circular, centered opening, called the pupil, which regulates the amount of light admitted to the interior of the eyeball. The iris has circular and radiating muscle fibers. In strong light and near vision, the circular muscles contract the pupils; in dim light and far vision the radial fibers dilate the pupils. This adjustment for near and distant vision is called accommodation.

The *retina,* the inner and photoreceptive layer of the eye, has no anterior surface, as it extends only to the ciliary body. The macula lutea retinae is an oval yellow depression at the center of the retina, about 2 mm from the optic nerve. It contains a pit, which is avascular, and the centralis fovea. The centralis fovea is the area of clearest vision; it is here that layers of the retina are spread apart to permit light to fall directly on elongated cones.

Cavities of the Eyeball

The eyeball has two cavities: anterior and posterior. The *anterior cavity* is divided into an anterior chamber and a posterior chamber. The anterior chamber is located in front of the lens and the iris. The posterior chamber is located between the lens and the iris.

Both chambers are filled with aqueous humor, which is secreted by the ciliary processes into the posterior chamber. From the posterior chamber, aqueous humor moves through the pupil into the anterior chamber. It drains from the anterior chamber into the canal of Schlemm (located within the sclera) and from there into small veins. Aqueous humor drains out of the anterior chamber at the same rate at which it drains into the posterior chamber; therefore, the amount of aqueous humor and the normal ocular pressure (20 to 25 mm Hg) remain constant.

The *posterior cavity* is located behind the lens, ciliary body, and ligaments. It is filled with vitreous humor, a soft, jellylike material, which maintains the spherical shape of the eyeball and bends light rays to focus on the retina.

Crystalline Lens

The lens is a transparent, encapsulated, biconvex structure suspended by ligaments. The ligaments extend radially to sites of attachment to an apex, where the ciliary body meets the choroid. Any change in tension on these ligaments alters the shape of the lens for the purpose of continually keeping the object of vision focused on the retina. The function of the lens is to portray distances accurately; to focus on near objects, the lens bulges; to focus on distant objects, the lens flattens.

Ocular Muscles

The ocular muscles, two oblique and four recti, are responsible for coordinated movements of the eyes. Additionally, the orbicular muscle closes the eyelids and the superior levator palpebrae muscle raises the upper eyelids (Figure 9–3).

The superior and inferior oblique muscles act synergistically (opposite each other) to turn the eyeballs downward and outward or upward and outward, respectively. The superior and inferior recti muscles move the eyeballs upward and downward, and the lateral and medial recti muscles abduct and adduct the eyeballs.

Accessory Structures

The accessory structures are the eyebrows, eyelashes, eyelids and lacrimal apparatus.

Eyebrows

Eyebrows are hairs growing on the transverse elevation, at the junction of the forehead and the upper eyelid.

Figure 9–3 Muscles

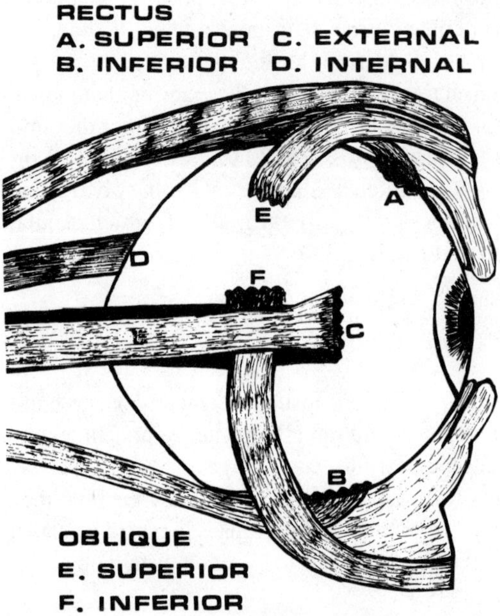

Eyelashes

The eyelashes are rows of cilia growing in double or triple rows on the border of the eyelids, in front of a row of ciliary glands, anterior to the meibomian glands. The ciliary glands located at the base of the lashes secrete a lubricating fluid. They may become infected, causing a sty.

Eyelids

The eyelids, or palpebrae, are two movable folds that protect the eyes from dust, trauma, and intense light.

The oval opening between the eyelids is called the palpebral fissure. Where the eyelids meet, on both ends of the palpebral fissure, they form the medial canthus and the lateral canthus.

A mucous membrane, the bulbar and palpebral conjunctivae, covers the outside of the eye and serves as a lining of the upper and lower eyelids.

The eyelids consist of a voluntary muscle and skin, with a border of free connective tissue on each lid, called the tarsal plate. The tarsal plate is the supporting connective tissue of the eyelid. The tarsal glands, located in the tarsal plate, are secretory follicles.

Lacrimal Apparatus

The lacrimal apparatus consists of the lacrimal gland, upper and lower canaliculi, lacrimal sac, and nasolacrimal duct (Figure 9–4). The function of the lacrimal apparatus is to produce and excrete tears. Tears excreted by the lacrimal gland flow through the lacrimal duct to a minute opening (punctum) in the upper and lower canaliculi and then to the lacrimal (tear) sac located on the medial wall of the orbit. Tears flow from the lacrimal sac into the nasolacrimal duct, which drains into the inferior nasal meatus.

Sight

In the normal eye, rays of lights from an object are reflected (bending of light rays) by the cornea, aqueous humor, lens, and vitreous humor and converge on the retina, where an inverted image is formed (Figure 9–5).

CONGENITAL AND HEREDITARY DEFECTS

Ptosis

In ptosis, the eyelids droop owing to weakness of the levator muscle or paralysis of the third cranial nerve. The condition, which is usually bilateral, may be corrected surgically by shortening the levator muscle.

Night Blindness (Nyctalopia)

Night blindness is the inability of the eyes to adapt to darkness. It may be caused by a hereditary anomaly, vitamin A deficiency, or retinal degeneration. This

Figure 9–4 The Lacrimal Apparatus

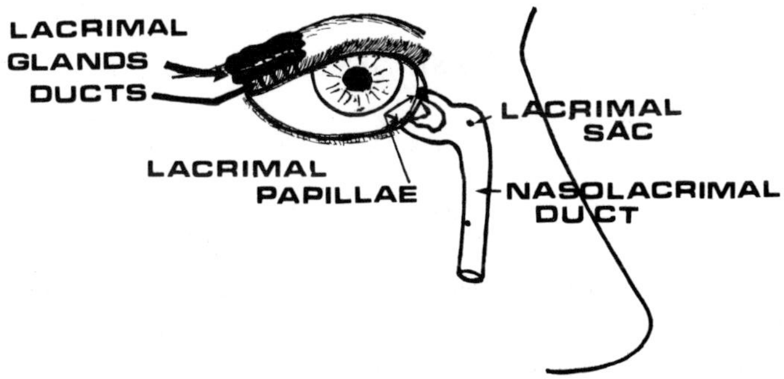

Figure 9–5 Vision—Right Eye (Normal)

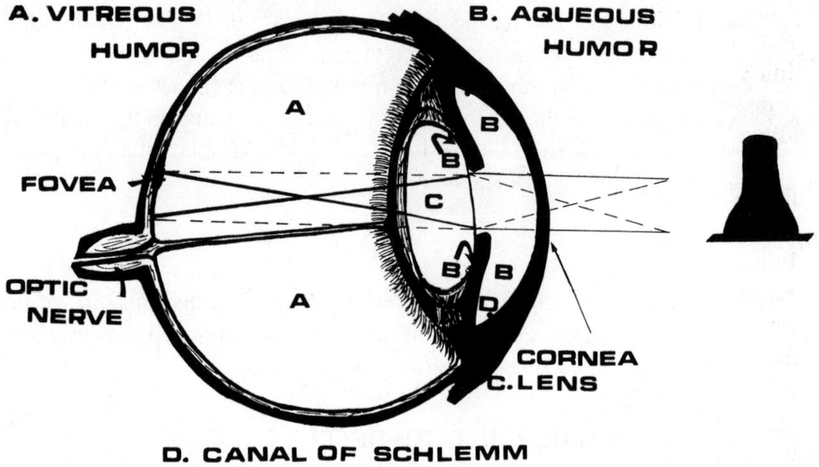

defect is most prevalent among children in underdeveloped countries owing to vitamin A deficiency. It is uncommon in the United States. Treatment consists of massive doses of vitamin A given intramuscularly. Caution must be exercised in administering vitamin A to children over a long period because of the possibility of their developing secondary hypervitaminosis.

Aphakia

Aphakia is the absence of the lens of the eye. This condition may be congenital or owing to trauma or cataract surgery. Refractive correction is accomplished by contact lens or surgical implantation of intraocular lens. The method used depends on the condition of the eye.

ACQUIRED DEFECTS AND DISEASES

Keratitis

Keratitis, inflammation of the cornea, may be associated with glaucoma, herpes simplex, or syphilis or may be due to a nerve lesion. Symptoms are impairment of vision, irritation, photophobia, nausea, vomiting, and pain in eye. Prognosis is guarded for possibility of prolapse of iris and perforation. Treatment depends on the primary cause of the infection.

Herpes Simplex Keratitis

Corneal herpes simplex is a viral infection of the cornea, which may result in a chronic inflammatory problem, scarring, ulcer, and loss of vision.

Initially, the patient will experience a foreign-body sensation in the eye, with lacrimation, photophobia, and conjunctival infection. Treatment consists of idoxuridine, vidarabine, and trifluridine.

Corneal Injury

Injury to the cornea is often caused by burn, foreign body, or laceration. Symptoms are pain in eye and impairment of vision.

Prognosis is uncertain, depending on the type and extent of the injury. Such complications as hemorrhage, infection, glaucoma, or detached retina may occur. Any injury to the eye needs to be treated immediately. Chemical burns should be irrigated with water or other fluids. Some foreign bodies, such as a dust particle, may be lifted out with a sterile cotton applicator; foreign body removal may require magnification. Application of ointments depends on the type and extent of injury.

Corneal Ulcers

Corneal ulcers involve degeneration of the cornea, which interferes with vision. They may be caused by hereditary keratitis, corneal erosion, nodular degeneration, or infection following trauma. Symptoms are impaired vision, irritation, photophobia, and eye pain.

Prognosis is uncertain; there may be scarring of the cornea, perforation, or prolapse of the iris as the disease progresses. Treatment depends on the etiology of the ulcer. In some cases a corneal transplant may be performed.

A corneal transplant (keratoplasty) is performed to improve vision in a person with otherwise normal eye structures. It is the grafting of corneal tissue from one human eye to another. Classification of grafts are (a) penetrating (whole-thickness), (b) lamellar (partial-thickness), or (c) keratectomy (peeling of the cornea). The type of graft used depends upon the patient's needs.

Anterior Uveitis

Anterior uveitis, inflammation of the uveal tract (iris, ciliary body, and choroid), may result from allergy, infection, syphilis, retinal detachment, and systemic diseases. If the flow of aqueous fluid between the posterior and anterior chambers becomes blocked, angle-closure glaucoma may develop. Untreated anterior uveitis may cause cataracts or corneal disease.

Symptoms include throbbing pain in the eye, which increases at night; photophobia; impairment of vision; redness; and lacrimation.

Treatment of the primary disease is foremost; atropine and dexamethasone may be prescribed initially. Prognosis is uncertain.

Cataract

A cataract is a gradually developing opacity of the lens of the eye. It may be bilateral or unilateral.

A common cause of vision loss, a cataract may be due to genetic and hereditary causes, aging, diabetes mellitus, accident, irradiation, and toxic condition. Congenital cataracts are generally hereditary but may be caused by a viral infection during the first trimester of gestation. Trauma may also result in a cataract. However, most cataracts accompany aging (senile cataracts).

Symptoms vary, depending on the cause of the cataract. General symptoms include progressive loss of vision with blurring images. On ophthalmoscopic examination, a gray-white opacity can be seen within the lens.

The mature cataract may be removed through aspiration or excision with implantation of intraocular lens.

Glaucoma

Glaucoma is abnormally increased intraocular pressure owing to the obstruction of aqueous humor flow. It may be congenital or secondary to trauma (contusion injury to eye), cataract extraction, retinal hemorrhage, inflammation (ciliary congestion), and unknown causes.

Acute angle-closure glaucoma occurs when the narrow angle between the iris and cornea dilates, causing the folded iris to block the exit of aqueous humor from the anterior chamber.[1] *Open-angle glaucoma* (chronic) is often asymptomatic. It is more common and develops slowly. The obstruction is believed to be within the canal of Schlemm.[2] The canal of Schlemm drains aqueous humor into the bloodstream.

Symptoms of acute glaucoma are extreme ocular pain, blurred vision, inflammation, and pupil dilation. Nausea and vomiting may be caused by increased ocular pressure. If untreated, blindness may result in a week. Chronic glaucoma may be asymptomatic except for progressive loss of peripheral vision.

Acute glaucoma is treated with eye drops to constrict the pupil and draw the iris away from the cornea. Such drugs as mannitol and glycerol are given systemically to lower the intraocular pressure. Iridectomy may be performed to produce a filtration for the aqueous humor. Treatment of chronic glaucoma includes carbonic anhydrase inhibitors and epinephrine eye drops.

Retinal Detachment

Retinal detachment is the separation of the retina from the choroid in the back of the eye. This separation usually results in a hole in the retina, which allows the vitreous humor to leak between the choroid and the retina. Predisposing factors include trauma, infection, and aging.

Symptoms are loss of vision in one part of the visual field, with dark spots floating in front of the affected eye. Retinal detachment usually begins slowly and progresses. If untreated, it may result in total blindness.

Surgical intervention is usually required to repair the hole in the retina and prevent the leakage of vitreous humor, which is the retina's source of nourishment. Sight restoration depends on the extent and duration of the detachment.

EARS

After the eyes, the ears may be next in importance to a person. The ear is composed of (a) the external ear, (b) the middle ear, and (c) the inner ear (Figure 9–6).

Figure 9–6 The Ear

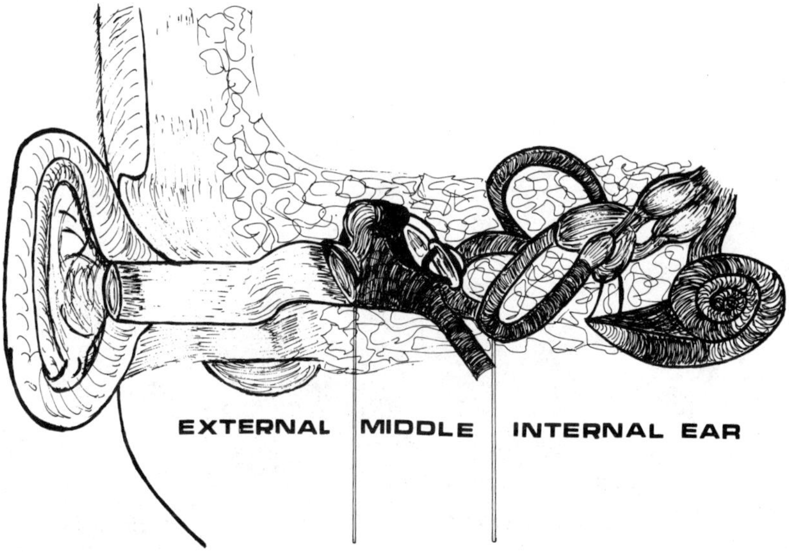

External Ear

The external ear consists of the auricle and the external acoustic meatus. The *auricle* is the appendage on the side of the head. The *external acoustic meatus* (ear canal) is the tube leading from the auricle into the temporal bone. This tube is approximately 3 cm long; it extends inward and forward and slopes downward. Modified sweat glands in the auditory canal secrete cerumen (waxlike substance); cerumen may become impacted, causing pain and deafness. The tympanic membrane (eardrum) stretches across the inner end of the auditory canal and separates the external ear from the middle ear.

Middle Ear

The tympanic cavity, lined with mucous membrane, contains three small bones, or ossicles: (1) malleus, (2) incus, and (3) stapes (Figure 9–7). The malleus attaches to the inside of the tympanic membrane (eardrum) at one end; at the other end, the head of malleus articulates with the incus; the incus articulates with the stapes; the opposite end of the stapes, the footplate, fits in the oval, or vestibular, window, an opening in the wall of the inner ear. The three little bones must be able

Figure 9–7 Middle Ear

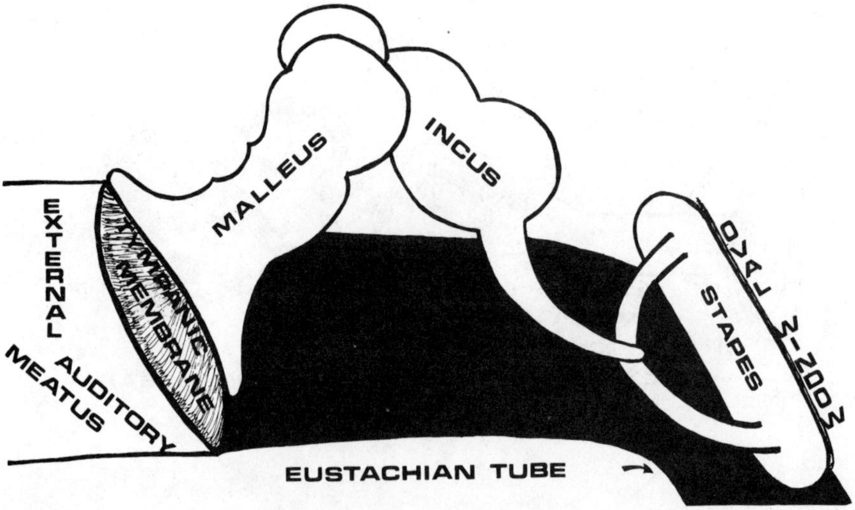

to move mechanically in order to conduct sound from the eardrum to the inner ear. Pressure is equalized by the cochlear window between the middle and the inner ear.

The middle ear opens into the nasopharynx through the eustachian tube, through which air enters the ear. The eustachian tube is essential for hearing. It is also the means by which throat infections may spread to the ears. Posteriorly, the middle ear exits to the mastoid process. It is through this opening that infection may spread to the mastoids.

The functions of the middle ear are (a) to transmit energy from sound vibration in the air column of the external acoustic meatus across the middle ear, into the fluid within the cochlea; (b) to reduce amplitude of vibrations accompanying loud sounds of low frequency; and (c) to equalize air pressure on both sides of the tympanic membrane.

Inner Ear

The inner ear contains bone lined with membrane, called labyrinths. The bony labyrinth is made up of (a) vestibule, (b) three semicircular canals, and (c) the shell-shaped cochlea (Figure 9–8). The function of the inner ear is hearing and balance. The organ of hearing within the cochlea is called organ of Corti. The organs of balance are the macula, located in the vestibule of the inner ear, and the crista, located in the semicircular canal. The auditory nerve extends to the brain.

Figure 9–8 Internal Ear

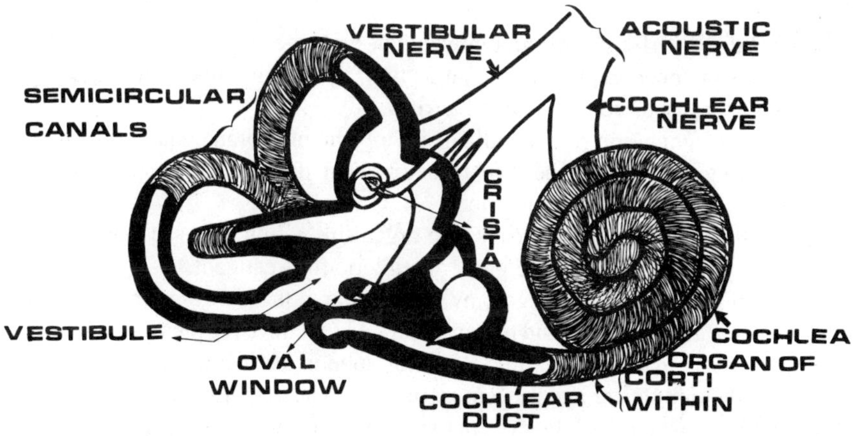

DISEASES AND DEFECTS OF THE EARS

Congenital Sensorineural Hearing Loss

One of the causes of congenital sensorineural hearing loss is the mother's infection with rubella during the first trimester. Other causes include anoxia during labor, bleeding in the inner ear from birth and delivery trauma, maternal ingestion of certain drugs, erythroblastosis fetalis, and hereditary factors.

Diagnosis requires observation of the child for language use and hearing test. Intervention with hearing aid should be commenced as early as age eight or nine months.

Atresia of External Auditory Meatus

Atresia of the external auditory meatus is the absence of the normal opening of the ear. Plastic surgery may be performed to open the external auditory meatus. Provided the remaining structures of the ear are present, the person would then be able to hear.

Myringitis

Myringitis is inflammation of the eardrum secondary to viral or bacterial infection. Symptoms are earache, tinnitus, impairment of hearing, and fever. Otoscopic examination of the ear reveals a tympanic membrane red with congestion and serous fluid. Treatment includes antibiotics for the primary infection and analgesics to relieve earache.

Otitis Media

Otitis media is a bacterial or viral infection of the tympanic membrane, usually secondary to an upper respiratory tract infection. Symptoms are earache, hearing deficit, fever, nausea, vomiting, and diarrhea.

Otoscopic examination reveals inflamed tympanic membrane that may or may not be bulging. There may be bloody or purulent drainage after spontaneous perforation of the tympanic membrane.

In otitis media to identify the causative organism, culture and sensitivity tests are necessary for selection of the proper antibiotic for treatment.

Treatment may include myringotomy, an incision of the eardrum for aspiration of middle ear fluid. The fluid and pus are aspirated to relieve the pressure and pain and to restore the patient's hearing. A plastic tube is often inserted to facilitate aeration of the middle ear and prevent recurrence. The operation may have to be repeated if the plastic tube comes out of the ear before the eustachian tube resumes its normal function.

Perforation of the Tympanic Membrane

Perforation of the tympanic membrane is a complication of otitis media. Symptoms are drainage, impairment of hearing, and tinnitus.

Otoscopic examination of the ear reveals perforation of the eardrum with drainage. There may be permanent hearing loss.

Tympanoplasty is a general term used for operations performed on the eardrum or ossicles of the middle ear to restore or improve hearing. It is preferable that the ear is no longer draining or infected at the time of surgery. Various types of autogenous materials—fascia, fat, vein graft, and others—are used to repair the perforated eardrum.

Otosclerosis

Otosclerosis is the slow formation of spongy bone within the labyrinth of the ear, often causing ankylosis of the footplate of the stapes. Symptoms include progressive conductive hearing loss and tinnitus. Treatment usually involves stapedectomy (removal of the stapes) and insertion of a prosthesis. The purpose of a stapedectomy is to restore hearing for patients with conductive deafness owing to stapedial ankylosis from otosclerosis. A stapedectomy involves the removal of the stapes and insertion of a vein graft, polyethylene tube, or other prosthesis in its place.

Meniere's Disease

Meniere's disease is characterized by severe dizziness, loss of hearing, tinnitis, nausea, and vomiting.[3] Its cause is unknown.

Examination by otoscope reveals dilation of the membranous labyrinth with hearing loss in both ears in 10 percent to 15 percent of patients with Meniere's disease.

Drug therapy with diazepam has been effective in relieving vertigo. Labyrinthectomy is sometimes performed when vertigo is disabling and hearing has degenerated.

NOTES

1. Neil R. Miller, Lawrence W. Hirst, and Arnall Patz, ''Ophthalmology in Medicine.'' In *The Principles and Practice of Medicine,* 11th ed., ed. A. McGehee Harvey et al. (New York: Appleton-Century-Crofts, 1980), 1460–1461.

2. Ibid., 1461–1462.

3. David S. Zee, ''Dizziness, Vertigo, and Hearing Loss,'' *Principles and Practices of Medicine,* 1266.

Chapter 10

The Cardiovascular System

Objectives

- Identify the structures of the cardiovascular system.
- Identify the structures of the heart.
- Trace blood through the cardiovascular system.
- Contrast the circulatory system of the fetus with that of the newborn.
- Explain the function of the cardiac cycle.
- Explain the mechanism of the cardiac cycle.
- Explain the function of the heart valves.
- Differentiate between a vein and an artery in structure and function.
- Name and explain three congenital heart anomalies.
- Differentiate between valvular stenosis and insufficiency.
- Explain the causes of ventricular hypertrophy.
- State how a myocardial infarction occurs.
- Explain the structural changes in an artery owing to an aneurysm.
- Contrast a thrombus with an embolus.
- Explain the circulation of blood through the body when the patient is on a heart-lung machine.

FUNCTION AND STRUCTURE

The cardiovascular system, including the heart, great vessels, arteries, veins, and capillaries, serves as a continuous system of vessels through which blood can circulate throughout the body.

THE HEART

Anatomy

The heart is a pear-shaped organ located somewhat to the left in the thoracic cavity, behind the sternum. The normal adult heart measures five inches in length (from the base to the apex) and three and one-half inches in width; it is two and one-half inches thick. The average man's heart weighs 10 to 12 ounces; the average female's heart weighs 8 to 10 ounces.[1]

The heart is enclosed in a saclike, fibroserous membrane, forming two layers known as the external fibrous pericardium and the internal serous pericardium. The pericardial fluid is found between these two layers.

The inner layer of the pericardium, the internal serous pericardium, is the first of three layers of heart tissue; it is known as the *epicardium*. The middle layer of tissue, the *myocardium,* is heart muscle. The third layer, the *endocardium* or inner lining of the heart, is continuous throughout the interior of the heart, lining the atria, ventricles, and valves. Figure 10–1 shows the three layers of heart tissue.

The interior of the heart contains four chambers, two atria and two ventricles, which are separated vertically by a septum, or wall. The *atria* are located in the upper portion of the heart—one on the right side of the atrial septum and the other on the left side. The *ventricles* are located in the lower portion of the heart—one on the right side of the ventricular septum and the other on the left side.

The *septum* dividing the right and left chambers of the heart is continuous, extending from the apex, or lower end of the heart, up to the base, or upper end of the heart. The function of the septum is to divide the left and right sides of the heart so that venous and arterial blood is separated.

The heart has four valves; two are located on the right side of the heart and two on the left side. On the right side of the heart, the *tricuspid valve* is located between the atrium and the ventricle; the *pulmonary valve* is located at the base of the pulmonary artery, where the right ventricle and pulmonary artery meet. On the left side of the heart, the *bicuspid,* or *mitral, valve* separates the atrium and ventricle; the *aortic valve* is located in the aorta, where the left ventricle and aorta meet. The structure of the heart is shown in Figure 10–2.

Figure 10–1 Layers of Heart Tissue

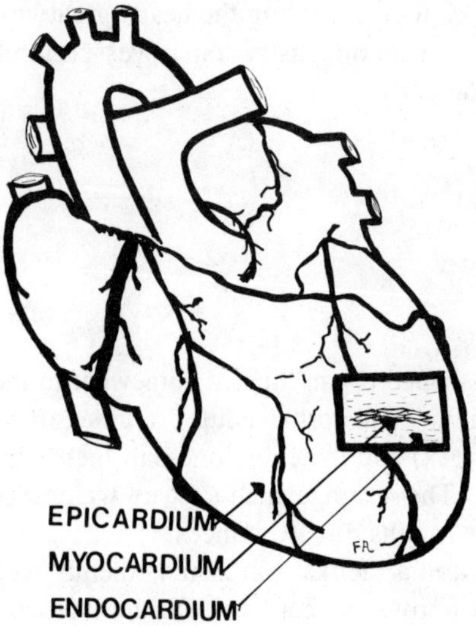

Figure 10–2 Heart Structures

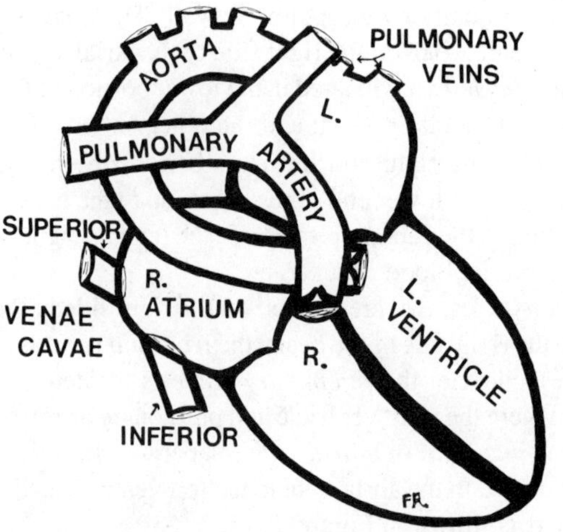

Physiology

The function of the heart is to pump venous blood into the lungs and to pump arterial blood returning from the lungs to all parts of the body. This pumping function is made possible by the conduction system of the heart, which (a) initiates the heartbeat, (b) conducts impulses throughout the system, and (c) coordinates the contractions of the atria and ventricles. The three components of the conduction system involved in the foregoing are (1) the sinoatrial (SA) node, (2) the atrioventricular (AV) node, and (3) the bundle of His (Figure 10–3).[2] The *SA node,* known as the pacemaker of the heart, is located at the base of the right atrium. The *AV node* is located just inside the right atrial septum, between the atrium and ventricle. The *bundle of His* extends down from the AV node and bifurcates into right and left branches in the ventricles, terminating in the Purkinje fibers located in the walls of the ventricles.

The SA node initiates the heartbeat by sending impulses through the right atrium to the AV node, located at the base of the atrium. The AV node transmits impulses to the bundle of His. The bundle of His sends these impulses to the Purkinje fibers. The cardiac cycle begins with impulses from the SA node causing the atria to contract and pump blood into the ventricles. The impulses from the Purkinje fibers cause the ventricles to contract and empty; this phase is called *systole*. The relaxation phase, called *diastole,* occurs when the ventricles are filling.[3] The cardiac cycle consists of one systole and one diastole. Because the cardiac cycle is the result of electrical impulses, the reaction takes place as rapidly as an eyelid blink.

Figure 10–3 Conduction System

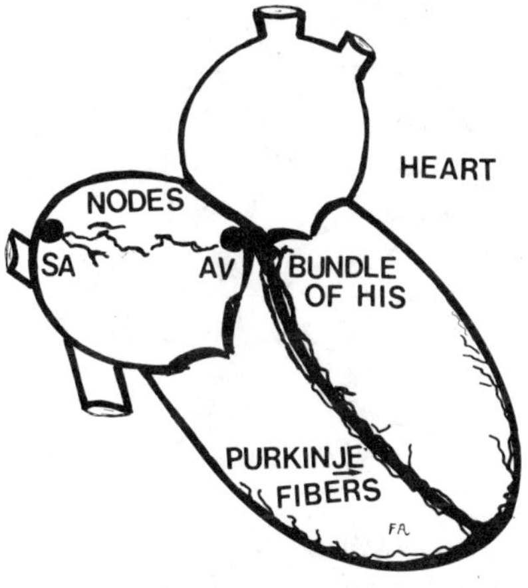

As a result of the cardiac cycle, venous blood from the upper part of the body enters the right atrium of the heart through the superior vena cava; blood from the lower part of the body enters the right atrium through the inferior vena cava. The right atrium's contracting pumps the blood into the right ventricle; the right ventricle's contracting pumps the blood through the pulmonary artery into the lungs, where the blood is oxygenated. The oxygenated blood is returned to the left atrium through the pulmonary veins. The left atrium's contracting pumps the blood into the left ventricle; the left ventricle's contracting pumps the blood through the aorta to all parts of the body.

Blood passes from the aorta to *arteries* and to microscopic vessels called *capillaries*. In the capillaries, nutrients and oxygen are exchanged for waste products from the cells. The oxygen-depleted blood flows from the capillaries into microscopic veins called *venulae,* to larger veins that empty into the superior and inferior venae cavae, and at last into the right atrium, where the process begins again. Figure 10–4 traces the blood through the cardiovascular system.

CONGENITAL DEFECTS OF THE HEART

Congenital defects of the heart are those which are present at birth. Such defects may result from inherited genetic disorders, chromosomal aberrations, or environmental causes, such as drugs, infection, radiation, and maternal diseases. The foregoing causes account for only about 10 percent of all congenital defects; the other 90 percent are due to unknown causes.

Figure 10–4 The Heart

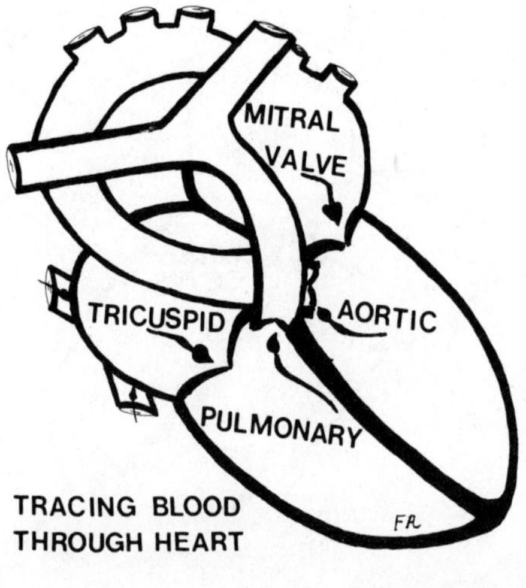

Before birth the fetus depends on the mother for cardiovascular circulation. Nutrients and oxygen from maternal blood enter fetal blood at the placental barrier, and waste products from fetal metabolism enter maternal blood. The foramen ovale, or oval-shaped window, in the atrial septum allows the mother's blood to circulate in the fetus. The ductus arteriosus, located between the pulmonary artery and the aorta, allows fetal blood to bypass the lungs. Normally, at birth, the membrane drops over the oval window to close it; the opening between the pulmonary artery and the aorta degenerates and closes within an hour after birth. Figure 10–5 shows the circulatory system of the fetus and newborn.

Patent Ductus Arteriosus

Patent ductus arteriosus occurs when the opening between the pulmonary artery and the aorta fails to close and degenerate after birth (see Figure 10–5). A newborn with patent ductus arteriosus reveals a systolic murmur until about age one, when a continuous murmur becomes audible. Other symptoms are congestive heart failure, pulmonary infection, and hypertension, and the baby does not gain weight according to age. Surgical intervention is generally indicated between ages 3 and 10. However, if symptoms are severe, correction is sometimes made before age three. Cardiac catheterization is recommended for diagnosis only, when there is an indication that other congenital anomalies are present.[4]

In the cardiac catheterization procedure a catheter is inserted through the brachial or femoral artery and vein directly into the area to be examined. Radi-

Figure 10–5 The Heart of an Unborn Child

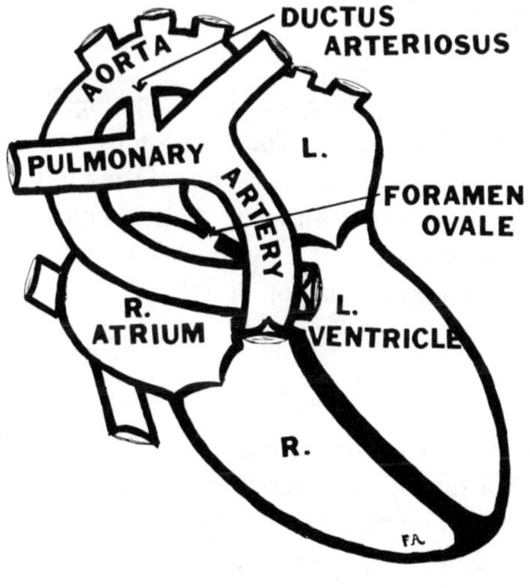

opaque contrast medium is injected through the catheter so that abnormalities or diseased areas of the heart may be visualized by fluoroscopy. Angiocardiography and aortography may also be used. During the procedure, the patient is monitored to detect any irregularities.

Surgical correction of patent ductus arteriosus is by ligation (short patent ductus) or by ligation and transection of the divided ends of a long patent ductus arteriosus.

Patent Foramen Ovale

Patent foramen ovale occurs when the membrane fails to close the foramen ovale entirely or partially after birth. Generally, this defect is associated with other congenital heart abnormalities, such as coarctation of the aorta, ventricular septal defect, and pulmonary stenosis. Symptoms depend on accompanying abnormalities. It has been found that children with an atrial septal defect are vulnerable to pneumonia.[5]

The heart-lung machine (cardiopulmonary bypass) allowing extracorporeal circulation (circulation of blood outside the body) for open heart surgery was developed during World War II. Regardless of the type or make of the heart-lung machine used, its purpose is to take over the function of the heart and lungs during open heart surgery. The tubes (cannulae) from the machine are inserted in the patient's body in the following two ways:

1. to the superior and inferior venae cavae so that the venous blood bypassing the heart is oxygenated by the heart-lung machine; and,
2. to the ascending aorta or femoral artery for return of oxygenated blood from the heart-lung machine to arterial circulation. Figure 10–6 shows the heart-lung machine.

Inserting the cannulae is called cannulation; removing the cannulae at the close of surgery is called decannulation. These two terms used in surgical reports describing heart-lung machine procedures are referred to in this book.

Surgical correction of a patent foramen ovale is carried out during extracorporeal circulation. The patent foramen ovale is closed by simple suture of the two edges; a larger defect requires a Dacron or Teflon patch.

Atrial Septal Defects

Atrial septal defects are named in relationship to the position and seriousness of the defect in the atrial septum. The persistent ostium primum is low in the atrial septum. It is serious because blood pumped into the left atrium will flow through the atrial defect into the right atrium (left-to-right shunt) causing congestive

Figure 10–6 Cardiopulmonary Bypass

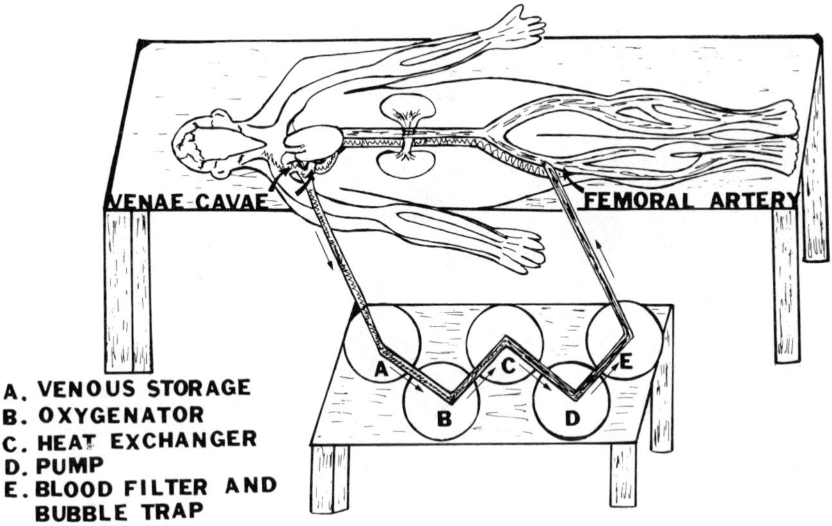

failure. Only a small number of infants and young children have symptoms of congestive failure that warrant surgical repair. Operations should not be carried out in patients with small defects or insignificant left to right shunt.

Surgery should be recommended for children 3 to 6 years old with uncomplicated atrial septal defects where there is evidence of significant left-to-right shunt.

The persistent ostium secundum is a defect high in the atrial septum. Because blood flows downward in the atrium, only a small amount of blood seeps through the defect in a left-to-right shunt. Asymptomatic in childhood, it is the most common congenital heart disease found in adults, especially females. Symptoms accompanying persistent ostium secundum include dyspnea on exertion, fatigue, and ventricular tachycardia.[6] Diagnosis is confirmed by cardiac catheterization. The surgical procedure is the same that is used for patent foramen ovale. Figure 10–7 shows atrial septal defects.

Surgical repair for closure of atrial septal defect is essentially the same as that described for patent foramen ovale. (See Figure 10–8.)

Ventricular Septal Defects

The embryonic development of the heart begins at the apex, or lower end, and continues upward to the base. Any type of small hole in the septum represents a defect. Such a defect is due to interruption in the growth process of the septum

Figure 10–7 Atrial Septal Defects

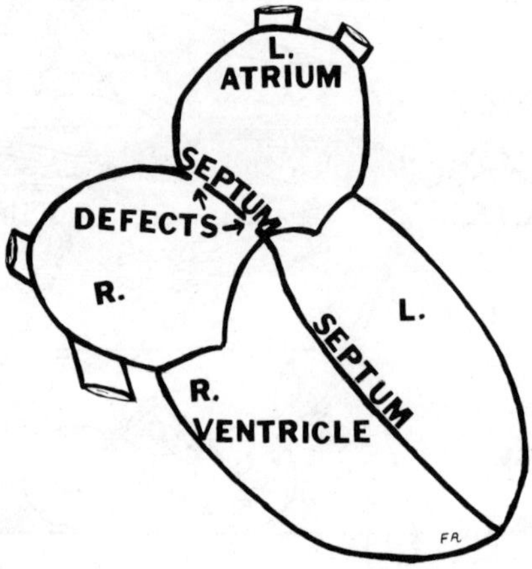

Figure 10–8 Surgical Repair of Atrial Septal Defect

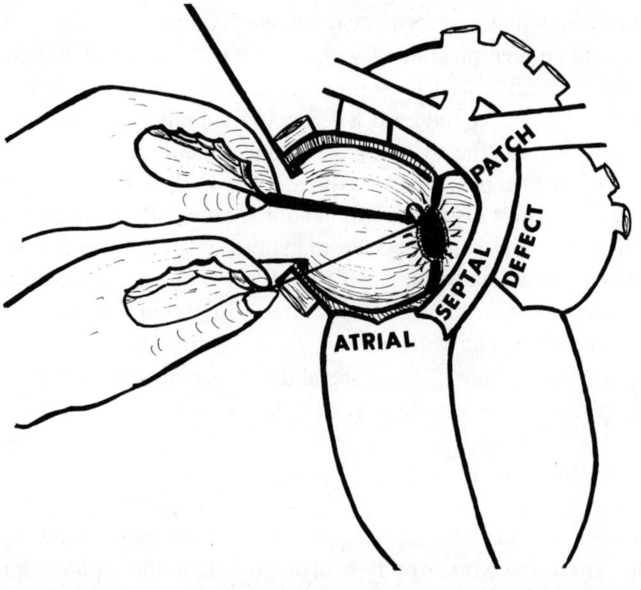

during embryonic development. A child with a small ventricular septal defect may be asymptomatic as an infant but develop pulmonary hypertension in early childhood. Less congenital ventricular defects are seen in adults today because many received successful surgical intervention during childhood.[7] Figure 10–9 shows a ventricular septal defect.

Surgical correction of a ventricular septal defect is performed using extracorporeal circulation. The defect is closed by simple end-to-end suture of a small defect or utilizing synthetic or pericardial graft to repair a large defect in the ventricle. Figure 10–10 illustrates this.

Coarctation of the Aorta

Coarctation is a narrowing of the aorta near the area where the ductus arteriosus joins the aorta (Figure 10–11). Because of the narrowing, a sufficient quantity of blood cannot be pumped through the aorta and circulated to all parts of the body.

To correct coarctation of the aorta, a thoracotomy is performed in the usual manner and the mediastinal pleura is incised. After the coarctation is identified and isolated, the area of aortic stricture is excised and an end-to-end anastomosis is performed (Figure 10–12). An aortic graft may be necessary when the coarctation is long and an anastomosis cannot be achieved.

Figure 10–9 Ventricular Septal Defect

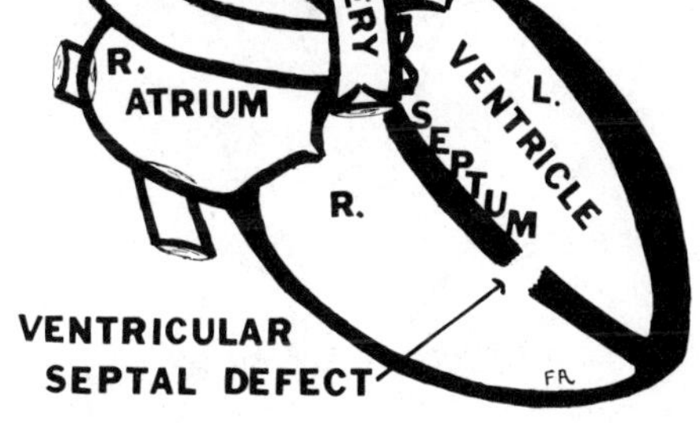

Figure 10–10 Surgical Repair of Ventricular Septal Defect

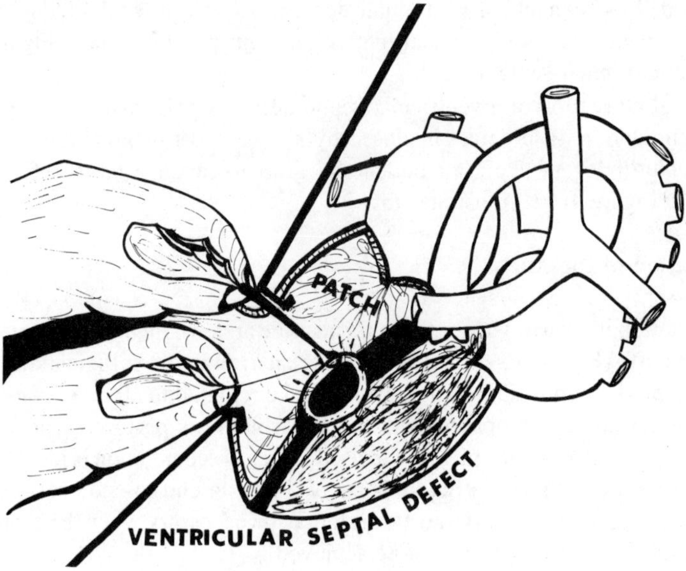

Figure 10–11 Coarctation

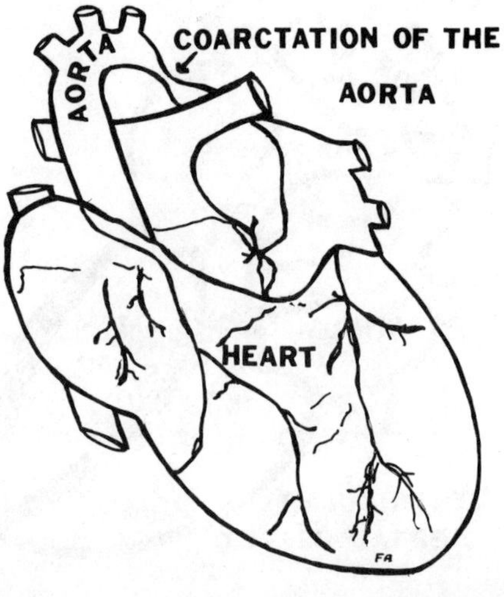

Figure 10–12 Anastomosis

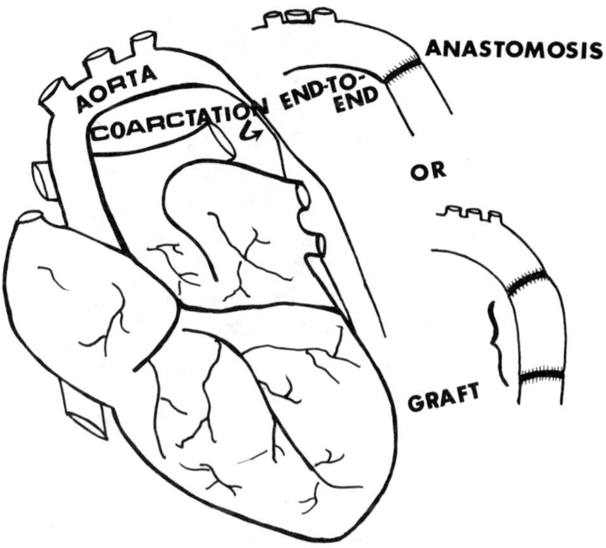

Valvular Stenosis

The functions of the pulmonary and aortic valves are to open and close properly to allow blood to flow away from the heart; the functions of the tricuspid and bicuspid valves are to open and close properly to allow blood to flow into the ventricles. Valvular stenosis does not permit the valves to open far enough to allow sufficient flow of blood through them. This condition occurs most often in the pulmonary valves. Symptoms are ventricular hypertrophy, owing to the requirement of the heart to work hard to pump an adequate amount of blood to the lungs and the body; cyanosis; weight loss.[8] Figure 10–13 shows a comparison between normal and stenosed valves.

Correction of the pulmonary or aortic valvular stenosis is performed under extracorporeal circulation. It is accomplished by separating the fused leaflets of the valve through an incision in the pulmonary or aortic artery.

Tetralogy of Fallot

Congenital defects of the heart generally do not occur singularly; when there is one defect, often multiple defects are found. Tetralogy of Fallot is a combination of four defects identified as (1) high ventricular septal defect, (2) pulmonary

Figure 10–13 Normal and Stenosed Valves

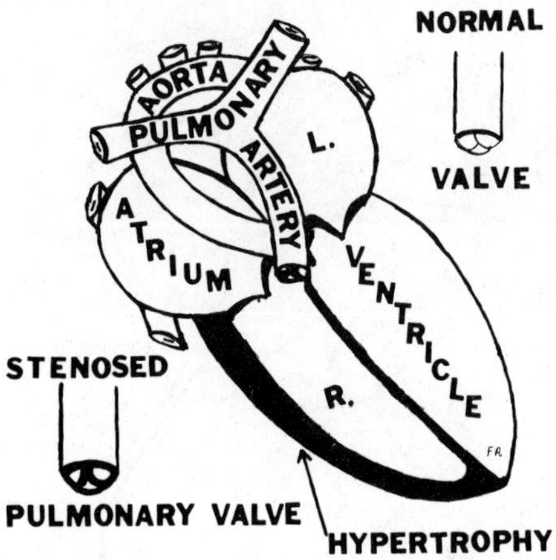

---

valvular stenosis, (3) right ventricular hypertrophy, and (4) dextroposition of the aorta—displacement of the aorta to the right (Figure 10–14).[9] Symptoms in an infant may include cyanosis, minimal weight gain owing to feeding problems, dyspnea on exertion, and clubbing of fingers and toes. Surgical intervention in infants between 3 and 12 months of age is successful; the preferred age for surgery is four or five years of age.[10]

The following describes the palliative Blalock-Taussig procedure for Tetralogy of Fallot. It is designed to send poorly oxygenated blood back to the lungs for reoxygenation to increase the blood flow in pulmonary circulation. An end-to-side anastomosis is performed between the subclavian and pulmonary arteries.

In corrective surgery at a later date under extracorporeal circulation, the anastomosis is reversed; the fused leaflets of the valve are separated, and the ventricular septal defect is closed with a synthetic or pericardial graft. Figure 10–15 illustrates correction of Tetralogy of Fallot.

ACQUIRED DEFECTS OF THE HEART

Bacterial Endocarditis

Endocarditis is a bacterial infection of the heart valves, with formation of pathogenic vegetation on the valves. Bacterial endocarditis may be subacute or acute.

Figure 10–14 Tetralogy of Fallot

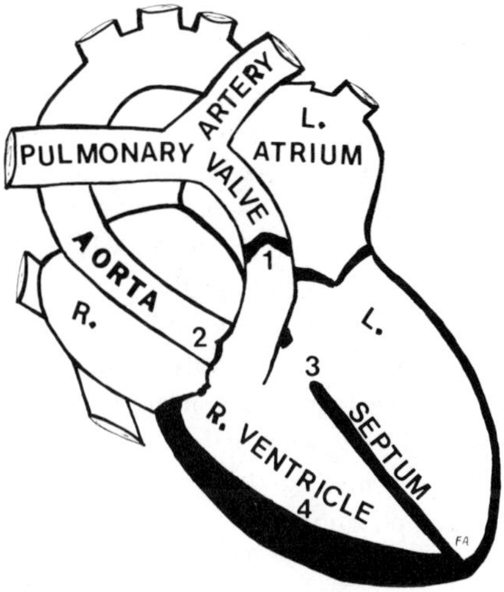

1. VALVULAR STENOSIS
2. DEXTROPOSITION OF AORTA
3. VENTRICULAR SEPTAL DEFECT
4. RIGHT VENTRICULAR HYPERTROPHY

Figure 10–15 Correction of Tetralogy of Fallot

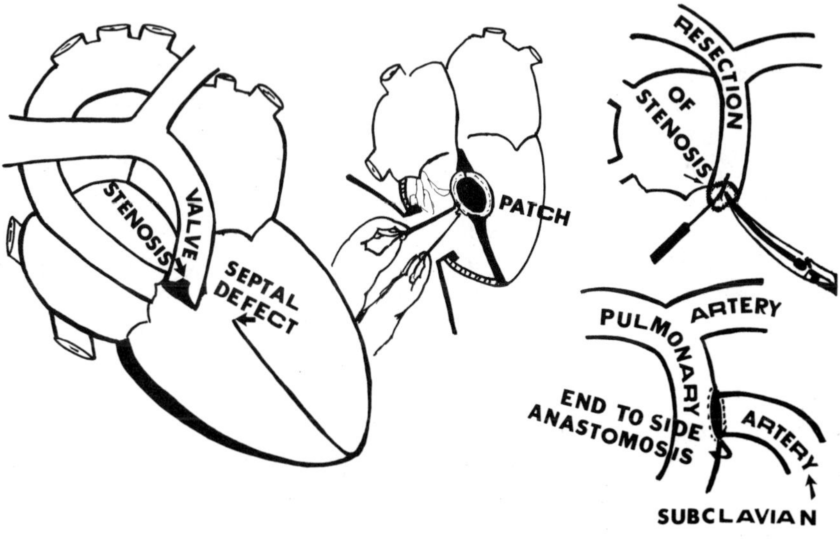

Subacute bacterial endocarditis develops slowly and does not progress rapidly. It generally occurs at the site of a previously infected or damaged cardiac valve, including congenital defective valves. Hemolytic streptococci that have been circulating in the bloodstream for some time are usually responsible for subacute bacterial endocarditis. Unlike acute bacterial endocarditis, the bacteria does not originate from a major systemic infection, but rather from its normal habitat, where injury has occurred. When injury occurs in the interior of the heart, or anywhere in the body, mechanisms in the body attempt to repair the injury. For example, when a person cuts a finger, the finger bleeds; next, a clear fluid appears and a scab is formed. However, during the healing process, the injury is vulnerable to infection. The circulation of agglutinin antibodies at the site of the sterile platelet fibrin thrombi on the injured heart valve attracts bacteria from the bloodstream. Over a period of time, bacterial concentration accumulates, forming a large amount of pathogen-laden vegetation, which interferes with the function of the valves to open widely or close tightly.

The most dangerous complication accompanying subacute bacterial endocarditis is the formation of blood clots. The smooth lining of the endocardium generally prevents clot formation, but the bacterial vegetation causes an irregular surface on the otherwise smooth endocardial lining, incorrectly setting off the blood-clotting mechanism in the tissue. The blood clots break off and drift in the bloodstream (embolism) until they reach a vessel that is too small for them to enter. At this point they lodge (thrombosis), preventing further circulation of blood to that part of the body. All tissues of the body depend on a continuous supply of blood and nutrients for nourishment and survival. When the tissues do not receive an adequate supply of oxygen and nutrients, they become ischemic, or undernourished. Over a period of time, they atrophy, or deteriorate, and finally become necrotic, or die. Sometimes collateral circulation takes place, when other vessels take over the function of supplying the area with oxygen and nutrients.[11] Figure 10–16 shows the diseased valve, a thrombus, an embolism, necrotic area, and collateral circulation.

Acute bacterial endocarditis develops quickly and progresses rapidly. The most common causative organisms are highly invasive organisms, such as *Staphylococcus aureus, Streptococcus pyogenes, Pneumococcus, Gonococcus,* and *Hemophilus influenzae*. Therefore, the infection occurs at the site of a normal healthy valve and pathogen-laden vegetation is not necessary for infection to occur. The invasive bacteria originate at the site of an active infection, such as in the integumentary, respiratory, or genitourinary systems.

Subacute endocarditis occurs in younger patients who have had rheumatic heart disease. The patient appears to be chronically ill. There is intermittent mild fever and a heart murmur (a raspy noise heard on auscultation). Petechiae may be seen under the skin.

Figure 10–16 Damage Resulting from Endocarditis

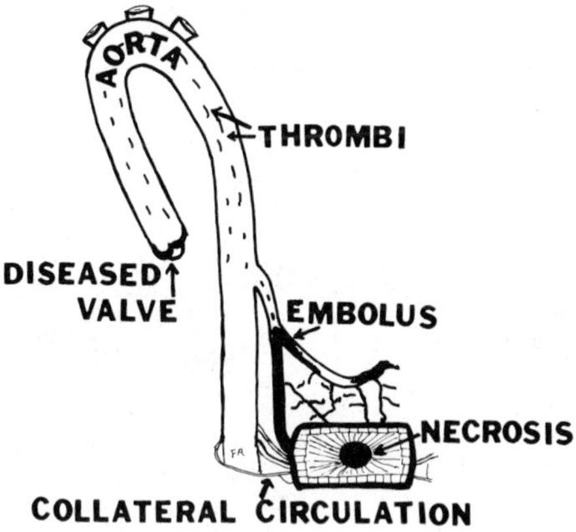

Acute endocarditis occurs in older people who have not had previous heart disease. Onset is abrupt, with intermittent fever, anemia, and slight leukocytosis. Later clinical effects include heart murmurs, emboli, and congestive heart failure. The patient complains of weakness, anorexia, malaise, and arthralgia.

In both subacute and acute endocarditis, blood cultures and sensitivity testing are necessary to identify the causative organism, enabling selection of the proper antibiotic for treatment. Such therapy usually lasts two to six weeks.[12] Clinical response to treatment is a good indicator of successful therapeutic regimen, along with repeated blood cultures negative for bacteria. Digitalis is a standard drug for cardiac problems. When digitalis alone is not effective, surgical removal of the infected valve is indicated. Cardiac catheterization and echocardiography can identify patients who would profit from prosthetic valve replacement.

Generally, patients with congenital or acquired heart disease should receive prophylactic antimicrobial drugs before, during, and after dental work and when upper respiratory tract infections or other infections are present.

Common causes for aortic valve and mitral valve replacements are valvular insufficiency owing to rheumatic fever, subacute bacterial endocarditis, and congenital anomalies. The diseased valve loses its ability to close tightly, allowing blood to leak back into the left ventricle. Over a period of time, the left ventricle develops hypertrophy; left ventricular failure occurs owing to the added strain placed on the ventricle to eject excessive blood into the aorta. Figure 10–17 shows aortic valve replacement.

Surgical correction of aortic valvular stenosis with valve replacement is performed using cardiopulmonary bypass. The aortic valve is examined to confirm

Figure 10–17 Aortic Valve Replacement

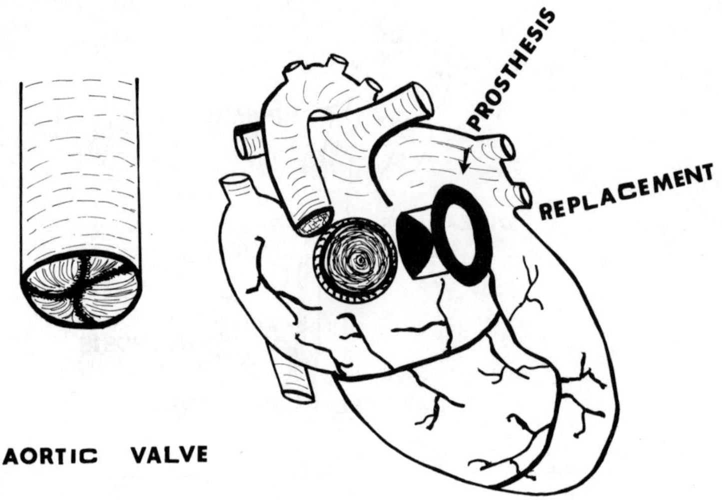

the extent of the damage. After the diseased valve is excised, a prosthetic valve is inserted.

Rheumatic Fever

Rheumatic fever is a febrile disease occurring as a sequela to a streptococcal infection. It may cause structural changes in the heart valves, blood vessels, and joints. Rheumatic fever occurs primarily in children aged 5 to 15.

The origin of the streptococcal infection is generally thought to be a sore throat. Onset may be gradual or abrupt and is characterized by fever, malaise, epistaxis, and sore throat. The patient complains of vague to severe joint discomfort, with varying degrees of redness, swelling, warmth, and tenderness. There may be chest pain with dyspnea on exertion or abdominal pain with nausea and vomiting.

Physical examination may reveal enlarged heart, muffled heart sounds, possibly accentuated pulmonic second sounds, soft diastolic murmurs at the left borders of the sternum, and blowing systolic murmurs at the apex of the heart.

Laboratory tests reveal Aschoff bodies in connective tissues of the heart and in the synovia of joints, capsules, tendons, and fascia. (Aschoff bodies, sometimes called Aschoff nodules, are submiliary collections of cells and leukocytes in the interstitial tissues.) Rheumatic fever may damage all three layers of heart tissue. Although damage of the endocardium may occur in any of the valves, the mitral and aortic valves are affected most often.

Treatment of carditis includes eight weeks of salicylates to suppress inflammation. Appropriate drug therapy should be prescribed for a patient with cardiac decompensation. Antistreptococcal prophylaxis should be maintained at all times after the first attack of acute rheumatic fever to prevent recurrence.[13]

Valvular Heart Disease

Mitral Stenosis

Rheumatic fever may bring about a thickening and fusing of the outer edges of the bicuspid, or mitral, valve's flaps. This structural change, known as mitral stenosis, prevents the valve from opening widely enough to maintain the normal blood flow from the left atrium to the ventricle. Owing to the restricted opening of the mitral valve, the left atrium is forced to pump hard to maintain adequate blood flow. The additional work required of the atrium causes hypertrophy of the atrial wall, and the atrium may revert to fibrillation or spasm. Trauma to the atrial wall may also trigger an embolus, which travels through the bloodstream only to lodge in a vessel as a thrombosis.

Mitral stenosis is more common in females than in males. The patient experiences tachycardia; dyspnea on exertion; coughing, possibly with hemoptysis; and general weakness. There may be abdominal discomfort and angina pectoris.[14] Cardiac catheterization and electrocardiography are necessary for diagnosis. (See Figure 10–12 for a comparison between a normal and a stenosed valve.)

Closed (without extracorporeal circulation) mitral commissurotomy is performed by breaking apart the stenosed leaflets of the mitral valve by inserting a finger, valvulotome, or transventricular dilator into the valve.

The valvuloplasty utilizing cardiopulmonary bypass is more common. Figure 10–18 illustrates a closed mitral commissurotomy.

Mitral Insufficiency

Another malfunction of the valves resulting from rheumatic fever is insufficiency of the mitral valve. In order to understand mitral insufficiency, it is necessary to review the function and structure of the valves between the atria and ventricles. The function of the mitral, or bicuspid, valve and the tricuspid valve is to permit blood to flow downward into the ventricles. The structures that assist the valves to work normally are the papillary muscles and the chordae tendinae; these are located along the ventricle walls. The papillary muscles are long, nipple-shaped muscles extending upward from the septum and the ventricle walls. The nipple-shaped end of the muscle is attached to tendinous cords extending from the flaps of the mitral and tricuspid valves. The valve flaps open easily when blood is forced from the atria into the ventricles. However, when the ventricles contract, the force of blood against the ventricular side of the flaps closes the valves. As the

Figure 10–18 Mitral Commissurotomy

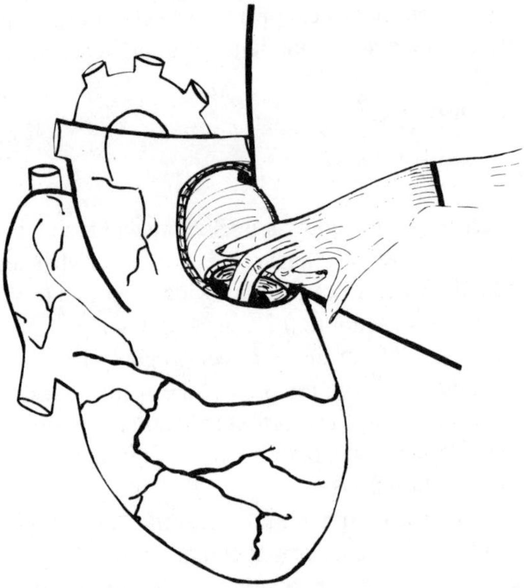

valves close, the chordae tendinae are stretched tightly to hold the valve flaps in place, preventing blood from flowing back into the atria. The valve with insufficiency does not close tightly, so blood from the ventricle regurgitates, or flows backward, into the atria. This may occur because of defective chordae tendinae, papillary muscles, or annular ring at the base of the valve. Figure 10–19 shows the structure of the valves, including chordae tendinae, papillary muscles, and annular ring.

The regurgitation of blood into the left atrium at the same time that the atrium is filling with blood from the lungs causes pressure in the atrium. This pressure is transferred to the lungs, raising the pulmonary pressure. The lungs, unable to empty properly into the left atrium, become congested.

Mitral valve insufficiency is more common in males than in females. It is initially asymptomatic, with progressive cough, weakness, nocturnal dyspnea on exertion, and orthopnea.[15] The patient experiences weight loss, fatigue, exhaustion, and cachexia. Cineangiographic studies are diagnostic of mitral insufficiency. Repair of the valve may be indicated. Figure 10–20 shows mitral insufficiency.

The insufficient mitral valve is corrected by mitral annuloplasty. In this procedure, sutures are taken in the annulus so that the leaflets come tighter together.

Figure 10–19 The Valves

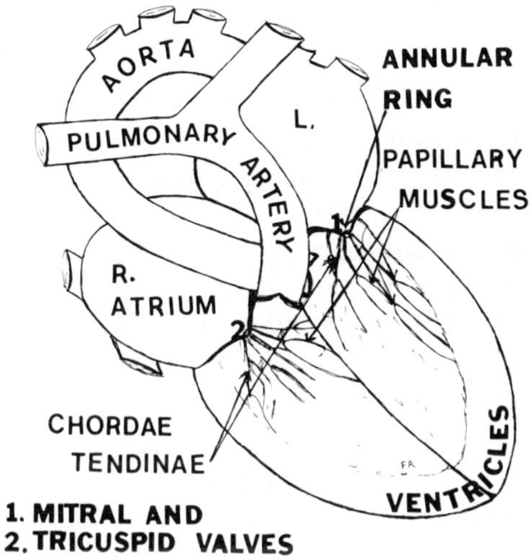

Figure 10–20 Mitral Insufficiency

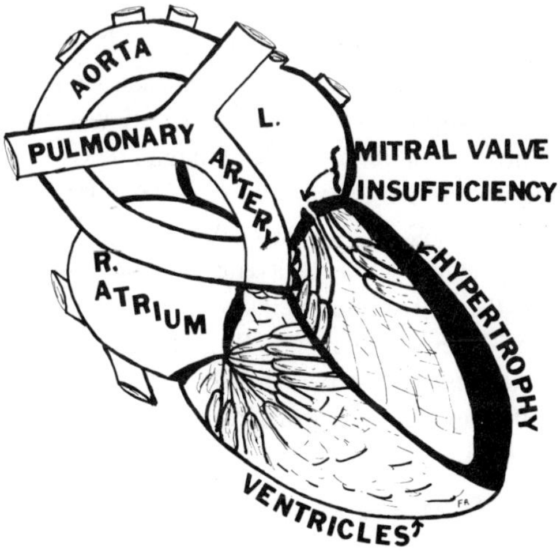

This procedure is preferred over a valve replacement, owing to the problem with rejection that accompanies a valve insertion.

Tricuspid Stenosis

Tricuspid stenosis is closely associated with rheumatic heart disease and accompanies rheumatic mitral stenosis. Because of this defect, the right atrium works hard to force blood through the ventricle. This strain on the atrium produces hypertrophy, or enlargement.

The patient complains of dyspnea on exertion and anorexia. There may also be vague complaints of abdominal pain. Electrocardiography may reveal atrial fibrillation. Fluoroscopy may suggest atrial hypertrophy.

Tricuspid Insufficiency

Tricuspid insufficiency is associated with enlargement of the annular ring owing to right ventricular hypertrophy. Enlargement of the ventricle stretches the annular ring, preventing the valve from closing tightly so that blood regurgitates into the right atrium. Tricuspid insufficiency, secondary to almost any pulmonary or heart disease, hastens ventricular failure.[16]

Aortic Stenosis

Problems with the semilunar valves occur less frequently than with the mitral valve. The aortic semilunar valve with stenosis presents a narrow orifice through which blood flows to the body (Figure 10–21). As a result, the left ventricle is required to work hard to maintain adequate blood flow. The muscle of the left ventricle enlarges and becomes stronger and the ventricular wall thickens and becomes hypertrophied. The space within the ventricle decreases. Although the ventricle is required to pump harder, it is never emptied of blood. An adequate circulation of blood throughout the body is not maintained, especially circulation of blood to the heart muscles. This condition is known as *decompensation*; it may lead to coronary insufficiency. There may also be ventricular fibrillation.

The patient with aortic stenosis may be asymptomatic until the late stages of the disease, at which time the patient complains of dyspnea on exertion, orthopnea, dizziness, syncope, and severe anginal pain. Physical examination reveals varying degrees of left ventricular hypertrophy. Cardiac catheterization is one diagnostic tool for determining the degree of stenosis and necessity for surgery.

Aortic Insufficiency

In aortic insufficiency, the aortic valve does not close sufficiently during diastole. This allows the blood to regurgitate into the ventricle. In order to

Figure 10–21 Aortic Semilunar Valve with Stenosis

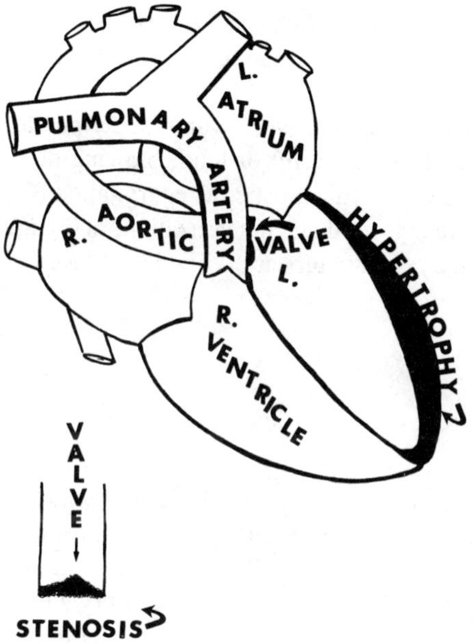

maintain an adequate blood supply, the left ventricle expands so that it can hold an additional amount of blood, which results in ventricular hypertrophy.

Aortic insufficiency in women is generally associated with rheumatic heart disease. The patient's complaints are similar to those of patients with rheumatic heart disease: dyspnea on exertion, orthopnea, severe anginal pain. Cardiac catheterization reveals aortic ventricular regurgitation. Aortic valve replacement is recommended for patients who are asymptomatic of aortic regurgitation.

Pulmonary Stenosis

Problems of the pulmonary semilunar valve are similar to those of the aortic semilunar valve. Pulmonary stenosis, or narrowing of the valve orifice, forces the right ventricle to work hard in an effort to maintain adequate blood flow to the lungs, which leads to hypertrophy of the right ventricle (see Figure 10–21).

The patient may be asymptomatic until early adulthood, at which time complaints consist of dyspnea on exertion, fatigue, chest pains, and syncope. Laboratory tests reveal elevated hematocrit, prolonged circulation time, and decreased carbon dioxide diffusing capacity. Electrocardiography and cardiac catheterization are tools for diagnosing pulmonary stenosis.

Pulmonary Insufficiency

Pulmonary insufficiency is of congenital origin rather than the result of rheumatic heart disease. The structural change is the same as that of any insufficient valve, in that it does not close tightly enough to prevent regurgitation into the right ventricle.

The patient experiences mild to severe cyanosis, peripheral edema, and fluid in the abdominal cavity. There is a soft or loud, blowing diastolic murmur in the second to third left interspace diagnostic of regurgitation (Graham Steell's murmur). Electrocardiography, cardiac catheterization, and angiography results are diagnostic of the primary disease process. Valvular replacement may be indicated.

ARTERIES

Anatomy

The artery is circular, with a hollow middle through which blood flows. Like the heart, the artery has three layers of tissue: (1) tunica adventitia, (2) tunica media, and (3) tunica intima (Figure 10–22). The *tunica adventitia,* the outer layer, is a thick covering of connective tissue that joins the artery with whatever structure it passes through. The *tunica media* is the middle layer of tissue. The *tunica intima,* the innermost layer, is continuous with the endocardium of the heart. Therefore, it has the same properties as the endocardium and readily clots blood at the site of an irregular surface on the tunica intima.

Figure 10–22 Layers of Tissue

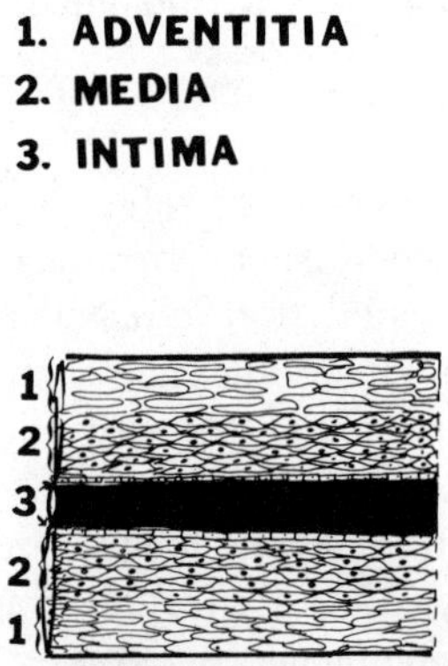

Physiology

The function of arteries is to carry blood and nutrients to all body tissues. From the heart, blood is pumped through the aorta, which supplies blood to the upper and lower extremities.

In addition, there are right and left arteries branching from the aorta that circle down around the heart, called coronary arteries. The function of the coronary arteries is to supply the heart muscles (myocardium) with blood and nutrients. This is accomplished through multiple division of the coronary arteries down to a microscopic network of capillaries that nourish the myocardium. Figure 10–23 shows the coronary arteries.

ARTERIAL DISORDERS

Arteriosclerosis

Arteriosclerosis is a generalized term for a group of diseases characterized by the thickening and loss of elasticity of the arterial walls. The three forms of arteriosclerosis are (1) atherosclerosis, (2) Mönckeberg's arteriosclerosis, and (3) arteriolosclerosis.

Atherosclerosis, the most common of the three forms, is characterized by deposits of yellow plaques containing cholesterol, lipoid (fatlike) material, and

---

Figure 10–23 The Coronary Arteries

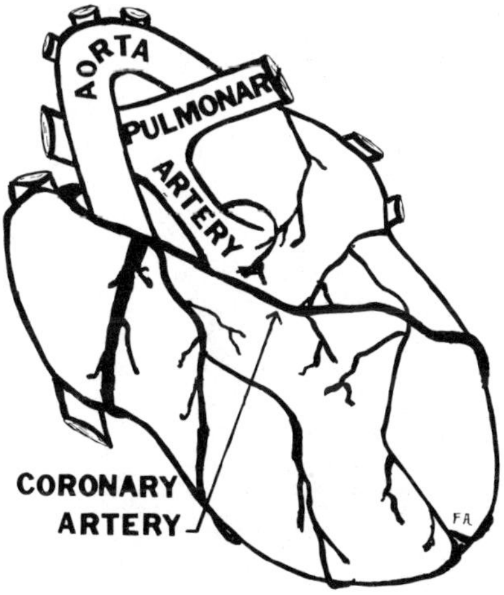

lipophages (cells that engulf fat) within the tunicae intima and media of the large and medium-sized arteries. In *Mönckeberg's arteriosclerosis,* deposits of calcium are found in the tunica media of the arteries. *Arteriolosclerosis* is characterized by the thickening and hardening of the walls of the arterioles; it is generally associated with hypertension. All three types of arteriosclerosis leave the arteries hardened and thickened owing to the deposits in the tunicae, which build up until they occlude the artery (Figure 10–24).

Myocardial Infarction

Coronary occlusions resulting from arteriosclerosis or from coronary embolism from thrombosis owing to rheumatic heart disease, endocarditis, or other diseases, have been found in most patients who have myocardial infarctions. The following description is based on the supposition that a myocardial infarction results from a coronary occlusion or an embolus. Strictly speaking, however, a distinction between a coronary occlusion and an embolus as a definitive diagnosis is usually made only on autopsy.

The irregular surface on the intima of the coronary artery attracts atherosclerotic plaque from the bloodstream, which builds up over time. The lumen of the coronary artery becomes narrow, thus curtailing the passage of blood through the artery. A *coronary occlusion* occurs when the lumen of the artery becomes partially or completely blocked, cutting off the blood supply to coronary tissue and depriving the myocardial tissue of oxygen and nutrients.

An *embolism* occurs when a blood substance breaks off from a diseased area to travel through the blood. When the embolus reaches an area in the artery that is too small for it to pass through, a *thrombus* (sudden blocking of an artery) is formed.

Both a coronary occlusion and thrombus cause *ischemia* (deficiency of blood in a part) to the myocardium. All body tissues depend on a continuous supply of blood

Figure 10–24 An Occluded Artery

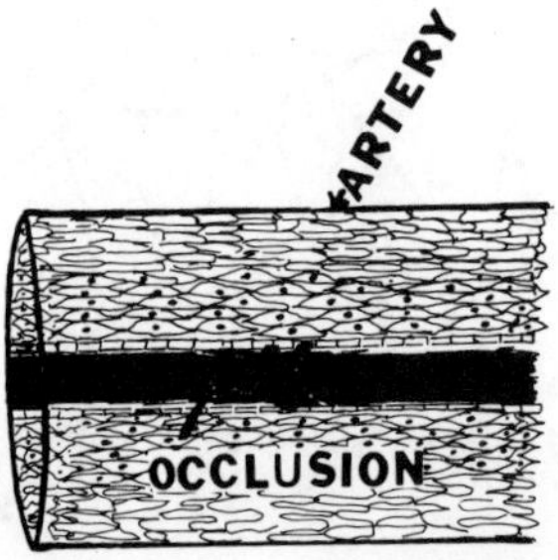

and nutrients for nourishment and survival. When the myocardium does not receive an adequate supply of blood through the coronary artery, the tissue becomes ischemic, or undernourished. Over a period of time, it atrophies, or deteriorates.

An *infarction* is an area of necrotic (dead) tissue owing to ischemia (lack of blood supply), resulting from an occluded blood vessel that has interrupted the blood supply to the myocardium.

In some instances smaller circulatory vessels, supplied with blood from another part of the coronary artery, take over the function of supplying blood to the area below the occlusion or embolus. This is called *collateral circulation*. If collateral circulation takes place, a patient may have an occlusion or embolus without a myocardial infarction. However, in cases in which a myocardial infarction has occurred, collateral circulation may take over to such an extent that the signs and symptoms of an infarction abate and the patient does not seek medical care. This is called a silent coronary. Figure 10–25 shows a coronary occlusion, thrombus, embolus, ischemia, myocardial infarction, and collateral circulation.

The patient with a myocardial infarction usually complains of crushing chest pain radiating down the left arm, cold perspiration, dyspnea, weakness, fainting, nausea, vomiting, and anxiety.

Physical examination may reveal increased heart rate, hypotension, and fever. Laboratory tests reveal an increase in the white blood cell count within a few hours from 12,000 to 20,000. Changes in the serum enzyme levels confirm myocardial infarction and help to evaluate the amount of myocardial damage. Serum aspartate

Figure 10–25 Myocardial Infarction

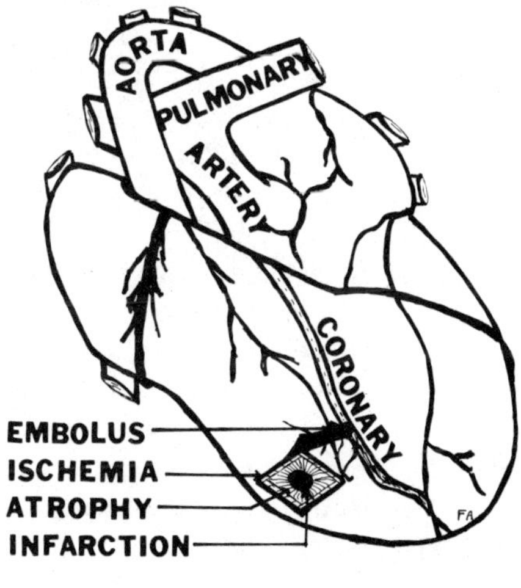

transaminase (AST, formerly SGOT) is elevated within 12 hours after the infarction, reaches two to four times the normal level in 24 hours, and returns to normal within four to seven days. Electrocardiography, diagnostic in 80 percent of the patients with myocardial infarction, traces the area of the infarction.

The goal of treatment is to relieve pain, reduce the heart's workload, and prevent or treat complications.

Generally, morphine is given for pain. It also depresses respiration. reduces myocardial contractions, and dilates vessels. Hypotension and bradycardia may occur with the use of morphine; these complications can be overcome by elevating the patient's legs. Unresponsive hypotension and bradycardia may be treated with atropine sulfate. A mild tranquilizer, such as diazepam, may also be given. The patient is placed in a cardiac care unit (CCU), with cardiac monitoring and maximal restriction of visitors, newspapers, and radios. New surgical procedures attempt to dissolve or remove the occlusion or embolus through cardiac catheter methods of chemotherapy or modified use of the laser.

Aneurysm

The cells of the arteries receive oxygen and nutrients from small blood vessels called vasa vasorum. These blood vessels arise from a branch of the artery or from another nearby vessel. When an artery becomes occluded by arteriosclerotic plaque or weakened by infection or trauma, the artery walls in that area are unable to obtain sufficient nourishment. The weakened walls stretch and bulge. Blood seeps in between the layers of arterial tissue, filling the defect and forming clots. This describes an aneurysm. An aneurysm may occur in the wall of an artery, vein, or the heart, but generally is found in an artery.

The three types of aneurysms are (1) saccular, (2) fusiform, and (3) dissecting (Figure 10–26). A *saccular aneurysm* is a distended sac that affects only a localized area of the circumference of the arterial wall. A *fusiform aneurysm* is a spindle-shaped enlargement that involves the entire circumference of the artery. A *dissecting aneurysm* is one resulting from hemorrhage, causing the longitudinal splitting of the arterial wall with a tear in the intima (inner layer of the vessel). This allows blood to flow between the layers of wall tissue.

Congenital aneurysms are found intracranially, on the circle of Willis (berry aneurysm). They usually occur around age 40, with a sudden, severe headache accompanied by intracerebral hemorrhage and demise.

Aneurysms located in the first portion of the aorta often result in aortic insufficiency. Such aneurysms are often associated with bacteremia, septicemia, or trauma. Syphilitic aneurysms generally occur in the descending thoracic aorta.

Abdominal aortic aneurysms are generally arteriosclerotic in origin and are experienced by the aged. They are often of the dissecting type and may rupture owing to pressure on the dorsal vertebrae.

Figure 10–26 Aneurysms

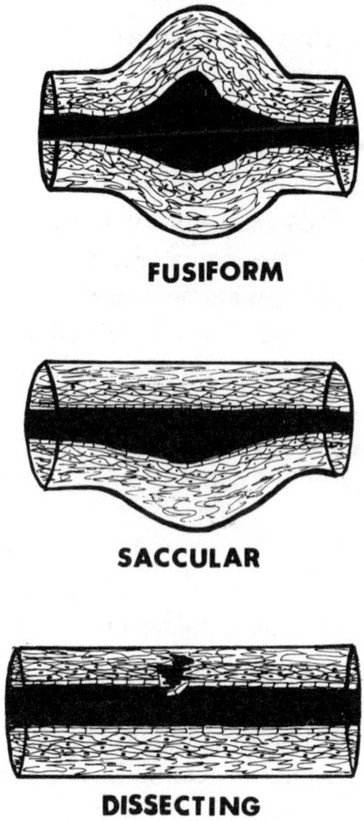

Symptoms include excruciating pain in the area of the aneurysm. Except for the intracranial aneurysm, physical examination reveals a pulsating mass indicative of an aneurysm. Further diagnostic evaluation includes a combination of laboratory findings and arteriography to determine the location and extent of the aneurysm. Such evaluation determines the need for surgery as well as the type of reconstruction to be done. A ruptured aneurysm demands immediate surgery owing to the danger from massive hemorrhage.

Resection of a thoracic aortic aneurysm is performed using extracorporeal circulation. The aneurysm is identified, ligated, and an end-to-end anastomosis is performed or prosthetic graft is sutured in place.

Thromboangiitis Obliterans (Buerger's Disease)

Thromboangiitis obliterans is inflammation of the tunica intima of a medium-sized artery below the elbows and knees where a thrombus is lodged as an embolus. This prevents circulation to the walls of the tunica intima. Ischemia occurs in the arterial walls, which eventually is debilitating to the patient, who develops necrosis and gangrene of the lower extremities. The disease often coexists with thrombophlebitis. It occurs predominantly in heavy cigarette smokers because nicotine is a vasoconstrictor.

The patient with Buerger's disease complains of severe pain in one or more toes during ambulation. The pain may become so severe that walking is impossible.

Physical examination reveals absent or diminished pulse in the dorsal pedal, posterior tibial, and possibly the popliteal arteries. Segmental occlusions of the distal arteries of the hands and feet are detected through arteriography.

Treatment consists of removing all causes of reduced circulation in the lower limbs, such as trauma from tight footwear. Bed rest is necessary when gangrene or ulceration is evident. Elevation of the head of the bed six to eight inches may improve circulation. In the presence of gangrene, amputation may be necessary. (Limb amputation is reviewed in Chapter 6.)

Raynaud's Disease

Raynaud's disease is a vascular disorder characterized by vasospasm of the arteries of the hands and feet when they are exposed to cold. Raynaud's disease, believed to be hereditary, is more common in females than in males. During the late stages of the disease, the tunica intima, or inner lining of the artery, thickens. Hypertrophy of the tunica media, or middle layer of arterial tissue, occurs with eventual thrombosis, sometimes developing into gangrene of the fingers and toes.

Patients with Raynaud's disease experience numbness, tingling, and cyanosis of the hands and feet when they are exposed to minimal coldness. The color of the fingers and toes changes from blue to deep red when the vasospasm ceases and circulation returns to the fingers and toes.

Physical examination reveals thickening of the skin of the upper extremities and difficulty in swallowing. Wrist pulses are positive, but pulses below the wrist are absent.

Treatment consists of protecting the body from extreme cold. Smoking is prohibited, since nicotine is a vasoconstrictor. If symptoms are severe, phenoxybenzamine may be given. Other drugs are prescribed at the discretion of the attending physician. Surgical intervention with sympathectomy gives only temporary relief.

Advanced Heart Diseases

Criteria for heart transplant are advanced heart disease with heart failure syndrome or congestive failure; inability to perform any activity without discomfort; and prognosis for one year survival. Additionally, the patient must have shown evidence of psychological stability and compliance with medical treatment prescribed.

Heart Failure Syndrome

A syndrome is a set of symptoms that occur together. Heart failure owing to the inability of the heart itself to function is called *primary heart failure*. Heart failure is characterized by distinctive signs and symptoms resulting from decreased cardiac output or from increased venous pressure. Decreased cardiac output means that the heart is unable to pump an adequate supply of blood to maintain body functions. This is due to an increased workload on the ventricles and hypertrophy, or enlargement, of the heart owing to vascular disease or defects. When hypertrophy of the ventricles is present, the cells of the ventricles enlarge, rather than the space within the ventricles that holds the blood. Increased workload on the ventricles over time also weakens their walls so that they fail to expand adequately to expel the blood. Therefore, when the ventricles do not expand sufficiently to allow an adequate amount of blood to enter, or when the ventricles are unable to expel the blood within, ventricular heart failure is imminent.

Congestive Heart Failure

Congestive heart failure is considered primary when the left ventricle is unable to empty adequately in order to accept blood from the left atrium during diastole. This condition results in a backup of blood. The left ventricle, because of its inability to empty adequately, has low output to the body. The left atrium, because of its inability to empty adequately into the ventricle, cannot accept blood from the lungs. The right ventricle cannot empty adequately into the lungs, which are already filled with blood. The right atrium is unable to empty into the right ventricle, which is already filled with blood. The result is left-sided backward failure and low-output syndrome; there is also right-sided and backward failure because the right atrium and ventricle are unable to fill with blood or empty adequately. The foregoing describes what often takes place when congestive heart failure occurs. This condition may be due to mitral insufficiency, left ventricular hypertrophy, or a combination of cardiac deficits. In addition, there is pleural effusion.

In the early stages of the disease, the patient may complain of dyspnea on mild exercise and fatigue on exertion. In the advanced stage, the patient complains of paroxysmal nocturnal dyspnea, cough with production of brown sputum, and wheezing.

Physical examination of the cardiovascular system may reveal left or right ventricular failure and acute pulmonary edema with frequent ventricular premature or atrial premature beats. There is increased water in the lung area and pulmonary venous hypertension is present.

Chest x-ray reveals the extent of congestive heart failure as well as its cause. Edema surrounding bronchioles and peribronchial cuffing may help to establish the presence of pulmonary infiltrates. Examination of cardiac silhouette may reveal enlargement of chambers and cardiac calcification.

Treatment consists of bed rest to reduce cardiac workload and heart rate. Sedation with diazepam and flurazepam is recommended. Diuretics and sodium restriction are prescribed on a long-term basis to reduce and control hypertension. Prazosin, an antihypertensive drug, is used to produce vascular relaxation. Some physicians no longer favor the use of digitalis because of its toxic effects.

The results of a cardiac examination using blood chemistry, cineangiocardiography (motion picture of the cardiac cycle), phonocardiography (record of heart sounds produced during cardiac cycle), arteriography, electrocardiography, and cardiac catheterization may determine whether the patient is a candidate for heart transplant. Criterion for heart transplant is end-stage cardiac disease resulting from repeated myocardial infarctions and advanced atherosclerosis.

Heart Transplant

Donor

The heart may be preserved in a brain-dead donor. Preservation of the donor's heart is of utmost importance if it is to resume full activity in the recipient's body after transplantation.

Teams

Two teams, in adjoining operating rooms, are needed for the procedure—one team for excision and transportation of the donor's heart at the precise minute and the other team to transplant the heart into the recipient.

Procedure

After institution of extracorporeal circulation (see Figure 10–6), the recipient's heart is removed by severing the atria leaving the posterior wall attached to their venous attachments; the aorta and pulmonary arteries are severed just above their semilunar valves.

The donor's heart is then placed in the recipient's pericardial cavity. The donor's atria are sutured to the portion of the recipient's atria that were not removed. The aorta and pulmonary arteries of the donor's heart are anastomosed to the recipient's arteries. A temporary pacing mechanism is attached to the right ventricle.[17, 18]

The patient is given prednisone, azathioprine, and antithymocyte (immunosuppressants) as indicated to guard against tissue rejection. The patient is monitored for 4 to 6 weeks for tissue rejection. In 1979, the current survival rate was reported to be one year for 70 percent of the patients undergoing heart transplantation.[19]

HYPERTENSION

Hypertension is measured by blood pressure. The normal blood pressure is 120 mm Hg during systole and 80 mm Hg during diastole, measured by a column of mercury in an instrument called a sphygmomanometer. This is written as 120/80. Blood pressure reading is an indirect measurement of the force of blood against the arterial walls as the heart contracts and relaxes. A person may be said to have hypertension when the systolic pressure persistently ranges from 140 to 200 mm Hg and diastolic pressure ranges from 90 to 110 mm Hg. Generally, the criterion for stating that a person has hypertension is diastolic pressure over 90 mm Hg in adults under age 60 and over 100 mm Hg in persons over age 60. After determining that the patient's blood pressure is not within normal limits, it is necessary to establish whether the patient has primary (essential) hypertension or secondary hypertension. It is also necessary to assess the degree of involvement of the central nervous system, eyes, heart, and kidneys.

Essential Hypertension

Essential, or primary, hypertension is persistently high blood pressure without known systemic cause. Blood pressure at onset, which may occur at any age, is not persistent, but rises and fluctuates in response to role overload in occupational and family situations.

During the early stage of hypertension, the patient is asymptomatic; hypertension is discovered during routine physical examination. Next, mild symptoms develop, including headache, vertigo, fatigue, nervousness, and flushing. A later stage of hypertension reveals heart, eye, cerebral, and kidney involvement. Left ventricular hypertrophy develops. Cerebral developmental symptoms are headache on awakening that gradually subsides during the day. There are transient periods of weakness, numbness, and tingling of the hands and feet.

Once essential hypertension is diagnosed, with the patient having a diastolic blood pressure higher than 90 mm Hg, antihypertensive drugs, such as a diuretic, are warranted. Additionally, the patient requires monitoring, with sedation, rest, weight reduction, and sodium dietary restrictions in an attempt to reduce the blood pressure.

Secondary Hypertension

This type of hypertension, or high blood pressure, is secondary to a known systemic disease. It is generally associated with renal or endocrine diseases, although there are many other known causes.

The patient may experience dyspnea on exertion, vision impairment, dizziness, epistaxis, or seizures. Secondary hypertension is curable when the underlying disease is treated.

Malignant Hypertension

The malignant phase of essential hypertension has an abrupt onset without respect to age and may be primary or secondary. It progresses rapidly, with an increase in arterial pressure. There may be marked damage to the blood vessels of the kidneys, pancreas, mesentery, adrenals, and retina, resulting in renal and left ventricular failure and stroke.

In addition to the rising blood pressure, the patient may experience vision impairment, nausea, and vomiting and may complain of the loss of feeling and use of an extremity. Prognosis is poor if not treated immediately.

Laboratory findings sometimes include proteinuria and hematuria with an occasional red cell cast. Renin and aldosterone levels are elevated. Diagnosis includes a persistent diastolic blood pressure higher than 120 mm Hg, as well as evidence of cardiac and renal involvement.

Treatment is necessary for survival. Hypertension is reduced with diet and appropriate drug therapy. Dialysis may be necessary owing to progressive renal insufficiency.

Pulmonary Hypertension

Pulmonary hypertension is primary when it is due to obstruction of the pulmonary artery by glomera. Glomera are microscopic neurovascular structures that are located near the main branches of arteries. they contain chemoreceptors that play a role in reflex regulation of respiration by responding to changes in oxygen, carbon dioxide, and hydrogen ion concentration in the blood.

Pulmonary hypertension may be secondary to pulmonary artery disease resulting from chronic obstructive pulmonary disease, arteriosclerosis, syphilis, and congenital hypoplasia of the pulmonary artery. It is characterized by increased left arterial pressure and evidence of right heart failure and is sometimes called cor pulmonale.

This type of hypertension occurs most often in women between ages 20 and 40. The patient complains of dyspnea on exertion, fatigue, and weakness. Physical examination reveals swelling of the face, puffiness of the eyelids, cyanosis, and enlargement of the heart. Electrocardiography is diagnostic of pulmonary hypertension by peaked P waves and delayed precordial transition. Increased right precordial voltage may also be indicative of congenital malformation. Echocardiography is useful in diagnosing cardiac etiology of pulmonary hypertension.

Therapeutic management depends on the underlying disease. Digitalis and diuretics have proved effective in persons with right-sided heart failure. Anticoagulants are used with patients who have a pulmonary embolism.

Hypertensive Cardiovascular Disease

Hypertension that does not affect the heart is called hypertensive vascular disease. When atherosclerosis or ischemic heart disease and ventricular hypertrophy are present, it is called hypertensive cardiovascular disease. Symptoms of hypertension are characterized by diastolic pressure consistently above 100 mm Hg in patients over age 60, or 90 mm Hg in patients under age 60. The World Health Organization specifies blood pressure of 160/95 as the upper limits of normal.

The patient, who is generally over age 40, may complain of dyspnea on exertion or rapid heartbeat.

Physical examination reveals enlargement of the heart with prominence in the left ventricle. The patient has a history of elevated blood pressure resulting from excitement, nervousness, or apprehension. Eye examination shows retinal vascular sclerosis. Urinalysis reveals albumin, casts, low specific gravity, and nitrogen retention.

Hypertension can be prevented, and treatment greatly reduces impending heart failure and incidence of cardiac failure. Public health studies show that only a small percentage of persons with hypertension are receiving antihypertensive treatment. Cardiovascular symptoms found in hypertensive cardiovascular disease can be reversed through timely treatment of hypertension.

VEINS

In order to understand diseases that affect the veins, it is necessary to understand the venous structure in relationship to function. There are two kinds of veins: pulmonary and systemic. Figure 10–27 shows two kinds of veins.

The *pulmonary veins* are concerned with circulation in the lungs; they carry arterial blood from the lungs to the left atrium. *Systemic veins* are concerned with general circulation throughout the body. They return deoxygenated (venous) blood from the body to the heart. Venous blood enters the heart through the

Figure 10–27 Types of Veins

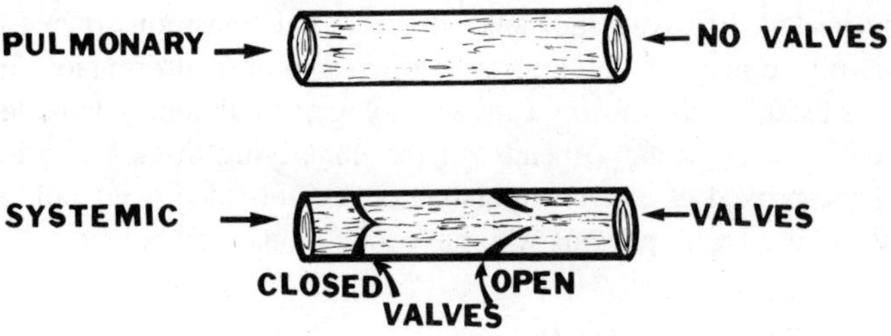

superior and inferior venae cavae from the upper and lower extremities of the body, respectively. Veins have the same three layers of tunicae as arteries, except that the layers are much thinner owing to the small amount of elastic and muscular tissues that they contain.

The systemic veins are divided into the (a) superficial, (b) deep, and (c) sinuses. The *superficial veins* are found between the superficial fascia layers, just beneath the integument. They return blood from the superficial fascia and communicate with the deep veins. *Deep veins* enclosed in the same sheath accompany the arteries, except for the veins of the skull, spinal canal, hepatic veins in the liver, and larger veins coming from the osseous tissue. *Sinuses* are venous channels found on the interior of the skull. They consist of channels formed by two layers of dura mater: fibrous tissue and endothelial layers.

The valves in veins are formed from the inner lining membrane, which prevents the backward flow of blood away from the heart. Figure 10–28 shows the structure of veins.

Figure 10–28 Structure of Veins

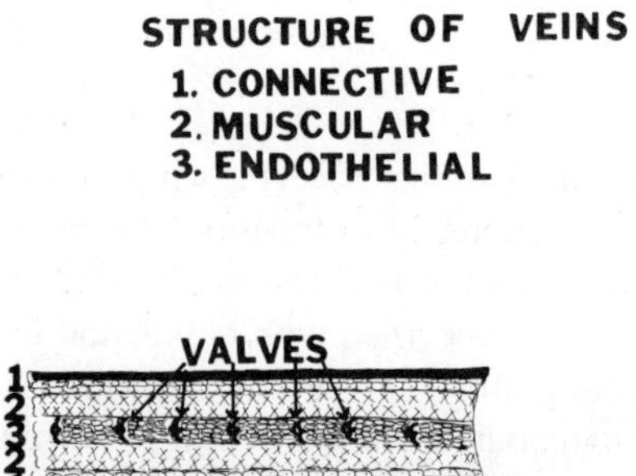

VENOUS DISORDERS

Varicose Veins

Varicose veins occur when the semilunar valves in the veins do not close properly, allowing the backward flow of blood. In other words, the valves are incompetent. The excessive blood in the venous system disseminates to the other layers of the vein, resulting in dilatation of the veins. Since the tunicae of the veins are thin and many of them are close to the skin surface, congested and dilated veins appear as bulged and twisted blue marks, especially in the areas of the legs and thighs.

Varicose veins are four times more common in women than in men; they may become evident in women after pregnancy. The patient may complain of soreness and burning in the region of the varicosity, accompanied by cramping of leg muscles. Physical examination reveals blue, tortuous veins protruding on the surface of the skin, generally in the areas of the thighs and calves. Surgical intervention may be indicated.

After the saphenous varicose vein is identified and ligated, surgical correction is carried out by ligation and division of the saphenous trunk with or without subsequent stripping and excision.

Thrombophlebitis

A thrombosis is a blood clot that forms on the intima, or inner lining, of the vein. This may occur when the wall of the vein weakens, bulging occurs, and blood pools to form a blood clot. When inflammation of the vein occurs at the site of the thrombus, it is called thrombophlebitis. This generally affects the deep veins of the calves. The condition may be associated with surgery, trauma, obesity, advanced age, drugs, malignancy, and infectious diseases.

The patient complains of slight fever, with pain and discomfort over the affected area. On examination, the skin over the area may appear red and feel warm on palpation. There may be cyanosis and edema of the lower extremity below the affected area. Venography is diagnostic of deep venous thrombosis. A serious complication of thrombophlebitis is a pulmonary embolism which is diagnosed by lung scan or pulmonary arteriography.

The goal of therapy is to prevent pulmonary embolism. Bed rest is ordered, with the foot of the bed elevated. Antibiotics should be used only to combat ulceration with cellulitis or other serious infection; causative microorganism should be identified by laboratory culture and sensitivity. Because of the danger from hemorrhage, anticoagulants should not be prescribed unless diagnosis of thrombophlebitis or pulmonary embolism is confirmed. After confirmation, drug therapy may consist of heparin for 7 to 14 days; oral coumarin is given to overlap the heparin; warfarin sodium should be given until the prothrombin time rises to a level of 1.5 to 2.5 times control, at which time the heparin should be discontinued. Surgery may be necessary when an ulcer is involved but is recommended on an individual basis.

Hemorrhoids

Varicose veins may occur in the rectal region; these are called hemorrhoids. They are classified as internal or external. Hemorrhoids develop owing to constipation and straining on defecation, or bowel movement.

The patient may complain of discomfort during defecation, such as pain, bleeding, and diarrhea. Internal hemorrhoids may protrude after defecation, giving discomfort on sitting. Barium enema and proctoscopy are indicated before surgery for diagnosis and to rule out cancer.

Surgical correction of hemorrhoids is carried out through excision and ligation of dilated veins in the anal region owing to rectal bleeding and discomfort.

LYMPHATIC SYSTEM

In Chapter 3, blood is discussed as a type of tissue, but no consideration is given to the lymphatic system. It is considered here as an accessory vessel system for the flow of fluid from tissue spaces into circulation.

Blood pumped by the heart passes through the aorta, into the arteries, into arterioles, and into capillaries. It is in the capillary where the exchange of oxygen and nutrients for carbon dioxide takes place. The capillary has an arterial end and a venous end. Pressure at the arterial end of the capillary is greater than at the venous end; therefore, the arterial end of the capillary passes oxygen and nutrients into the extracellular fluid, and the venous end of the capillary receives carbon dioxide and waste products from the fluid.

Normally, more fluid is released from the arterial side of the capillary than is absorbed on the venule side. Therefore, additional fluid is constantly being left behind. This means that if the additional fluid is not disposed of in some way, interstitial edema occurs. The function of the lymphatic capillary is to carry excessive interstitial fluid so that a constant fluid level is always maintained in the body. Once inside the lymphatic capillary, the interstitial fluid is called *lymph*. The lymphatic capillary is about the same size as the vascular capillary. Like the vascular capillary, the lymphatic capillary forms a branching pattern that eventually joins with larger lymph vessels, known as *lymph nodes*. Lymph vessels, like veins and arteries, contain valves to prevent the backward flow of lymph. Lymph nodes filter lymphatic fluid, removing waste materials, such as dead blood cells, cancer cells, and microorganisms, which they empty into the venous system. They also add blood cells, called *lymphocytes,* and antibodies to help ward off infection.

Lymph nodes are clustered throughout the body to service the various areas. The major groups of lymph nodes are named after the area in which they are located. For example, in the neck area are cervical lymph nodes, and in the armpits are axillary lymph nodes. Figure 10–29 outlines the lymphatic channels throughout the body.

LYMPHATIC SYSTEM DISEASES

Lymphedema

Lymphedema is characterized by unilateral or bilateral edema of the lower extremities. It may be either primary or secondary in origin.

Figure 10–29 Lymphatic System

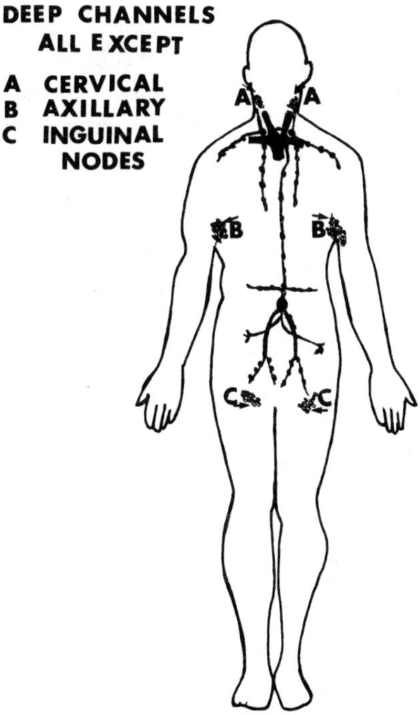

Primary Lymphedema

Milroy's disease, a congenital hereditary lymphedema, is characterized by obstruction of the lymphatic channels, resulting in edema of the legs, trunk, and face. Lymphedema praecox is another form of congenital lymphedema, which first appears at puberty with puffiness of the face and extremities. When the first appearance of lymphedema occurs beyond age 35, it is called lymphedema tarda. Lymphedema occurs primarily in females. The patient complains of swelling or puffiness of the feet and ankles, which often extends upward, with progressive enlargement from the lower extremities to the trunk.

Secondary Lymphedema

Acquired lymphedema is secondary to occlusion of the lymphatic channels by malignancies; it also occurs after surgery in which the lymph nodes have been removed.

Lymphadenitis

Lymphadenitis is inflammation of the lymph nodes associated with a bacterial, viral, fungal, or other pathogenic infection. The infection may be a generalized systemic infection or confined to regional lymph nodes, which drain the infection locally. It may also be due to a skin infection, with cellulitis or abscess formation that ruptures and drains through a sinus. Lymph node enlargement itself may be asymptomatic or accompanied by pain and tenderness in the area of the lymphadenitis. Treatment depends on the primary cause and its resolution. However, hot wet applications may relieve symptoms of painful lymph nodes.

NOTES

1. Henry Grey, *Anatomy, Descriptive and Surgical,* 15th ed. (New York: Bounty Books, 1977), 460.

2. Ibid., 458–459.

3. American Heart Association, *Heartbook: A Guide to Prevention and Treatment of Cardiovascular Diseases* (New York: E.P. Dutton, 1980), 132.

4. Eugene Braunwald, *Heart Disease: A Textbook of Cardiovascular Medicine,* vol. 1 and 2 (Philadelphia: W.B. Saunders Co., 1980), 996.

5. Ibid., 986.

6. Ibid., 1060–1061.

7. Ibid. 1057.

8. Ibid., 1004–1005.

9. Ibid., 245.

10. Laurence Urdang et al., *Mosby's Medical and Nursing Dictionary* (St. Louis: C.V. Mosby Co., 1983), 1064.

11. Braunwald, *Heart Disease,* 1181–1185.

12. American Heart Association, *Heartbook,* 252.

13. Patrick A. Murphy, ''Upper Respiratory Infections.'' In *The Principles and Practice of Medicine,* 11th ed., ed. A. McGehee Harvey et al. (New York: Appleton-Century-Crofts, 1980), 985–987.

14. J. O'Neal Humphries and Richard S. Ross, ''Cardiac Murmurs and Other Manifestations of Valvular Heart Disease,'' *Principles and Practices of Medicine,* 213–215.

15. Ibid., 215–217.

16. A. Kitchin et al., ''Diagnosis and Treatment of Tricuspid Stenosis,'' *British Heart Journal* 26 (1964):354.

17. Chester N. Barnard, ''The Operation: A Human Cardiac Transplant.'' *South African Medical Journal* 41 (1967):1271.

18. Chester N. Barnard, ''What We Have Learned About Heart Transplants,'' *Journal of Thoracic Cardiovascular Surgery* 56 (1968):457.

19. J.S. Schroeder, ''Current Status of Cardiac Transplantation—1978,'' *Journal of the American Medical Association* 241 (1979):2069.

Chapter 11

The Respiratory System

Objectives

- Name the structures of the respiratory system.
- Contrast internal and external respiration.
- Explain the relationship between the cardiovascular and respiratory systems.
- Explain the purpose and use of the Apgar scoring system.
- Name and explain three congenital anomalies.
- Explain the effect that cranial birth trauma has on the respiratory system.
- Contrast intrinsic and extrinsic substances that may result in asthma.
- Differentiate between empyema and emphysema.
- Differentiate between pneumonia and pleurisy.
- Differentiate between primary and secondary pneumothorax.
- Explain the structural phenomenon of inactive pulmonary tuberculosis.

FUNCTION AND STRUCTURE

The respiratory system, including the nose, pharynx, larynx, trachea, lungs, bronchi, bronchioles, alveoli, ribs, intercostal muscles and diaphragm, functions through the process of internal and external respiration. Internal respiration takes place in the capillaries, where oxygen and nutrients are exchanged for carbon dioxide and waste products, as discussed in Chapter 10. External respiration takes place in the lungs, where venous blood pumped from the right ventricle to the lungs is oxygenated through the chemical reaction of carbon dioxide in the blood with oxygen from air taken into the body. Figure 11–1 shows the respiratory system.

THE NOSE

External respiration begins with the nose, through which air is breathed into the lungs. The nose is an external organ consisting of bone and cartilage protruding from the center of the face. The top ridge of the nose and the connected sinus framework are composed of bone. The nares or nostrils open an area called the vestibule. The skin in the vestibule contains course hairs (vibrissae), sebaceous glands, and sweat glands. Posterior to the vestibule is the respiratory portion of the nasal cavity. The mucous membrane contains many mucous glands. The superior respiratory nasal cavity has a specialized membrane containing olfactory nerve cells.

Figure 11–1 The Respiratory System

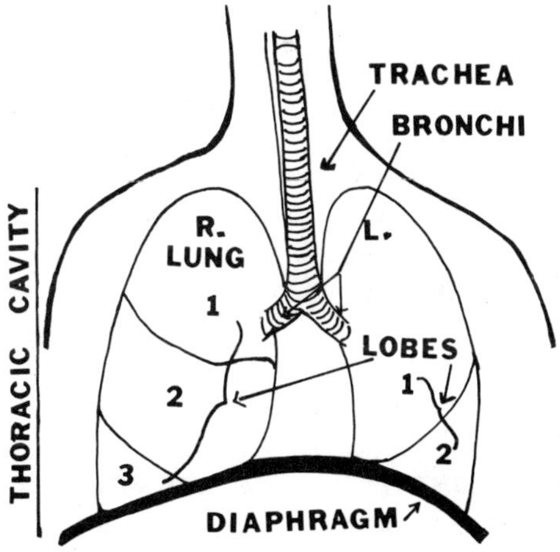

Air entering the vestibule is filtered of impurities by the hairs. The mucosa in the respiratory nasal cavity produces large amounts of mucus that moistens and warms the air. Olfactory nerve cells in the superior mucosa provide discrimination of odors. In summary, air entering the lungs through the nose is filtered of impurities, warmed, moistened, and chemically examined for material that may be harmful to the membrane of the lungs.

SINUSES

There are four pairs of nasal sinuses (cavities filled with air). They are named after the skull bones that surround them—frontal, maxillary, ethmoidal, and sphenoidal. The functions of the sinuses are (a) to equalize air pressure in the nasal cavity, (b) to reduce the weight of the skull and (c) to contribute to the sound of the voice. The mucous membrane lining the nasal cavity is continuous with the sinuses so that infection of the mucous membrane of the nose may diffuse to the sinus membrane. Figure 11–2 shows the location of the sinuses.

PHARYNX

The pharynx, a muscular tube of the alimentary canal, is divided into the nasal, oral, and laryngeal areas because it passes down behind the nose and mouth and connects with the larynx. The adenoids are located on the wall of the nasopharynx; the tonsils are located on the wall of the oropharynx.

Figure 11–2 The Location of the Sinuses

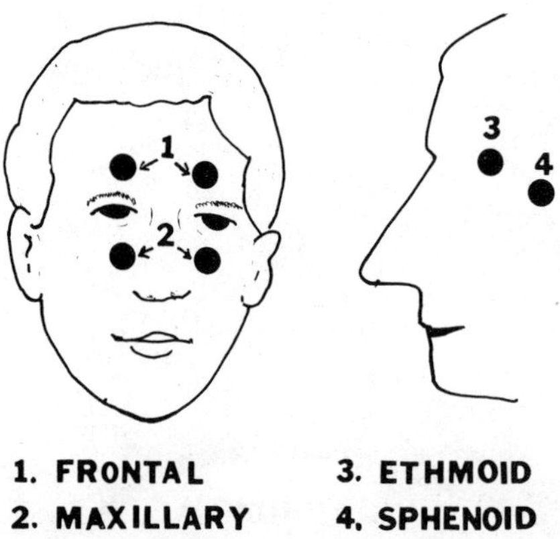

LARYNX

The mucous membranes of the pharynx are continuous with the larynx. The larynx, located between the lower portion of the pharynx and the trachea, houses the vocal cords. The epiglottis, located at the opening of the larynx, prevents food from entering the larynx.

TRACHEA

The trachea, commonly called the windpipe, is a tube of cartilaginous rings extending from the lower part of the larynx down to the level of the fourth or fifth vertebrae, where it bifurcates into two bronchi. The right and left bronchi extend into the right and left lungs, respectively.

LUNGS

The two lungs, essential for respiration, are separated by the mediastinum, which functions as a septum between the lungs and houses the heart and other structures. The three layers of lung tissue, from the outside in, are (1) the external serous coat, (2) the internal subserous areolar tissue, and (3) the parenchyma, or lung tissue (Figure 11–3). The external serous tissue, derived from pleura, is thin and transparent. It envelops the entire lung. The internal subserous areolar tissue,

Figure 11–3 The Three Layers of Lung Tissue

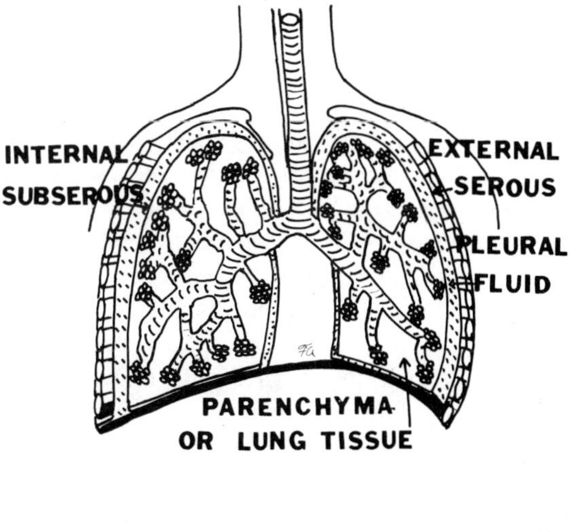

containing elastic fibers, covers the entire surface of the lung and extends between the lobules. The parenchyma are composed of various shaped lobules; each lobule contains branches of a bronchial tube, with terminal air sacs, pulmonary and bronchial vessels, lymphatics, and nerves connected by areolar tissue. Pleural fluid is found between the external serous coat and the internal subserous areolar tissue.

The lungs together weigh approximately 42 ounces; the left lung weighs about 2 ounces less than the right lung. The right lung has three lobes and the left lung has two lobes, owing to the anatomical position of the heart to the left.[1]

BRONCHI

On entering the lungs, the bronchi divide into a bronchial tree, which further divides into bronchioles. The division and subdivision of the bronchioles terminate in alveoli.

ALVEOLI

The alveoli found in the lungs are small, bulblike air sacs with ducts through which the chemical exchange of oxygen for carbon dioxide in the pulmonary capillaries takes place.

RESPIRATION

The two types of respiration, internal and external, are constantly going on in the living body. Internal respiration takes place in all parts of the body through the capillaries of the cells. It also takes place in the lungs through the capillary network of the lungs. External respiration occurs only in the lungs with the chemical exchange of carbon dioxide in the venous blood for oxygen in the air.

External respiration is carried out through the synchronization of the ribs, intercostal muscles, and diaphragm with breathing. The lungs are protected by the rib cage; the intercostal muscles are located between the ribs. The diaphragm is a musculomembrane that separates the thoracic and the abdominal cavities. The lower part of the lung rests on the diaphragm. During inspiration, the inspiratory muscles contract, the chest expands, and the diaphragm descends, allowing the lungs to expand with air. During expiration, the muscles relax, the diaphragm returns to normal position, and the lungs contract. The rib cage, inspiratory muscles, and diaphragm are shown in Figure 11–4.

Figure 11–4 The Rib Cage, Inspiratory Muscles, and Diaphragm

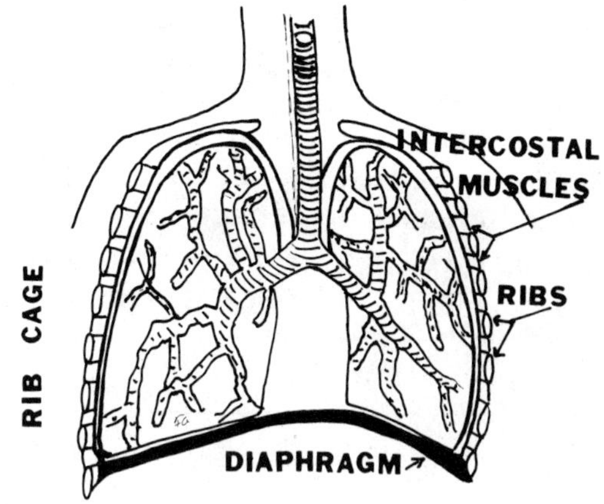

CONGENITAL RESPIRATORY DEFECTS

Congenital abnormalities of the respiratory system are discovered immediately after birth by using the Apgar scoring system to assess the infant. Observations are made within 1 minute after delivery and are repeated in 5 minutes. The Apgar score includes heart rate, respiratory effort, muscle tone, reflex irritability (stimulation of feet), and color as signs to observe in the newborn. These signs are recorded on a scale from 0 to 2, signifying absence at 0 and fully present at 2. To illustrate the use of the Apgar scoring system, a newborn with heart rate, respiratory effort, muscle tone, reflex irritability, and color of 2 would receive a rating of 10, two points for each sign.[2] Figure 11–5 shows the Apgar rating chart.

Choanal Atresia

Choanal atresia is an obstruction of the postnasal cavity (Figure 11–6). It is characterized by a growth of a membrane or bone structure that partially or entirely closes off the passageway between the nose and the pharynx. This obstruction may be unilateral or bilateral. Signs and symptoms of choanal atresia in the newborn are breathing through the mouth, choking on milk or water (therefore unable to take bottle), cyanosis, and weight loss. Surgical removal of the membrane or bone is necessary.

Figure 11–5 The Apgar Rating Chart

APGAR NEWBORN RATING CHART

	SCORE		
CRITERIA	0	1	2
COLOR	BLUE	SOME PINK	ALL PINK
HEART RATE	ABSENT	<100	≥100
RESPIRATION	ABSENT	IRREGULAR	STRONG
REFLEXES	NONE	SOME MOTION	GOOD CRY
MUSCLE TONE	LIMP	SOME FLEXION	ACTIVE

NORMAL NEWBORN SCORES 10

Figure 11–6 Choanal Atresia

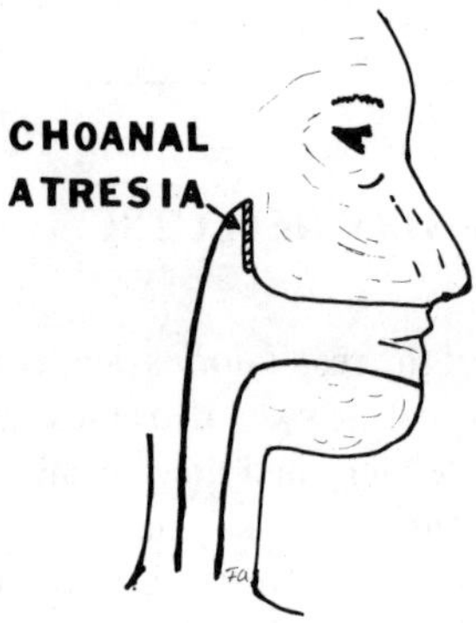

Deviated/Perforated Nasal Septum

The wall separating the nares in the nose is the nasal septum. The normal, straight septum allows air to flow freely through the nose into the lungs. If the septum is deformed—either crooked or perforated—at birth, the infant cannot breathe properly. Depending on the severity of the defect, corrective surgery may be warranted. Figure 11–7 shows a deviated and a perforated nasal septum.

Laryngeal Web

A laryngeal web is a thin membrane that has grown across the larynx, causing a stricture, or narrowing, of the trachea (Figure 11–8). This growth can occur in any

Figure 11–7 A Deviated and a Perforated Septum

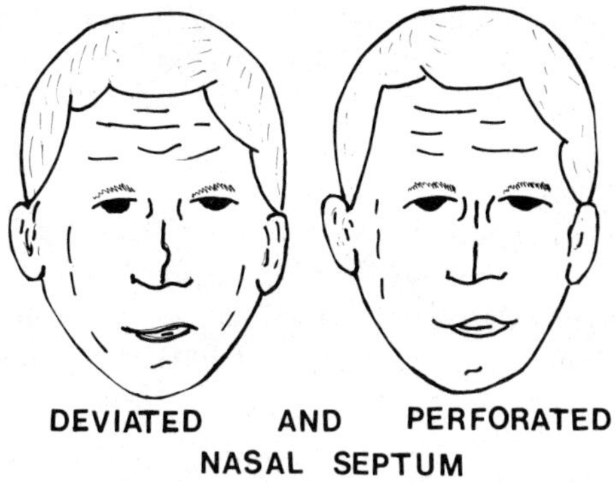

Figure 11–8 A Laryngeal Web

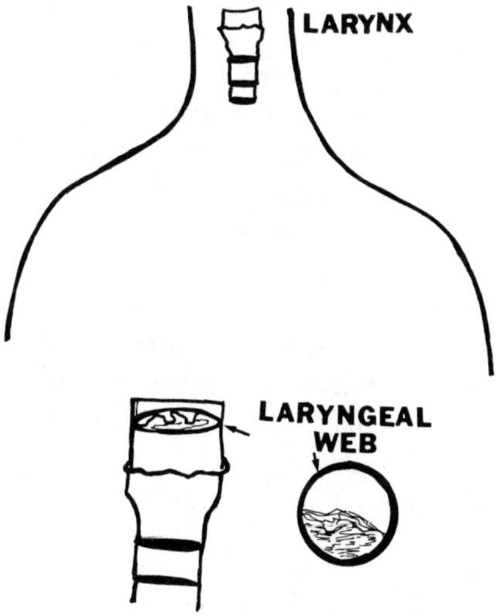

area of the larynx. This is a rare anomaly. Symptoms include cyanosis, hypoxia, and inability to take a bottle. Barium swallow is diagnostic. Surgical intervention consists of excision of the webbed area and an end-to-end anastomosis of the larynx.

PRENATAL CONDITIONS

Infants may be born with respiratory defects that are not considered congenital. These conditions are attributed to the prenatal period.

Respiratory Distress Syndrome

Respiratory distress syndrome (RDS), which occurs primarily in mature infants, is characterized by the newborn experiencing difficulty in breathing, with cyanosis, inability to take the bottle, and weight loss. The leading cause of infant mortality, RDS accounts for approximately 20,000 newborn deaths in the United States each year.[3]

Pulmonary Hyaline Membrane Disease

Hyaline, a glassy, transparent, fluid forms a film or membrane along the walls of the bronchioles, alveoli, and alveolar ducts, blocking the airways into the alveoli and alveolar ducts. After birth, as the mucus continues to be deposited, the alveolar airways are obstructed, preventing the exchange of oxygen for carbon dioxide in the blood. The infant reveals symptoms of dyspnea, cyanosis, nasal flaring, expiratory grunt, and pronounced movements of the chest.

Management consists in maintenance of adequate oxygenation to prevent acidosis and respiratory failure. Oxygen sufficient to maintain arterial tensions 50 to 80 torr (the pressure necessary to support a column of mercury 1 mm. high at 0 degrees centigrade and standard gravity) should be delivered into a hood or respirator through an oxygen-air blender to allow exact control over oxygen concentration. Frequent blood gas sampling is required to assure arterial oxygen tension (PO_2) at 50 to 80 torr.

Acute complications accompanying hyaline membrane disease are pneumothorax, pneumonia, and infection. Long-term complications include chronic lung disease, neurological impairment due to oxygen therapy, and family adjustment problems.

Supportive care of the critical infant includes constant monitoring for maintenance of oxygen flow, adequate fluids, and nutritional intake. Parental support is given through frequent reports about the progress of the infant. Parents should be encouraged to visit the nursery and taught how to care for the infant prior to discharge from the hospital.

Atelectasis

RDS occurs in atelectasis. A mature infant is born with the ability in its lungs to manufacture pulmonary surface-active agents consisting mainly of lecithin. The lungs of an infant born to a diabetic mother have been known not to develop the ability to manufacture pulmonary surfactant until 40 weeks of gestation.[4] (Surfactant is a mixture of lipoproteins—lecithin and sphingomyelin—secreted by the alveolar cells into the alveoli and respiratory air passages that functions to keep the alveolar ducts expanded during breathing.) Therefore, premature infants and infants of diabetic mothers are sometimes born before the lungs have developed the capacity to manufacture pulmonary surfactant.

An Apgar score at birth of less than 4 indicates respiratory distress. The child appears cyanotic, has slow or absent heart rate, irregular or slow respiration, and rib cage retractions. Respiratory distress may increase within the next 2 days and the baby expires or the infant's condition may improve within 5 days of birth.

Supportive treatment includes suction of meconium, administration of oxygen, and tracheal entubation. Continuous monitoring is required for maintenance of fluid balance through glucose and electrolyte concentrations in intravenous fluids. The chance of survival has improved greatly owing to premature neonatal intensive care centers.

BIRTH TRAUMA

Many injuries occurring at birth are due to traumatic delivery. For example, there may be a brachial plexus, spinal cord, or cranial nerve injury during delivery. However, brain injury is likely to result from cerebral anoxia.

Intracranial Hemorrhage

Intracranial hemorrhage, the escape of blood from a ruptured blood vessel within the skull, may result from birth trauma. This condition may affect the vital control centers, one of which is the respiratory center. The function of the respiratory center in the brain is to maintain adequate oxygen supply throughout the body. The respiratory center is notified when, for a specific reason, part of the body requires more oxygen than is generally necessary for function. In response, the respiratory center speeds up respiration. Trauma to the respiratory center may depress respiration or slow up the response for adequate oxygen supply to part of the body. As a result, breathing may be delayed and inadequate. Hypoxemia, anoxemia, and hypercapnia may occur.

Asphyxia Neonatorum

Asphyxia neonatorum refers to a newborn who does not breathe spontaneously at birth. A number of conditions may cause asphyxia, for example, premature labor, multiple births, or prolapsed cord. It may occur in utero or during labor and delivery. Perinatal asphyxia may be anticipated and prepared for in 70 percent of premature births, multiple births, and other high-risk pregnancies.[5] Asphyxia may occur during labor because of placental dysfunction in the mother or because of pulmonary dysfunction and intracranial hemorrhage in the newborn. Asphyxia in utero may be caused by placenta previa or insufficiency, so at the time of birth, the infant may not breathe because of asphyxia before birth. Narcosis from drug or anesthetic administration may also cause asphyxia. On the Apgar scale, asphyxia may be measured from severe (0 to 3) to moderate (4 to 7).

ACQUIRED DEFECTS AND DISEASES

Defects and diseases may be acquired through trauma and infection.

Nose Fracture

Perhaps the most common traumatic defect is a broken nose, which, depending on the severity, may or may not require surgical intervention. Surgery for cosmetic purposes may also be desired.

Reduction of a nasal fracture should be performed as soon as the edema subsides. Under anesthesia, intranasal manipulation is necessary to elevate depressed bone or cartilage that is pushed into the paranasal sinuses.

Deviated/Perforated Nasal Septum

The septum is a straight, cartilaginous partition separating the nostrils. However, owing to trauma, the septum may be perforated by a broken bone or bent by a blow on the nose. Severe deviation or perforation may obstruct the air passageway. Surgery may be indicated. Figure 11–7 shows a congenital deviation of the nasal septum.

Rhinoplasty with submucous resection is performed to correct a deviated nasal septum resulting from infection, trauma, or congenital causes. No two operations are the same, but generally the surgeon lays back a flap of mucous membrane in the area of the nose to be repaired. Then a portion of the deflected nasal septum is removed and the flap of mucous membrane is replaced, using sutures.

Rhinitis

Simple Acute Rhinitis (Common Cold)

Simple acute rhinitis is a generalized infection of the mucous membrane of the nose, characterized by profuse clear mucus discharge. The mucous membranes of the nose swell to the extent that the nasal passageway may be entirely closed.

Acute Bacterial Rhinitis

Acute bacterial rhinitis is a generalized infection of the mucous membrane of the nose owing to bacterial infection.

The patient complains of fever, loss of appetite, and aching all over. Bed rest and fluids are prescribed. The infected area is cultured for identification of the bacteria; antibiotics are prescribed according to the results of the sensitivity test.

Chronic Rhinitis

Chronic rhinitis may occur in patients with syphilis, tuberculosis, blastomy-ocosis, or other pathogenic and fungal diseases in which granuloma formation is present along with destruction of soft tissue, cartilage, and bone. Symptoms are nasal obstruction, purulent discharge, and nosebleed. Identification of causative organism is made through culture and sensitivity tests. Antibiotics are prescribed accordingly.

Allergic Rhinitis (Hay Fever)

Allergic rhinitis is seasonal; it is generally caused by airborne pollen from trees, grass, and weeds and fungal spores. Symptoms are itching of the nose, roof of the mouth, and eyes. There is clear discharge from the nose, watery eyes, and bouts of sneezing. The patient may experience headaches, irritability, and anorexia. Mucous membranes become acutely swollen. Skin tests are recommended for identification of the allergic agent; oral antihistamines are prescribed. The patient's condition improves after avoidance of offending irritants.

Acute Sinusitis

Because the mucous membrane lining of the sinuses is continuous with that of the nasal cavity, infection from the nasal cavity may easily spread to the sinuses. Sinusitis is infection of the mucous membranes of the sinus cavities. Since there are four sets of sinuses, sinusitis is identified by location, for example, maxillary sinusitis or ethmoidal sinusitis. Acute sinusitis may be caused by an invasion of microorganisms, such as streptococci, pneumococci, and staphylococci, causing purulent, or pus, drainage.

Symptoms may be headache, malaise, fever, chills, and yellow purulent drainage from the nose. Culture and sensitivity tests are indicated for identification of the causative organisms and the antibiotic most effective in treating the infection. Treatment includes antibiotic control of infection, improved drainage from the sinuses, bed rest, and fluids.

Acute Pharyngitis

Acute pharyngitis, although usually viral in origin, may result from streptococci or staphylococci. Symptoms include a sore throat and pain on swallowing, with the presence of purulent exudate and infected mucosa. Chills, fever, cervical adenopathy, and leukocytosis are also present. Culture and sensitivity tests are necessary to isolate microorganisms and to institute antibiotic therapy. Treatment includes bed rest with forced fluids, saline gargles, and antibiotic therapy.

Tonsillitis

Acute Tonsillitis

Tonsils are a small mass of lymphoid tissue in the oropharynx, bilaterally. They function as filters to protect the body from microorganism invasion. Acute tonsillitis, inflammation of the tonsils, is generally caused by a streptococcal or viral infection. For reasons not known or understood, rheumatic fever is sequela to acute tonsillitis owing to hemolytic streptococci (see Chapter 10, Rheumatic Fever).

The patient complains of sore throat with pain on swallowing and referred pain to the ears. Symptoms may also include fever, chills, malaise, headache, and purulent exudate.

Culture and sensitivity tests are indicated for identification of microorganisms and appropriate antibiotic therapy. Treatment consists of bed rest, forced fluids, warm gargle, analgesics, and antibiotics as required.

Chronic Tonsillitis

Chronic tonsillitis, the result of recurrent acute tonsillitis, is manifested by edema and scarring of the tonsils. Symptoms include cough, fetid breath, and pharyngeal exudate.

For children, treatment is surgical excision. In older patients, in whom an operative risk exists, medical treatment is given consistent with acute tonsillitis.

Hypertrophy of Tonsils

Enlargement of the tonsils often results from recurrent acute and chronic infections. It is often accompanied by hypertrophy of the adenoids.

Hypertrophy of Adenoids

The adenoids (pharyngeal tonsils) are lymphoid tissue located on the back upper wall of the nasopharynx. Because lymphoid tissue functions as a repository for infection in the body, nasosinusitis drains into the adenoids, which become swollen and, over a period of time, enlarged.

Tonsillectomy and Adenoidectomy

The surgical excision of tonsils and adenoids is controversial as to the appropriate age and the indications for surgery. Strong indications for surgery are evidence of malignancy; acute and chronic recurrent tonsil and adenoid infections that do not respond to antibiotic therapy and are accompanied by ear infections; and recurrent streptococcal infections with risk of rheumatic fever, rheumatic heart disease, or nephritis. Enlarged tonsils or adenoids do not warrant surgery.

Contraindications for surgery are acute infection; a cleft palate that would bring further speech impairment to a child; systemic diseases, such as uncontrolled diabetes, tuberculosis, and heart disease; and a hemorrhagic disease, such as hemophilia.

Acute Laryngitis

Infections from the pharynx, nose, sinuses, and tonsils easily spread to the larynx because the mucous membrane lining the larynx is continuous throughout the area.

Symptoms are change in tone of voice, dysphonia, dysphagia, and aphonia. The patient complains of fever, malaise, and sore throat. Acute laryngitis is associated with, and many times secondary to, such infections as bronchitis, pneumonia, influenza, and diphtheria. Culture and sensitivity tests are necessary to identify the pathogen and prescribe appropriate antibiotic therapy.

Tracheal Stenosis

Tracheal stenosis is the narrowing of the trachea owing to scar tissue from a previous tracheostomy, vocal cord paralysis, enlarged lymph nodes, tumors, or burns (Figure 11–9). The patient complains of shortness of breath. Physical examination reveals wheezing and inspiratory stridor. Pulmonary function tests and fluoroscopy are necessary for diagnosis of stenosis.

Acute Infectious Bronchitis

Acute infectious bronchitis, inflammation of the tracheobronchial tree usually occurs after pharyngitis or laryngitis. Bronchitis may be caused by a virus or bacteria. The patient complains of fever, malaise, cough, and vague chest pain. Physical examination reveals rhonchi and wheezing without evidence of lung consolidation confirmed by chest x-ray. Treatment consists of bed rest, forcing fluids, expectorants, and appropriate antibiotic. Acute infectious bronchitis is life threatening for young children, people over age 65, and those sustaining chronic lung disease.

Figure 11–9 Tracheal Stenosis

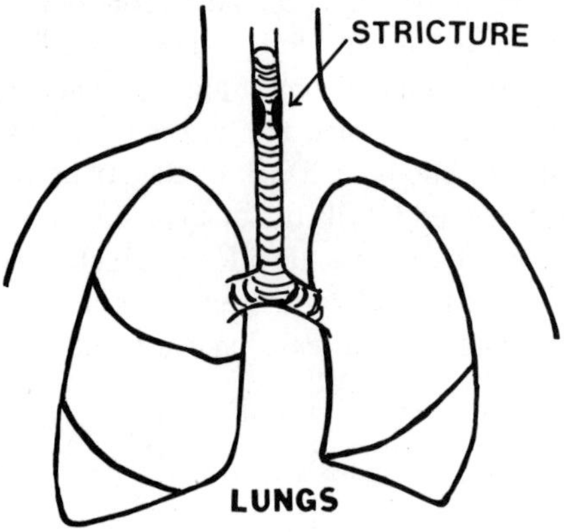

Chronic Obstructive Pulmonary Disease

Chronic obstructive pulmonary disease (COPD) is a term applied to at least two lung diseases of long duration characterized by progressive resistance to airflow. Two examples are chronic bronchitis and emphysema.[6]

Chronic Bronchitis

The early stage of chronic bronchitis is characterized by cough; then there are recurrent attacks of bronchitis with mucopurulent, foul-smelling sputum; later the airways become obstructed as the patient experiences dyspnea as well as productive cough. Chronic bronchitis is defined as bronchitis continuing over a three-month period in two consecutive years, accompanied by attacks of coughing and lung changes that are documented by chest x-ray. In later stages of the disease, the patient's history reveals patterns of repeated colds, acute bronchitis, and upper respiratory tract infections.

The patient complains of fever, dyspnea, productive cough, and respiratory distress.

Bronchograms reveal, on inspiration, cylindrical dilatation of the bronchi and, on forced expiration, bronchial collapse and thickening of the bronchial walls. Laboratory findings reveal secondary polycythemia. The sputum may be mucoid and nonpurulent, or it may reveal *Hemophilus influenzae* and *Streptococcus pneumoniae*.

Treatment consists of discontinuance of cigarette smoking and avoidance of other hazardous inhalants. Immunization for pneumococci and influenza are recommended to control respiratory failure. Antibiotics are not given except for acute bronchitis. Oral aminophylline and inhaled bronchodilators are used to open airways and increase breathing capacity.

Emphysema

Pulmonary emphysema, thought to be inherited, is considered a common cause of death in the United States. It is caused by a deficiency of alpha$_1$-antitrypsin, which activates trypsin. Owing to the deficiency of alpha$_1$-antitrypsin, trypsin and other enzymes decrease the elasticity of the tissues and finally engulf the elastic tissue in the alveolar airways. The course of pulmonary emphysema may be described as the distention of alveolar ducts and spaces forming cystic or bulbous areas in the alveoli spaces through which gas exchange cannot take place. It is characterized by increased size of the alveoli owing to the trapping of air behind bronchioles and alveoli. More air enters on inspiration than leaves at expiration. Therefore, the alveoli become stretched, grow larger, and become distended. Over a period of time the lungs become enlarged and the chest bulges to accommodate them. The chest deformity that results is known as barrel chest. The overdistended alveoli, after a period of time, lose elasticity, burst, and degenerate; the lungs function less and less in the exchange of carbon dioxide for oxygen. As the disease advances, more strain is placed on the heart, which tends to compensate by increasing the amount of blood pumped into the lungs; cor pulmonale (pulmonary heart disease) or hypertrophy of the right ventricle of the heart develops in the terminal stage of the disease. Figure 11–10 shows cor pulmonale and emphysema.

Figure 11–10 Cor Pulmonale and Emphysema

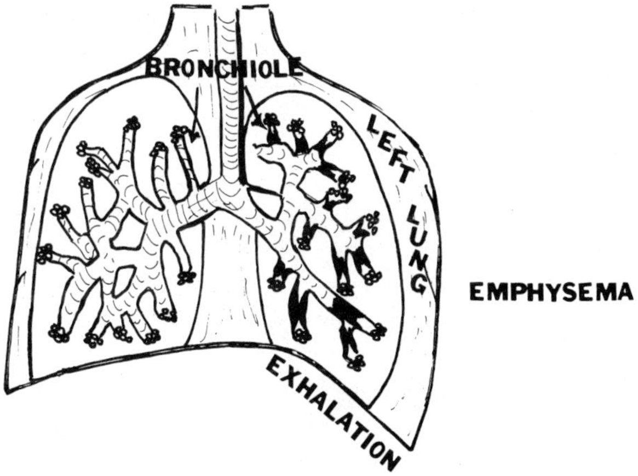

The findings on physical examination depend on the stage of the disease. Generally, there is increased chest diameter; overinflation of the lungs, with diaphragmatic depression and little motion on respiration; decreased breath sounds, with increased expiratory phase; and wheezing. In the advanced stage, there is clubbing of the fingers and toes, pedal edema, hepatomegaly, ascites, and right ventricular hypertrophy.

Emphysema cannot be cured, but patients are cautioned to avoid all toxic inhalants, especially fumes and cigarettes. Because emphysema patients are at high risk for respiratory tract infection, inoculation against influenza virus is recommended.

Bronchiectasis

Bronchiectasis is chronic dilatation of the bronchi and bronchioles, characterized by attacks of coughing that produce purulent, blood-tinged mucus. The patient complains of sporadic coughing in the morning, producing foul-smelling, purulent, blood-tinged mucus.[7] Past history reveals repeated pulmonary infection, which may include tuberculosis, pertussis, or COPD. Auscultation of the chest reveals rales and rhonchi over the affected area of the lungs. Late stages include emaciation, cyanosis, and hemoptysis. Laboratory tests are not significant. Bronchoscopy is diagnostic of saccular, cylindric, or fusiform dilatation of the bronchi. Saccular dilatations are indicative of permanent damage from the disease. Cylindric changes caused by complications of pneumonia will revert to normal after the pneumonia is resolved. Fusiform dilatations of the terminal bulbus also indicate permanent damage to the bronchi. Treatment consists of avoidance of exposure to all kinds of fumes. Cigarette smoking is forbidden. Postural drainage may give temporary relief. Antibiotic therapy is prescribed to treat specific microorganisms identified through culture of sputum and sensitivity tests. Surgical intervention, lobectomy, may be recommended in severe cases after all other treatment has failed. Figure 11–11 shows saccular, cylindric, and fusiform dilatation of the bronchi and bronchiectasis.

Bronchial Asthma

Asthma may be classified by origin according to (a) nonallergic or intrinsic substances and (b) allergic or extrinsic substances.

Nonallergic asthma has its genesis in pathophysiological disturbances in the body, such as, an upper respiratory tract infection or bronchitis.

Allergic factors causing asthma are subdivided into organic and inorganic substances. Organic substances triggering asthma are those derived from living organisms, such as trees, cotton, flowers, and animals. Inorganic substances causing asthma are dusts created by industrial occupations related to the mining of

Figure 11–11 Dilatation of the Bronchi or Bronchiectasis

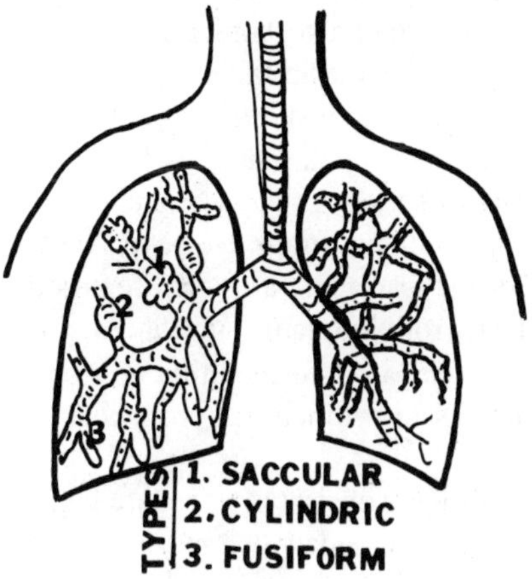

rocks and metals. Allergic organic and inorganic substances are summarized in Figure 11–12.

Bronchial asthma begins with the release of histamine and other activating substances into the mucous membrane of the bronchi. Histamine, a chemical substance derived from protein, is found in all body tissues. These substances bring about mucosal edema of the bronchi, which blocks the normal air passageways.[8]

Bronchial asthma is described as recurrent attacks of paroxysmal shortening of breath with wheezing owing to bronchospasms. Triggered by a nonallergic condi-

Figure 11–12 Allergic Organic and Inorganic Substances

ORGANIC (LIVING ORGANISMS)	INORGANIC (NON-LIVING ORGANISMS)
ANIMALS	DUST
	COAL
FLOWERS	METALS
	WOOD
TREES	FUMES
	CHEMICALS

tion or an allergic substance, bronchospasms are crampy contractions of muscle bands that wrap around the bronchiole and, on contraction, close the airways (Figure 11–13). The lungs attempt to compensate for the closing airways by overinflating, and breathing becomes difficult.

The patient complains of recurrent shortness of breath, wheezing, and mucoid productive cough. In cases in which the cause is intrinsic, asthma may occur only during a respiratory tract infection, such as bronchitis, or another infection, or when the patient is under emotional strain. However, when the cause is extrinsic, bronchial asthma may occur seasonally as plant life produces pollen or when the person is exposed to dusts from inorganic substances.

Laboratory tests reveal increased eosinophilia. Chest x-ray usually shows no abnormality. Severe attacks are sometimes complicated by pneumothorax, or collapse of the lung.

In the acute stage, treatment consists of adequate bed rest with psychological support to relieve apprehension, sedatives, and drug therapy with epinephrine. Aerosol therapy drugs include isoproterenol and isoetharine with phenylephrine. Sedation should be given with caution in severe asthmatic attack.

Status Asthmaticus

Status asthmaticus occurs when an acute asthmatic attack becomes severe and prolonged and does not respond to medication. Elevation of blood gas $PaCO_2$ indicates the need for immediate hospitalization owing to the risk of hypoxia, cyanosis, and unconsciousness.

The ability of the lungs to exchange oxygen for carbon dioxide through diffusion of the capillary membranes is assessed by blood gas analysis. An unclotted arterial blood sample is put into a chamber of a computerized instru-

Figure 11–13 Bronchospasms

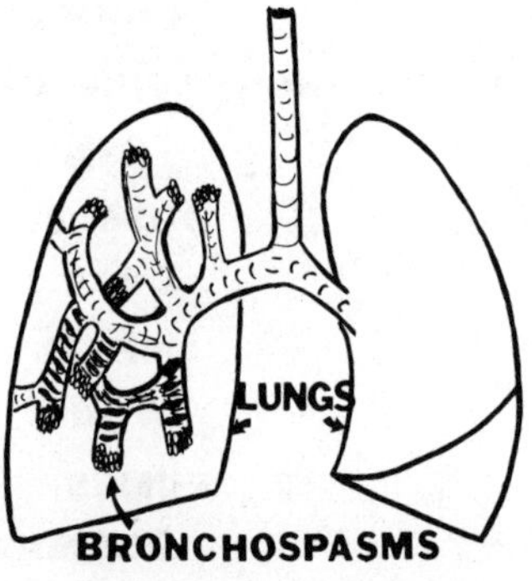

ment, where the blood sample is in contact with electrodes for measuring the blood's pH, or acid-base index; PO_2, or oxygen pressure; and CO_2, or carbon dioxide pressure.

Treatment includes intravenous aminophylline and hydrocortisone sodium succinate. Nasal oxygen should be given for hypoxemia and bronchodilators may be given through inhalation.

After the acute stage has subsided, an attempt should be made to identify the causative factor or substance.

Pneumoconiosis

Pneumoconiosis is a general term for a group of chronic lung diseases caused by inhalation of various dusts, usually of occupational or environmental origin. Some types of pneumoconiosis are anthracosis, asbestosis, and silicosis.

Anthracosis

Anthracosis, or black lung disease, is developed through inhalation of soot and coal dusts. Over a long period of exposure to coal dusts, black nodules develop on the bronchioles; this may result in emphysema. No specific treatment is recommended other than change in occupation, preventing further exposure to coal dust.

Asbestosis

Asbestosis is a lung disease caused by the inhalation of asbestos fibers. It occurs mainly in miners and those who are exposed to asbestos building materials. Asbestos used in the ceilings of elementary school classrooms has been a threat to children. Over a period of time asbestosis may lead to alveolar, interstitial, or pleural fibrosis.

Chest x-rays reveal small linear opacities spread throughout the lungs and diffuse pulmonary fibrosis. Sputum test reveals the presence of asbestos.

The patient complains of progressive dyspnea on exertion, with cyanosis, cough, and weight loss that is aggravated by continued exposure to asbestos. The disease may be halted by avoiding further exposure to asbestos. There is no treatment.

Silicosis

Earlier, under bronchial asthma, it was explained that external inorganic materials interfere with respiration. Silica is the most common inorganic dust particle that is hazardous to workers in lead, coal, copper, and silver industries. Inhaled dust particles from silica stone and sand are carried to the alveoli. In the alveoli, a foreign-body tissue reaction is set off against the silica dust. The dust becomes surrounded by phagocytes that carry it through the lymph vessels to regional lymph nodes. There the dust-filled phagocytes contribute to the formation of nodules, or solid masses of fibrous or scar tissue. Gradually, the fibrous tissue replaces normal tissue. As the fibrous nodules increase in size, they also increase airway resistance. In the early stage of the disease, the patient experiences cough. As the disease advances, the cough becomes productive and there is dyspnea on exertion, with reduction of vital capacity. Emphysema develops in the late stages. The patient becomes increasingly disabled, with susceptibility to pulmonary infections, tuberculosis, and pneumothorax. Gross pathology reveals thickened, gray, subpleural nodules with black discoloration of the lungs. There are fibrotic nodules of varying sizes in the lungs, and the tracheobronchial lymph nodes are enlarged. Although no cure is known, change in employment is recommended to slow down the progress of the disease.

BRONCHOPNEUMONIA

Bronchopneumonia is inflammation of the bronchioles secondary to an infection in the pharynx, trachea, or larynx that has spread to the lower respiratory tract. It may result from bacterial pneumonia, viral infection, aspiration of vomit, or debilitating terminal disease. Bronchopneumonia, primary in infants and the aged, may be fatal.

The patient may complain of productive cough with blood-tinged sputum, fever, chills, and malaise. Auscultation reveals increased breath sounds and rales. Chest x-ray shows patchy areas of increased density. Sputum culture reveals the presence of bacteria.

Treatment includes antibiotics and oxygen therapy. Supportive measures include keeping the bronchi clear of secretions and analgesics for relief of pleural pain.

Influenza

Influenza is an acute respiratory infection of viral origin, striking sometimes as an epidemic. It is characterized by acute inflammation of the mucous membrane of the respiratory tract. Influenza begins with an incubation period, when the patient complains of headache, nasal stuffiness, and sore throat; chills and fever follow, accompanied by myalgia. There may be nausea, with or without vomiting, and a nonproductive cough. Influenza predisposes the patient to secondary bacterial infection, and often acute sinusitis, otitis media, acute bronchitis, or pneumonia develops.

Laboratory tests reveal a low white blood cell count; hemagglutination inhibition test is positive. Chest x-ray may or may not show vascular markings.

Antibiotic therapy is not recommended unless an organism can be identified and the sensitivity test can be completed. Bed rest, forced fluids, analgesics, and cough mixture are recommended.

Pneumonia

Simply stated, pneumonia is an acute microorganismal infection of the parenchyma of the lung with consolidation. When it involves an entire lobe, it is called lobar; when it involves only a segment of the lung it is called segmental. It may be viral, bacterial, fungal, protozoal, myobacterial, mycoplasmal, or rickettsial in origin. Pneumonia may be either primary, when it originates in the lungs, or secondary to an upper respiratory tract infection.[9]

Signs and symptoms are sudden chills with rising fever, chest pain, productive cough, and headache. In addition to the foregoing, the patient may complain of nausea, with or without vomiting, dyspnea, cyanosis, and perspiration. On auscultation, there may be fine rales and decreased breath sounds over the infected area. As the lungs consolidate, tachycardia, tachypnea, and cyanosis are found on physical examination. Chest x-rays will confirm lung consolidation. Laboratory sputum test for culture will isolate the microorganism, and sensitivity test will confirm the drug most likely to resolve the infection. Recommended treatment includes bed rest, forced fluids, oxygen by nasal catheter, and analgesics. Penicillin may be given initially until culture and sensitivity test results are available. Mortality is high in infants and in those over age 65.

Pleurisy

Pleurisy is inflammation of the pleura, with exudation into the pleural cavity. It may be secondary to pneumonia, infection, trauma, or inhalation of noxious agents.

The pleura is the serous membrane surrounding the lungs. The visceral layer adheres to the lung and the parietal layer lines the thoracic cavity. Pleural fluid is found between the visceral and parietal layers of membrane and covers the pleural surface (Figure 11–14). It enables the lung to move smoothly. When there is an inadequate amount of pleural fluid, the lungs cannot move freely; pleural friction rub results. When the pleura is inflamed, transudate or exudate can seep into the pleural cavity, causing pleural effusion, and the lung may collapse.

Hemothorax

A hemothorax is a collapsed lung owing to blood in the pleural cavity. This may occur if there has been injury to the rib cage and one of the broken or fractured ribs punctures the lung.

Figure 11–14 The Pleural Cavity

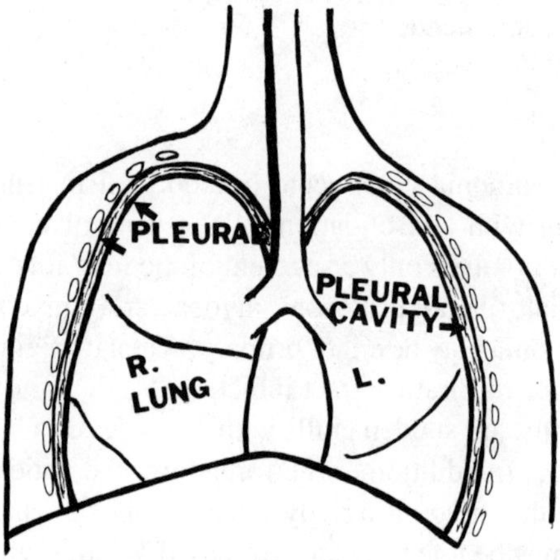

Pneumothorax

A pneumothorax is a collapsed lung owing to air in the pleural cavity. It may be secondary to a traumatic injury to the lung or to an infection, such as pneumonia or tuberculosis.

Pyopneumothorax

A pyopneumothorax occurs when a lung abscess ruptures, with pus and gas entering the pleural cavity.

The patient complains of sudden chest pain, which may be present only with deep breathing and coughing, after trauma to the chest area or during infection. Physical examination reveals rapid, shallow respiration with diminished breath sounds and pleural friction rub. Pleural effusion resolves the chest pain, but physical examination reveals percussion dullness, absent tractile fremitus, and decreased or absent breath sounds.

Chest x-ray does not confirm pleurisy. Thoracentesis is the preferred diagnostic procedure. In this procedure a surgical hollow needle is inserted in the chest wall and fluid is aspirated from the pleural cavity for analysis.

Pulmonary Tuberculosis

Pulmonary tuberculosis (TB) is contracted through inhalation of airborne organisms —usually *Mycobacterium tuberculosis* or other strains of mycobacteria—

produced by the cough of an infected person. The primary infection begins with the germ invading the lungs. The body sets up a mechanism whereby the TB germs are surrounded and walled in by other cells that form nodules around them, called tubercles. The tubercles render the tuberculosis inactive. Tuberculosis may be reactivated when the person's resistance is low because of age or infection or as a result of environmental factors, such as high humidity.

The patient complains of fatigue, weight loss, malaise, productive cough, dull aching chest pain or pleurisy and night sweats.[10]

Percussion reveals dullness over the involved area, bronchial breath sounds, rales, and fremitus.

Tests to rule out TB are the Mantoux, Tine, Heaf, and purified protein derivative (PPD). The PPD test is the most reliable. Sputum smear and guinea pig inoculation are also positive for TB.

In most instances, initial hospitalization is recommended for isolation, laboratory, radiographic techniques, and institution of chemotherapy. In the hospital environment the patient's response to treatment is easily monitored through laboratory evaluation of the persistence of bacilli in the sputum. In addition, adequate drug dosage and the patient's psychological attitude are handled more efficiently.

As soon as the diagnosis of active tuberculosis has been verified, the patient should be informed. The risk of infection for others should be emphasized as well as the need for investigation of the family and associates for infection.

The basic plan for treatment includes a regimen of chemotherapy with daily oral doses of isoniazid and rifampin for 9 to 18 months or longer. Once fever and night sweats are gone, cough is diminished, and sputum is negative for tubercule bacilli on three consecutive cultures, the patient is discharged to home. Follow-up visits to the doctor's office or clinic including repeat sputum tests and x-rays vary depending upon the response of the lesion to chemotherapy. Few persons die of tuberculosis today.

NOTES

1. Henry Gray, *Anatomy, Descriptive and Surgical,* 15th ed. (New York: Bounty Books, 1977), 975.
2. Robert Berkow, ed., *The Merck Manual of Diagnosis and Therapy,* 14th ed. (Rahway, N.J.: Merck Sharp and Dohme Research Laboratories, 1982), 1757.
3. Ibid., 1759.
4. Ibid.
5. Ibid.
6. Richard E. Brashear and Mitchell L. Rhodes, *Chronic Obstructive Lung Disease* (St. Louis: C.V. Mosby Co., 1978), 11.
7. Ibid.

8. Ibid.

9. Patrick A. Murphy, ''Pneumonia.'' In *The Principles and Practice of Medicine,* 11th ed., ed A. McGehee Harvey et al. (New York: Appleton-Century-Crofts, 1980), 995–1013.

10. John J. Mann, ''Infections without localizing manifestations,'' *Principles and Practices of Medicine,* 962–963.

Chapter 12

The Gastrointestinal System

Objectives

- Name the structures of the digestive system.
- Trace food through the digestive system from the mouth to the anus.
- Explain the change that takes place in food as it passes through the digestive system.
- Compare incompetency and insufficiency of a gastric sphincter and a heart valve.
- Describe the three types of anastomosis.
- Differentiate between intussusception and volvulus.
- Compare the differences between myocardial, pulmonary, and mesenteric infarctions.
- Explain the differences between a stricture and a fistula.

FUNCTION AND STRUCTURE

The digestive system consists of an alimentary canal and accessory organs (Figure 12–1). The alimentary canal, a musculomembranous tube 30 feet in length, extending from the mouth to the anus, includes the mouth, pharynx, esophagus, stomach, and small and large intestines. It functions by digestion, or chemically converting food into a form that can be absorbed into the body. The accessory organs—the teeth, salivary glands, liver, gallbladder, and pancreas—assist the process of digestion with the manufacture and distribution of enzymes and hormones.

MOUTH

Food entering the alimentary canal at the mouth is chewed, or masticated. One of the first signs of growth that parents look for in their child before he or she is one year of age is teeth protruding through the child's gums. These first teeth are called deciduous teeth; they are replaced by permanent teeth.

Figure 12–1 Alimentary Canal with Accessory Organs

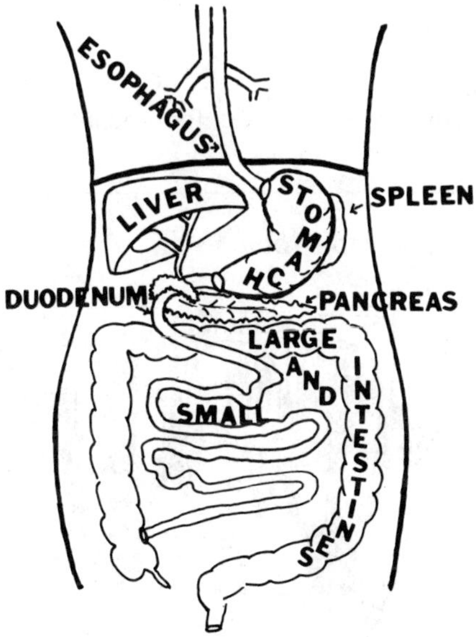

Examination of a tooth reveals a crown protruding above the gum. The parts of the tooth below the gum, in the socket, or alveolus, are the neck and the root. The five primary parts of the tooth are:

1. the enamel or outer layer
2. the cementum, continuous with enamel but below the gum, covering the root and the neck in the socket
3. the periodontal membrane lining the socket
4. the dentine, resembling bone, which is the bulk of the tooth
5. the pulp or innermost part of the tooth, which contains the blood supply and nerves.

Figure 12–2 shows the parts of a tooth.

Food entering the mouth undergoes mastication. Mastication is aided by saliva, which contains enzymes secreted by the salivary glands. The saliva speeds up the breakdown of starch to bolus before the food is swallowed.

SALIVARY GLANDS

The salivary glands—parotid, sublingual, and submaxillary—produce saliva containing enzymes, water, and other substances. This acts as a catalyst in starting the food digestion.

PHARYNX

The pharynx is a common passageway for food and air (see Chapter 11).

Figure 12–2 The Parts of the Tooth

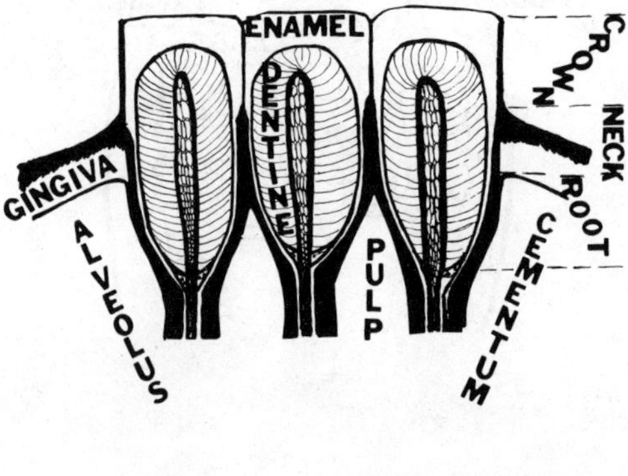

ESOPHAGUS

The bolus is carried through the esophagus, a musculomembranous tube, by rhythmiclike muscular action, called peristalsis, to the cardiac sphincter, or opening, where bolus enters the stomach. The orifice is called the cardiac sphincter because of its proximity to the heart.

STOMACH

A circular muscle called the cardiac sphincter is located on the superior end of the stomach. The function of this sphincter is to move the bolus from the esophagus into the stomach. The three parts of the stomach are (1) the fundus (upper part), (2) the corpus (the body), and (3) the pylorus (lower part). Figure 12–3 shows the parts of the stomach.

The four layers of stomach tissue are:

1. the outer peritoneal, or serous, layer
2. the longitudinal, oblique, and circular fibromuscular layer
3. the submucous layer
4. the mucous membrane (inner layer) in folds called rugae.[1]

Figure 12–3 The Parts of the Stomach

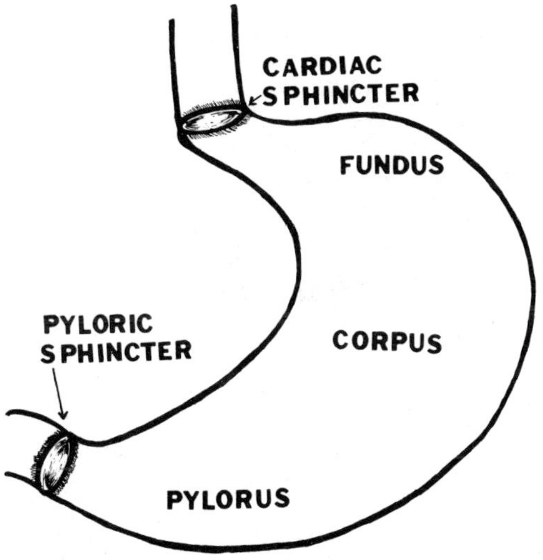

Figure 12–4 shows the tissue layers of the stomach.

The mucous membrane, or inner layer of stomach tissue, contain glands that secrete four substances:

1. mucus, a lubricant
2. intrinsic factor for absorption of vitamin B
3. enzyme pepsin for protein breakdown
4. hydrochloric acid for protection against bacteria and maintenance of proper pH for pepsin reaction.

When the bolus in the stomach is further digested through secretions, the pyloric sphincter opens for the chyme to be pushed into the small intestines.

SMALL INTESTINES

The three parts of the small intestine are (1) the duodenum, (2) the jejunum, and (3) the ileum (Figure 12–5). The small intestine is lined interiorly with minute projections called villi, which contain a network of blood vessels and lymph capillaries through which absorption takes place into the blood and cells of the body.

The 1-foot-long *duodenum* receives bile from the liver and gallbladder and enzymes from the pancreas. Bile breaks down fats so that digestive juices can act on them. The pancreatic enzymes—amylase, lipase, and trypsin—continue digestion begun in the stomach by acting on chyme to break down fat, protein, and carbohydrate.

Figure 12–4 Tissue Layers of the Stomach

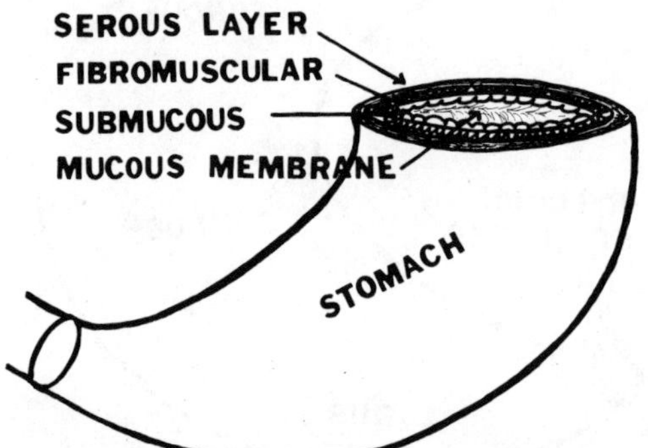

Figure 12–5 The Small Intestine

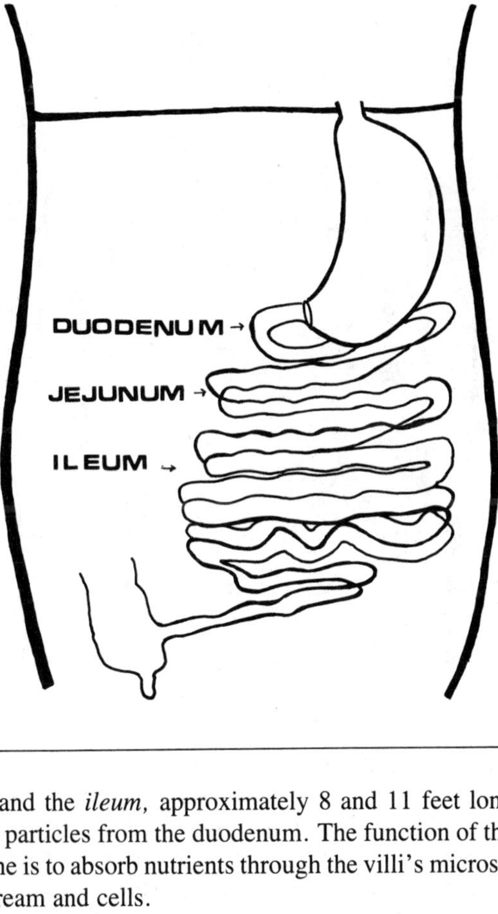

The *jejunum* and the *ileum,* approximately 8 and 11 feet long, respectively, receive digested particles from the duodenum. The function of these two parts of the small intestine is to absorb nutrients through the villi's microscopic capillaries into the bloodstream and cells.

The small intestine is 20 feet long; it is called small because it is smaller in diameter than the large intestine.[2]

LARGE INTESTINE

The four parts of the 5-foot-long large intestine, extending from the ileum to the anus, are (1) the cecum, (2) the colon, (3) the sigmoid colon, and (4) the rectum (Figure 12–6). The cecum connects the colon to the ileocecal sphincter. The three sections of the colon are the ascending, transverse, and descending colons. The descending colon is connected to the sigmoid colon, which terminates with the rectum and the anus.[3]

Figure 12–6 The Large Intestine

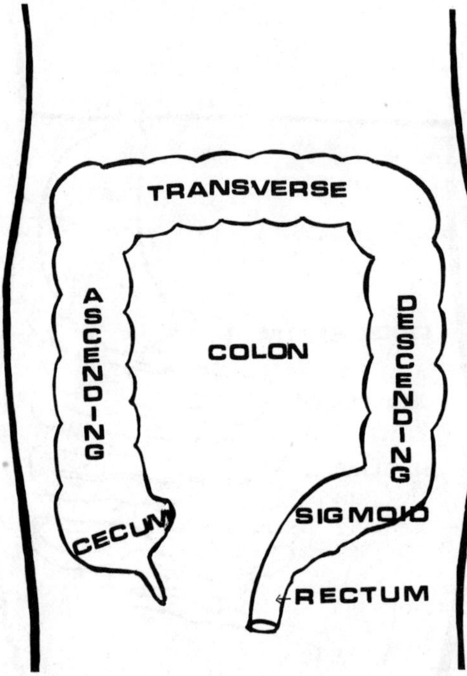

The functions of the large intestine are to store waste products for defecation and to regulate the balance of water in the body. The moving along of waste products in the maintenance of water balance is performed by peristalsis. Peristalsis is the rhythmic movement of the musculature that moves waste materials through the intestines. When peristalsis is decreased, waste material is not moved through the large intestines and constipation occurs.

LIVER AND GALLBLADDER

The liver and gallbladder, through the manufacture, storage, and dispensing of bile, play an important part in digestion.

The liver is located in the right upper quadrant of the abdomen; the gallbladder is conveniently located under the cleft of the liver. They are connected by a system of ducts. Figure 12–7 shows the position of the liver, the gallbladder, and the ducts.

The liver functions in digestion through the manufacture of a thick, green fluid called bile, which is stored in the gallbladder. Bile reaching the gallbladder by way

Figure 12–7 The Liver, Gallbladder, and Ducts

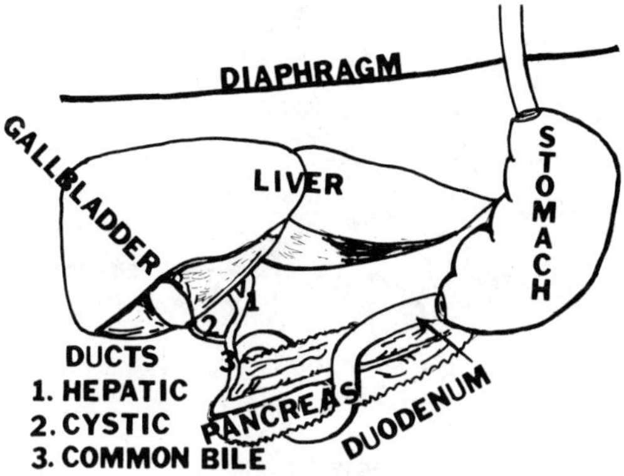

of a system of ducts contains cholesterol, bile acids, and pigments, one of which is bilirubin. Bilirubin, a waste product from red blood cells that are destroyed in the liver, is combined with bile in the liver, stored in the gallbladder, dispensed to the duodenum in the bile, and finally leaves the body through defecation with other feces. The function of bile is to emulsify fats in the duodenum so that they can be broken down by pancreatic enzymes.

PANCREAS

The head of the pancreas, as seen in Figure 12–7, lies next to the middle of the duodenum. The primary function of the pancreas is to manufacture pancreatic juice, which aids in digestion, and insulin, a hormone that maintains the sugar balance in the body.

PERITONEUM

The peritoneum is the serous membrane lining the abdominal cavity. The parietal layer, the outermost portion of the membrane, lines the abdominal wall. The visceral layer, the innermost portion of membrane, covers the abdominal organs and holds them in place. Between the parietal and visceral layers of peritoneum is the abdominal cavity. Within the abdominal cavity are two more complex layers of peritoneum: folds of greater and lesser omentum, which cover the organs to protect them. The mesentery, the last fold of peritoneum, attaches the intestines to the posterior aspect of the abdominal wall to support and hold them in place. Figure 12–8 shows the layers of peritoneum.

Figure 12–8 The Layers of Peritoneum

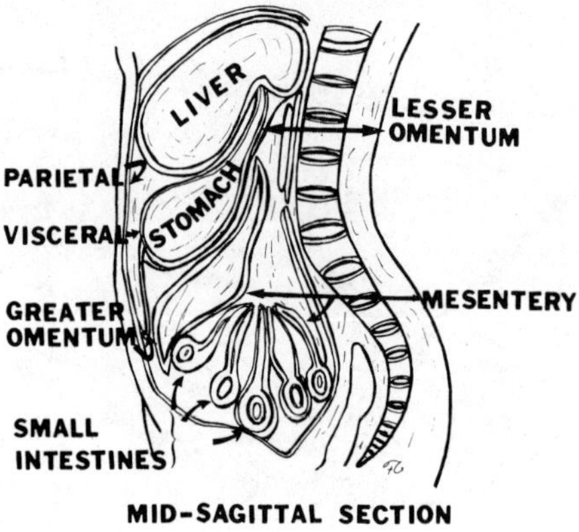

CONGENITAL DEFECTS OF THE DIGESTIVE SYSTEM

External congenital defects are easily recognizable at birth, but defects occurring to internal organs either in formation or in their relationship to other organs are often undetectable.

Cleft Lip and Palate

Cleft lip and palate may occur one without the other; however, the cleft lip, often associated with the cleft palate, is found in one of every 1,000 births.[4]

The cleft lip, lateral or bilateral, is a congenital vertical fissure of the upper lip. The cleft palate is a fissure in the roof of the mouth. The mouth with a cleft palate lacks separation between the nasal and oral cavities. An infant with a cleft lip or a cleft palate or both has difficulty eating and breathing. Later, during childhood, speech is difficult. The newborn with cleft lip and palate requires tube feeding to keep him or her from aspirating milk into the lungs. Plastic repair needs to be done as soon as possible. Figure 12–9 shows a baby with cleft lip and palate.

Depending on the extent of the defect, the plastic repair of the cleft lip is performed when the child is approximately three to four months old and weighs 12 to 15 pounds. Cheilorrhaphy is the plastic repair of a cleft lip in which the two edges of the lip are sutured together. Figure 12–10 illustrates a cheilorrhaphy performed for cleft lip.

The plastic repair of the cleft lip is followed with reconstruction of the cleft palate (palatoplasty) when the child is 18 months old, just before the time when he or she begins to speak (Figure 12–11).

Figure 12–9 Baby with Cleft Lip and Palate

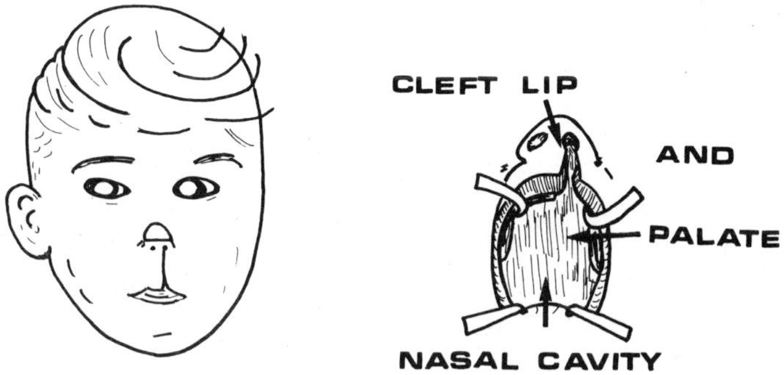

Figure 12–10 Cheilorrhaphy

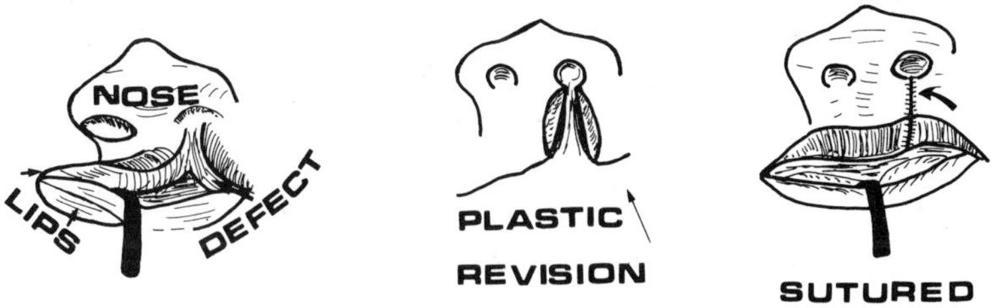

Figure 12–11 Palatoplasty

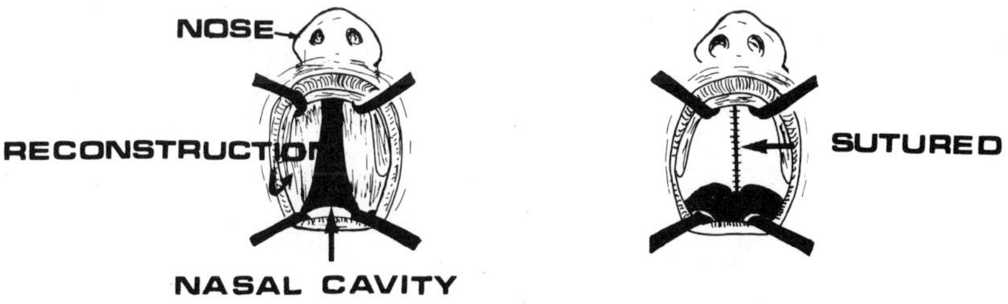

Esophageal Atresia

Early in preembryonic development the esophagus and trachea are one tube. During embryonic development a wall, or septum, forms, dividing the tube into two. Atresia of the esophagus is a congenital closure of the esophagus somewhere along the tube owing to nondevelopment. Figure 12–12 shows esophageal atresia.

Symptoms in the newborn are regurgitation, owing to the inability of food and liquid to reach the stomach, and constant weight loss. Diagnostic procedures for verification of esophageal atresia include an upper gastrointestinal radiographic series.

Surgery must be performed on the newborn as soon as possible, carrying out an end-to-end esophageal anastomosis or, in other words, sewing together the two ends. The procedure (esophagoesophagostomy) is shown in Figure 12–13.

Figure 12–12 Esophageal Atresia

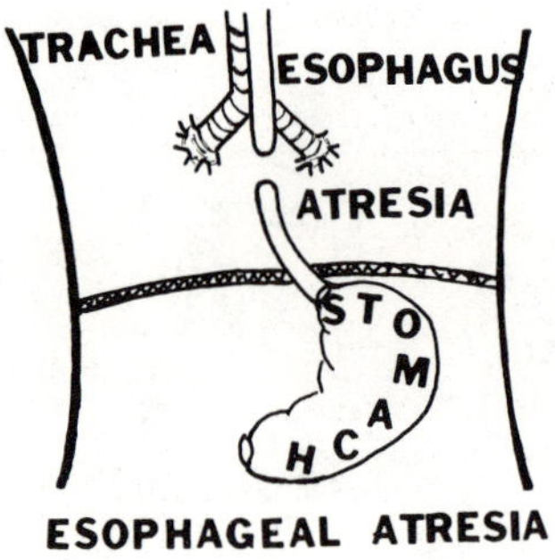

Figure 12–13 Esophagoesophagostomy

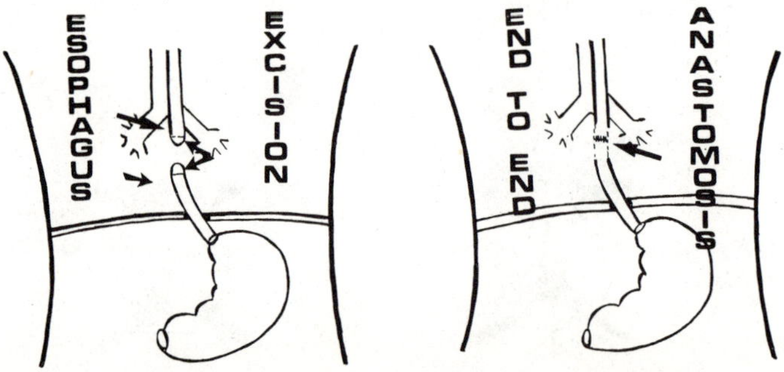

Tracheoesophageal Fistula

A congenital anomaly often found with atresia is tracheoesophageal fistula. A fistula is an abnormal passageway between two hollow organs, in this case the trachea and the esophagus. The fistula may occur either in the upper or lower end or middle of the esophagus or the entire esophagus may be connected to the trachea. Figure 12–14 shows the various types of fistulae that may occur.

Symptoms of tracheoesophageal fistula appearing shortly after birth are vomiting, choking spells, and cyanosis at feeding. The infant is unable to regain birth weight. Colic results when air enters the abdomen. Danger occurs when the infant aspirates milk into the lungs and pneumonia develops. Results from upper gastrointestinal radiographic series are diagnostic and surgery is a must for survival.

A newborn with esophageal atresia and a tracheoesophageal fistula must have immediate surgery (tracheoesophageal fistulectomy) for excision of the fistula; an additional procedure (esophagoesophagostomy) is necessary to attach the two ends of the esophagus by an end-to-end anastomosis. Figure 12–15 shows a tracheoesophageal fistulectomy and esophagoesophagostomy for tracheoesophageal fistula with esophageal stenosis.

Figure 12–14 Types of Fistulae

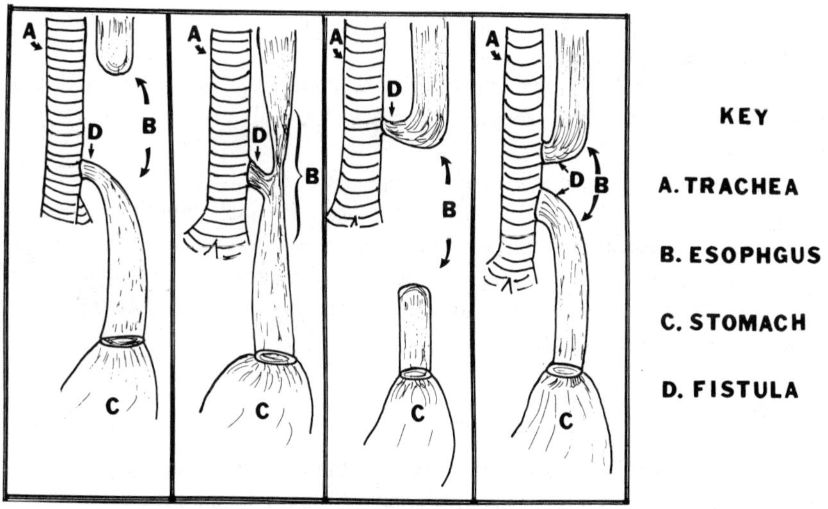

Figure 12–15 Tracheoesophageal Fistulectomy and Esophagoesophagostomy for Tracheoesophageal Fistula

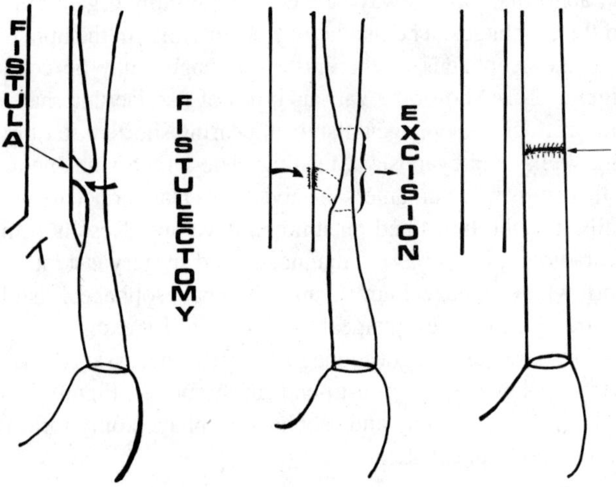

Esophageal Web

The laryngeal web is discussed in the congenital abnormalities section of Chapter 11, The Respiratory System. The esophageal web is a partial membranous stricture grown across the esophagus. It occurs in the lower half of the esophagus. Figure 12–16 shows an esophageal web.

Symptoms of esophageal web are consistent regurgitation with the inability of the newborn to regain birth weight. Upper gastrointestinal (GI) x-rays are diagnostic.

Esophagectomy for the excision of an esophageal web, stricture, or other lesion is performed with excision of the diseased esophagus, including the lesion. An esophagoesophagostomy is then performed with an end-to-end anastomosis of the esophagus. A small web or lesion may require only repair by esophagoplasty with graft. An esophagectomy and esophagoesophagostomy for removal of an esophageal web, stricture, or lesion are shown in Figure 12–17.

Stenosis

Congenital stenosis, a partial narrowing of the esophagus, may occur at any level (Figure 12–18). Surgery may or may not be required. An artificial opening in the esophagus may be created by dilating the esophagus.

Figure 12–16 Esophageal Web

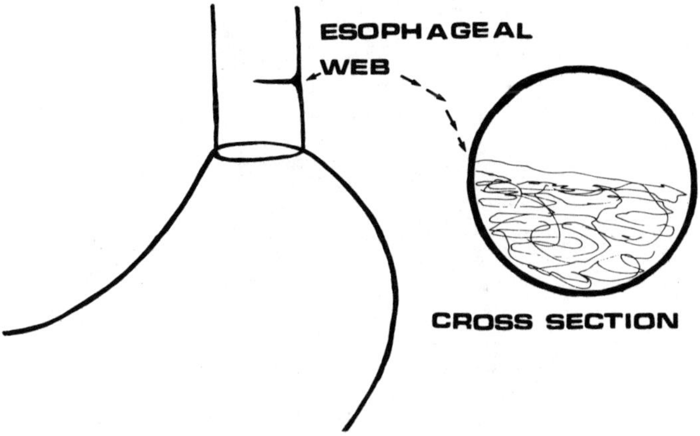

Figure 12–17 Esophagectomy and Esophagoesophagostomy for Esophageal Web

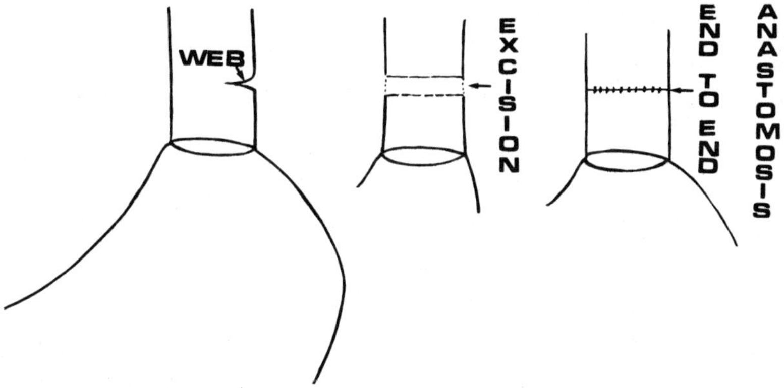

Hernia

A hernia is the abnormal protrusion of an organ through an opening.

A *diaphragmatic hernia* is the protrusion of abdominal organs or intestines through a congenital defect in the diaphragm. Physical examination reveals the absence of organs in the abdominal cavity. Surgery is necessary to replace the organs in the abdominal cavity.

Figure 12–18 Stenosis of the Esophagus

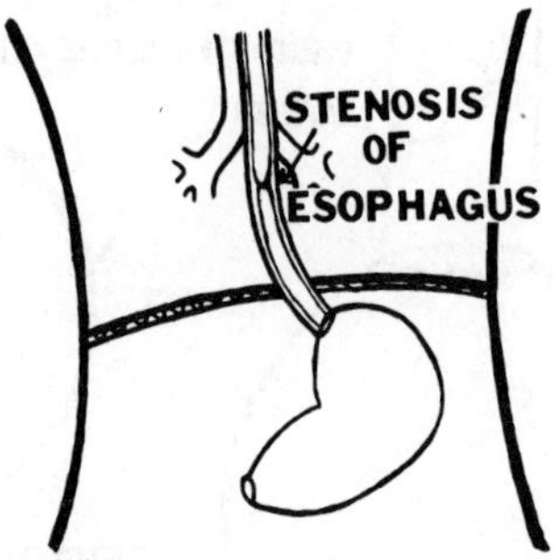

A *hiatus hernia* is the protrusion of part of the stomach through the esophageal hiatus (opening) in the diaphragm when the infant or adult is in a horizontal position. Symptoms in the infant are regurgitation, weight loss, and colic. Upper GI x-rays are diagnostic. Elevation of the upper part of the body and soft foods may be recommended. According to the severity of the abnormality, surgery may or may not be required. Surgical correction requires the replacement of the displaced viscera into the abdominal cavity and surgical repair of the defect. Figure 12–19 shows diaphragmatic and hiatal hernias; Figure 12–20 shows a diaphragmatic/hiatus hernia repair.

Figure 12–19 A Diaphragmatic and a Hiatal Hernia

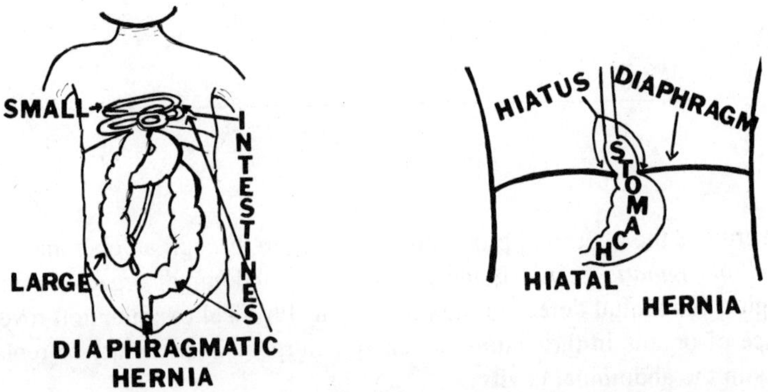

Figure 12–20 Hernia Repair

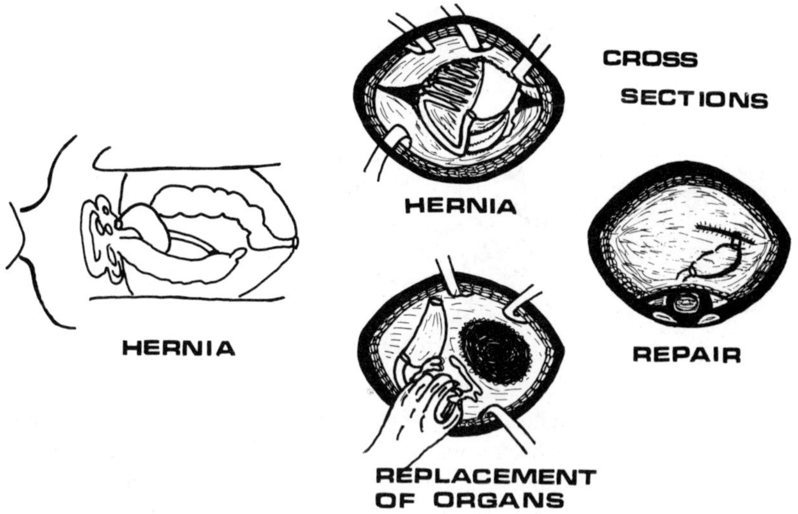

Chalasia

Chalasia is weakness or relaxation of the cardiac sphincter so that food flows through the esophagus to the stomach and gastric juices and acids regurgitate. The sphincter fails to close after food enters the stomach. This is often the cause of vomiting in infants.

Symptoms are regurgitation and weight loss. Growth is inhibited. Upper GI x-rays are diagnostic. Surgical repair of the cardiac sphincter may be indicated.

Agastria

Agastria is the congenital absence of the stomach. This condition may require surgery. If the esophagus and duodenum are not attached, an end-to-end anastomosis will be necessary. However, if the esophagus and duodenum are attached, the duodenum may take on the function of the stomach.

Hypertrophic Pyloric Stenosis

Hypertrophy is an abnormal enlargement of an organ or part owing to increase in cell size. Pyloric stenosis is the narrowing of the pylorus (lower end of the stomach) owing to enlargement or overgrowth of the pyloric muscle of the valve, which creates an obstruction (Figure 12–21).

Figure 12–21 Hypertrophic Pyloric Stenosis

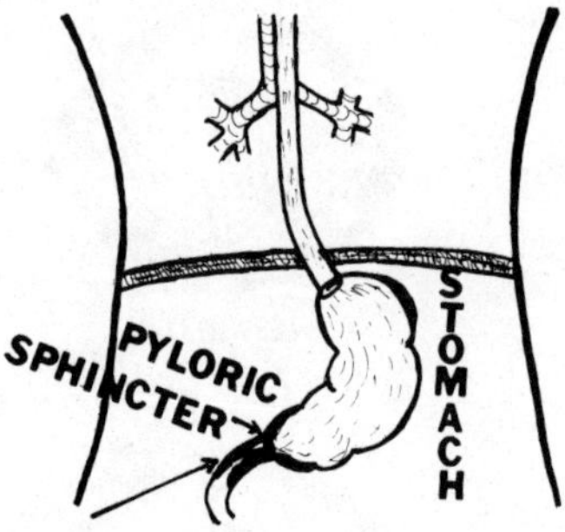

Incidence of pyloric stenosis is 3:1,000 infants, with a 1:4 ratio of females to males.[5] In infants, onset occurs with projectile vomiting and weight loss. On physical examination a palpable hard mass may be found in the right epigastrium. GI x-ray series are diagnostic. Treatment of choice is the surgical excision of the pylorus.

Diverticulosis

A diverticulum is a pouch or sac of mucous membrane caused by a defect in the muscular coat of the organ. Gastric diverticulum is found on the posterior wall of the stomach (Figure 12–22). It is not known at which stage of fetal development this defect occurs. All that can be said is that on x-ray, diverticula have been observed in the stomachs of fetuses.

Figure 12–22 Gastric Diverticulosis

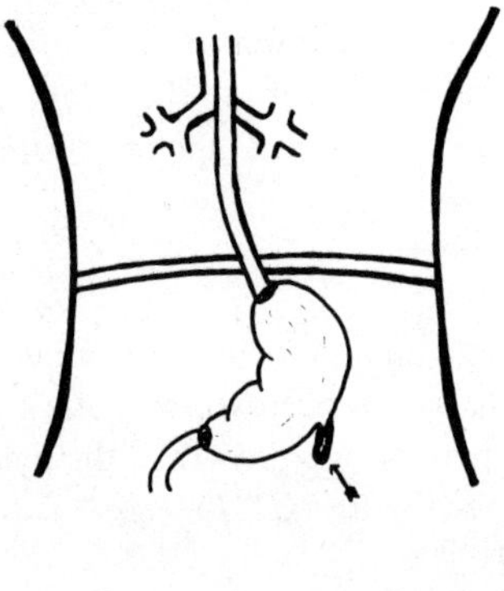

Gastric diverticula are generally asymptomatic; however, in some cases the stomach contents are caught in a diverticulum, causing discomfort. Inflammation and infection may also occur.

Biliary Atresia

Biliary atresia is hypoplasia of the bile ducts owing to impaired fetal development (Figure 12–23). Symptoms are jaundice appearing two to three weeks after birth, clay-colored stools, and dark urine. Urinalysis reveals positive bilirubin in the urine. Blood tests show increased alkaline phosphatase and prolonged bleeding and clotting time and prothrombin time.

If symptoms persist and a liver transplant in not performed, prognosis is poor.[6]

Atresia of Small Intestine

Atresia may occur in many parts of the body. Generally, it is a congenital absence or complete closure of a normal body orifice. Partial closure of a normal body orifice is called stenosis.

Symptoms of small-bowel atresia in the newborn are vomiting, loss of weight, and lack of stool. Surgery is required, consisting of the excision of the atresia with an end-to-end anastomosis of the two ends of the small bowel. Figure 12–24 shows atresia of the small intestine.

Omphalocele

At birth, sometimes the intestines protrude through the umbilicus owing to improper embryonic development. The protruding intestines are generally cov-

Figure 12–23 Biliary Atresia

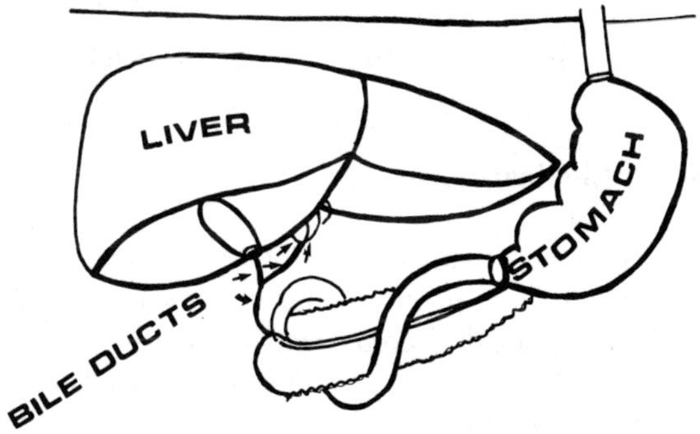

Figure 12–24 Atresia of the Small Intestine

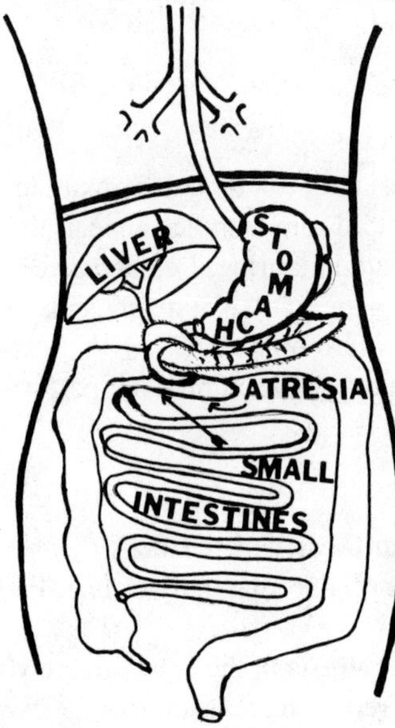

ered with a thin membrane, but they may not be covered at all. This is called an omphalocele (Figure 12–25). Precaution must be taken in the delivery room to keep the exposed viscera sterile. Surgery is urgent.

Umbilical Hernia

The umbilicus is the area to which the umbilical cord is attached in the fetus. An umbilical hernia is a protrusion of part of the intestines at the umbilicus; unlike the omphalocele, the protrusion and defect are covered with skin.

Repair of an umbilical hernia consists in reconstructing the abdominal wall by closing the defect in layers, beginning with the fascia through to the subcutaneous tissue.

Direct and Indirect Inguinal Hernia

The *direct inguinal hernia* is the bulging of peritoneum through an acquired weakness in the abdominal wall in the area between the rectus abdominis muscle and the inguinal ligament in the groin area. The peritoneal sac may contain abdominal viscera. The direct hernia is generally acquired in later life by straining or heavy lifting and is corrected by surgery.

Figure 12–25 Omphalocele

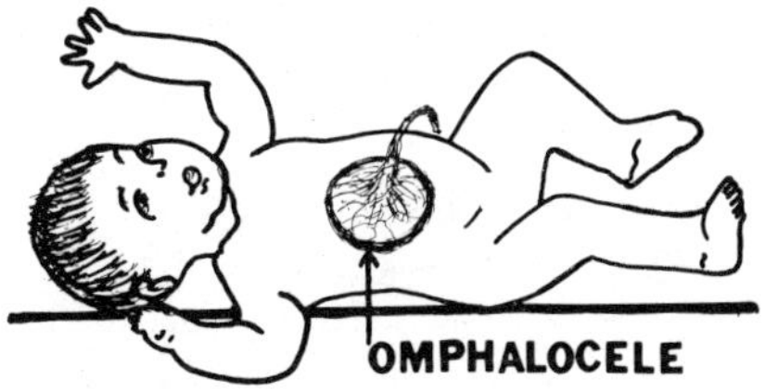

The *indirect inguinal hernia* is the protrusion of the peritoneal sac through a defect in the internal inguinal ring, from which it passes down along the spermatic cord in the inguinal canal. The peritoneal sac may also contain abdominal viscera. This defect is most common in premature male infants. Surgery is warranted when the baby has reached approximately five pounds in weight.

Hernias are surgically classified as reducible or irreducible. In reducible hernias the contents of the sac can be returned to the normal intra-abdominal site; whereas in irreducible hernias the contents of the sac are trapped (incarcerated). Patients with incarcerated hernias show signs of intestinal obstruction characterized by nausea, vomiting, and abdominal distention. The risk presented by incarceration is loss of blood supply to the area and eventually necrosis (strangulation) of the intestines. Emergency surgery is warranted.

Meckel's Diverticulum

Meckel's diverticulum is a sac or pouch occurring normally and found in the ileum near the cecum (Figure 12–26). It is thought to be a remnant of fetal structure that, before birth, connects the sac with the embryo's intestinal cavity. Generally, it is asymptomatic in the infant but may become a problem in the adult.

The patient complains of nausea and vomiting with vague abdominal pain; there may be rebound tenderness from left abdomen to right inguinal region. Signs and symptoms may mimic those of acute appendicitis. The intestinal obstruction resulting from Meckel's diverticulitis cannot be differentiated from appendicitis or other processes except through exploratory surgery.[7]

Meconium Ileus

Meconium ileus is an intestinal obstruction experienced by the newborn owing to the ileum being filled with a gray, sticky, thick substance called meconium.

Figure 12–26 Meckel's Diverticula

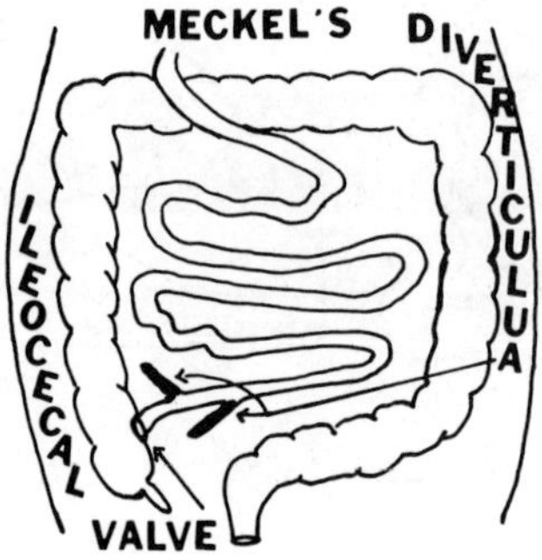

Meconium ileus has been found to occur in approximately 15 percent of the infants later diagnosed as having cystic fibrosis of the pancreas or Hirschsprung's disease.

Symptoms are vomiting and loss of weight. On examination, the spongy ileum can be palpated. The presence of undigested albumin in the meconium and GI x-ray series confirm the diagnosis. Enemas for relief of the obstruction may be tried before surgical intervention.[8]

Hirschsprung's Disease (Congenital Megacolon)

Hirschsprung's disease is the enlargement of the colon owing to the absence of ganglionic cells of the myenteric plexus of Auerbach. The nerves of the small intestines branch from the plexus of sympathetic nerves to the myenteric plexus of Auerbach. From the plexus of Auerbach, the nerves are distributed to the muscular coat of the intestines. The lack of ganglionic cells, which are parasympathetic innervators, results in the lack of peristalsis in the portion of the colon that is involved. Sympathetic overactivity in the area that is aganglionic results in mechanical obstruction and hypertrophy of the colon owing to the work required to move fecal material through the colon. Generally, the rectum, anus, and sigmoid colon are involved, with parts of the colon skipped.

Symptoms are vomiting, abdominal distention, and lack of peristalsis in the sigmoid area of the colon. GI x-ray series is diagnostic. Biopsy of the rectal wall revealing the absence of ganglia confirms the diagnosis. Because of the risk of obstruction, surgery is indicated.

There are several types of surgery that can be performed. Swenson's resection of the entire aganglionic portion of the colon by an abdominoperineal pull-through technique with an anastomosis at the anus is one method. Two modifications of the

Swenson's resection—the Duhamel's technique and the Soave procedure—have gained favor.

In the Soave procedure, the aganglionic rectal musculature is left in place, the rectal mucosa is removed, and the normal peristaltic ganglionic segment is brought down through the rectal muscular cuff. This procedure is completed through the rectum.

In the Duhamel's operation, the ganglionic proximal colon is pulled through posterior to the aganglionic rectum; the ganglionic and aganglionic are connected by a side-to-side anastomosis of the small bowel and colon respectively. Therefore, the small bowel provides peristalsis and the colon provides absorptive surface.

Anastomosis

The three types of anastomosis are end-to-end, end-to-side, and side-to-side. The Swenson's procedure demonstrates end-to-end anastomosis; the Duhamel's procedure illustrates the side-to-side anastomosis; and, the end-to-side anastomosis will be shown in the area of gastric resections. Figure 12–27 illustrates the three types of anastomoses.

Imperforate Anus

Imperforate anus is the congenital absence of the rectal opening. It is diagnosed by inspection of the perineum. The height of the rectal pouch that has not

---

Figure 12–27 Types of Anastomoses

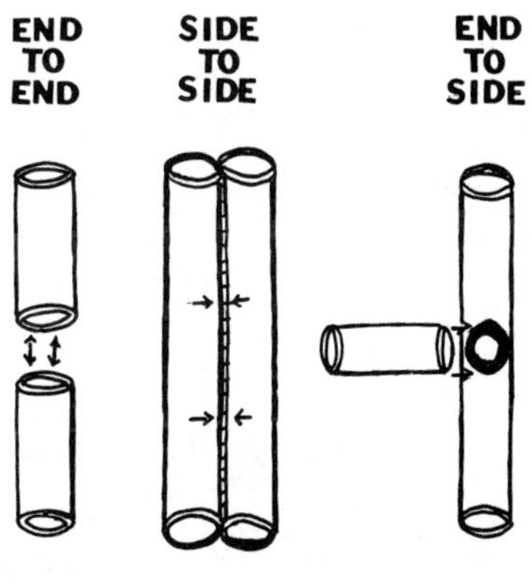

descended is determined by x-ray. Some type of fistula is generally found. This defect can be corrected by surgery.

A *rectovaginal fistula* in a female is an abnormal passageway between the rectum and the vagina (Figure 12–28). Symptoms are constipation and defecation through the vagina with recurrent vaginal infection. This defect may be found through rectovaginal inspection.

A *rectourethral fistula* in the male is an abnormal passageway between the rectum and the urethra (Figure 12–29). Defecation is impossible owing to the absence of the rectal orifice. This defect is discovered on examination of the newborn.

A *rectovesical fistula* is the presence of an abnormal opening between the rectum and the bladder (Figure 12–30). Defecation is impossible owing to the absence of the rectal orifice.

A *rectoperitoneal fistula* is an abnormal opening between the rectum and peritoneum (Figure 12–31). Symptoms are abdominal distention and bleeding with defecation. Examination of the newborn reveals the absence of the rectal orifice. Imperforate anus is repaired through establishing colorectoanal continuity through the external sphincter and closing the fistulas.

Figure 12–28 Rectovaginal Fistula

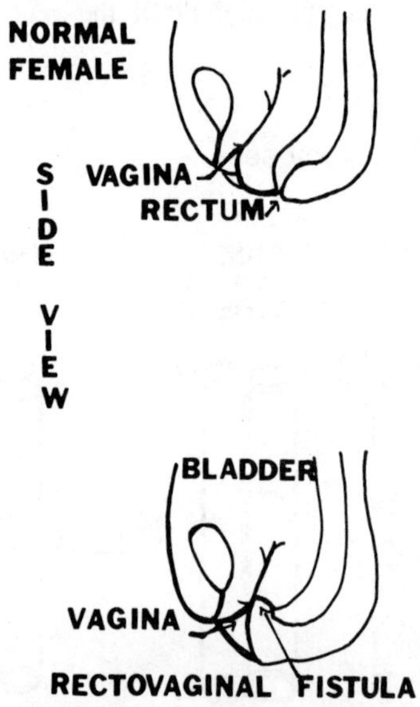

Figure 12–29 Rectourethral Fistula

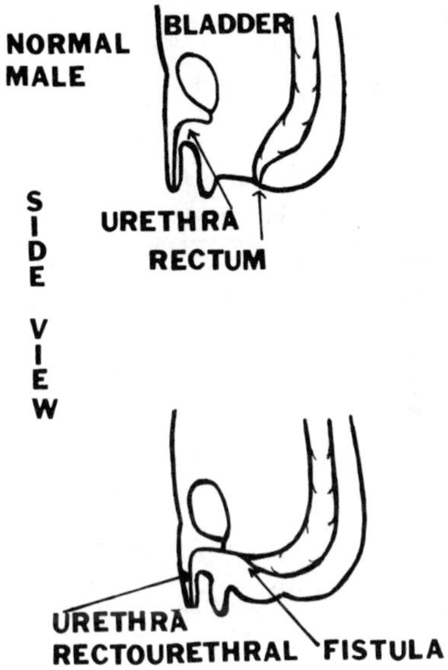

Figure 12–30 Rectovesical Fistula

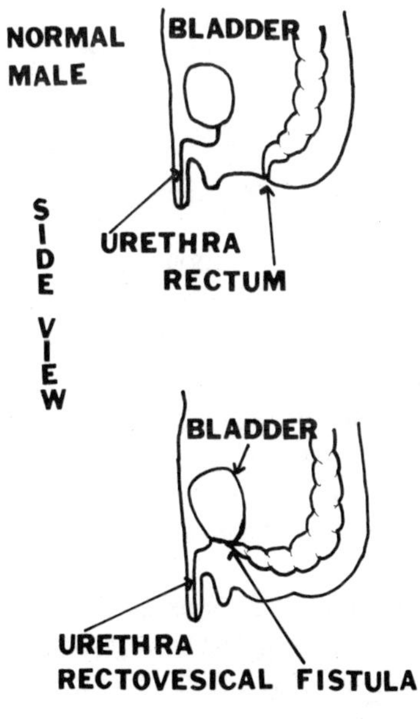

Figure 12–31 Rectoperitoneal Fistula

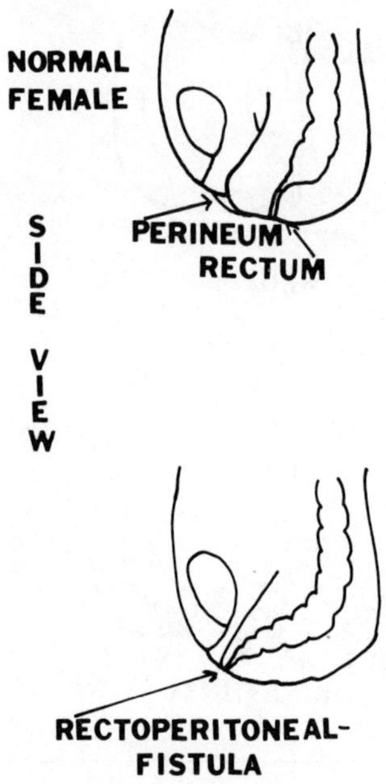

ACQUIRED DEFECTS AND DISORDERS OF THE DIGESTIVE SYSTEM

Esophagitis

Esophagitis, or inflammation of the esophagus, may result from many causes, for example, from ingestion of chemicals such as lye, from the presence of a foreign body such as a chicken bone, and from irritation from smoking.

The patient complains of substernal burning pain, difficulty in swallowing, esophageal spasm, and vomiting. Esophagoscopy may reveal mucosal hyperemia, tissue édema, and superficial ulceration. Prognosis depends on the cause and duration of esophagitis. Treatment depends on the extent of injury to the esophageal mucosa. Stenosis and fibrosis may be so severe that the esophagus may need to be dilated periodically.

Peptic esophagitis is a common disorder of the esophagus owing to the regurgitation of gastric secretions from the stomach into the esophagus. Such regurgitation may be caused by a defective cardiac orifice that does not close properly or by a defect in which there is intussusception of the gastric mucosa through the cardiac valve. Regurgitation of stomach acids may result in esophageal ulcers. Symptoms are heartburn shortly after eating, increased pressure in the regional area, pain on swallowing, and dysphagia. Upper GI x-ray series with fluoroscopy is diagnostic.

Chronic esophagitis is inflammation of the esophagus occurring over a long period. After the acute and recurrent phases, fibrosis, or scar tissue, may form. Chronic inflammation occurs owing to stagnation of food particles in the fibrotic area of the esophagus. Symptoms are dysphagia and a burning sensation in the esophagus, with sour eructation. Upper GI x-ray series with fluoroscopy is necessary for diagnosis.

Cardiospasm (Achalasia)

Chalasia, the relaxation of a bodily opening, such as the cardiac sphincter, is discussed earlier in this chapter. Achalasia is the general term used to describe the failure of smooth muscle fibers of the digestive system to relax at any point in the system where one organ joins another.

Cardiospasm is not a heart disease; it is the failure of the esophageal muscles at the cardiac sphincter to relax. The cardiac sphincter is located at the esophagogastric junction. Failure of the esophageal muscles to relax results in accumulation of food in the esophagus; the retention of food in the esophagus dilates the esophagus. Over a period of time the esophagus becomes enlarged. There is also danger of pneumonia owing to aspiration of food. Although a definitive cause is unknown, anxiety and tension may aggravate the condition.

The patient complains of dysphagia and a feeling of fullness in the sternal region, along with the tendency to choke or vomit. Any of the foregoing may be precipitated by anxiety and emotional tension.

Diagnosis may be confirmed by an upper gastrointestinal series of x-rays with fluoroscopy. Initial treatment consists of eating a low-bulk diet and acquiring slow eating habits. Surgery may be warranted. Surgical correction (Heller's cardiomyotomy) is a myotomy of the esophagogastric junction to correct the obstruction resulting from cardiospasm.

Esophageal Diverticulum

An esophageal diverticulum is a defect owing to infection or pressure, forming a progressive outpouching in the wall of the esophagus. The most common type is found in the elderly, in the upper end of the esophagus, between the transverse fibers of the cricopharyngeus muscle and the oblique fibers of the inferior constrictor muscle of the pharynx.

Symptoms are dysphagia, regurgitation, and noisy swallowing. Aspiration pneumonia may occur from swallowing when supine. Diagnosis may be confirmed with an upper GI series of x-rays, including fluoroscopy. Treatment consists of eating a soft diet and acquiring slow eating habits. Large diverticula may require excision.

Esophageal Varices

Varices are enlarged and twisted veins, arteries, or lymphatic vessels. Esophageal varices are enlarged and tortuous veins that anastomose with tributaries of the portal vein in the lower esophagus owing to portal hypertension in cirrhosis of the liver. Pressure builds up in the veins, which causes them to enlarge and become twisted. Sometimes the veins rupture, hemorrhage, and require emergency treatment. Splenomegaly often accompanies esophageal varices.

Symptoms are hematemesis of bright red blood, melena in the stool, and, sometimes, splenomegaly. Condition is improved through treatment of portal hypertension in cirrhosis of the liver.

Blood transfusion and vitamin K are supportive measures used in the treatment of bleeding esophageal varices. Measures to stop the bleeding consist of gastric ice water lavage and administration of vasopressin in 5% dextrose in water intravenously over one-half hour. If bleeding continues, Sengstaken-Blakemore intubation may be used. This procedure entails the insertion of a balloon catheter into the stomach and esophagus. The pressure of the inflated balloon on the varices may stop the bleeding.

Portacaval shunt is preferable when all other treatment fails to stop bleeding.[9] The objective of this operation is to reduce portal hypertension, which has been increased by obstruction to the flow of blood from the portal vein to the liver, resulting from cirrhosis, hepatitis, or thrombosis. Increased portal hypertension exacerbates venous distention and dilatation in the esophagus and risks hemorrhage. Figure 12–32 shows the anastomosis of the vena cava and the portal vein.

Foreign Body in the Esophagus

A foreign object wedged in the esophagus is painful and dangerous. It is painful because rough edges of an object lodged in the esophagus irritate the mucosa. It is dangerous because of the possibility that the foreign body will be passed through the esophagus to the stomach.

Symptoms may be gasping for breath and choking. Esophagoscopy may be necessary for removal of the foreign body. If the foreign object passes into the stomach, surgery may be necessary.

Figure 12–32 Anastomosis of the Vena Cava and the Portal Vein

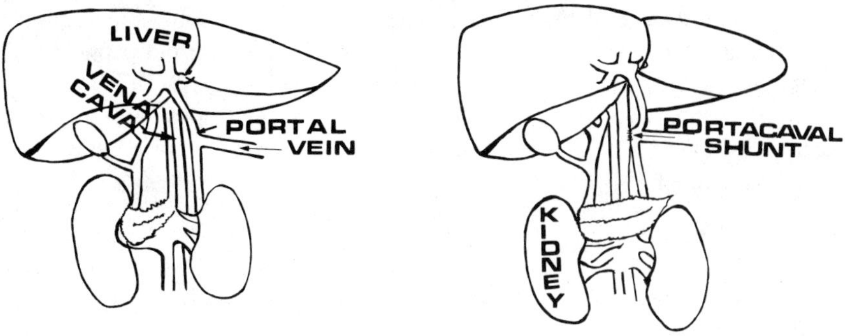

Gastritis

Acute Gastritis

Acute gastritis is a brief, severe occurrence of inflammation of the inner lining of the stomach. Causes include contaminated foods, bacterial or viral infections, ingestion of medicine, and excessive alcohol.

Symptoms are severe and sometimes prolonged vomiting, nausea, fever, discomfort in the epigastric region of the abdomen, and anorexia.

In a mild attack, diagnosis is often obscure. However, in severe attacks, hematemesis may occur, and melena may be found in the stool on laboratory examination. Bacterial infection requires culture and sensitivity testing in order to identify the bacteria and prescribe proper antibiotics.

Treatment is specific to the type of infection. Nothing is given by mouth until the acute phase has subsided (pain and nausea). Diet progresses from liquids to soft food as tolerated. Sedatives, phenothiazine tranquilizers, or an opiate (opium-derivative drug) may be prescribed as indicated. Symptoms generally subside within seven days.

Chronic Gastritis

Gastritis becomes chronic when it recurs frequently or persists over a long period. The cause of chronic gastritis is often unknown, but it has been known to exist in people with patterns of ingestion of alcohol, drugs, tobacco, and coffee. Other conditions associated with chronic gastritis are cancer, pernicious anemia, diabetes mellitus, and chronic iron deficiency.

Chronic gastritis is often asymptomatic. However, symptoms may be anorexia, feeling of fullness in epigastrium, heartburn, nausea, and vomiting.

Physical findings on examination and laboratory findings are often not remarkable. Laboratory studies may show macrocytic anemia. Gastric analysis may show achlorhydria (absence of hydrochloric acid). X-ray findings may show gastric folds that are thin or absent. Differential diagnoses must rule out peptic ulcer, carcinoma, cholecystitis, and pancreatic disease.

Treatment consists of a peptic ulcer diet and recommendations to refrain from the use of alcohol, salicylates, and caffeine. A mild tranquilizer may give symptomatic relief.

Toxic Gastritis

Toxic gastritis is severe inflammation of the stomach with injury to the mucosa owing to ingestion of poison or a corrosive agent.

Symptoms are severe epigastric pain with vomiting of blood-stained material and hematemesis, resulting from the destruction of the gastric mucosa. Preferred treatment is gastric lavage and administration of antitoxin reagent as prescribed by a poison control center.

Gastric Retention

When the normal functioning stomach empties, the cardiac sphincter opens, allowing bolus to pass from the esophagus to the stomach; the stomach muscles contract in rhythm as the bolus is reduced to chyme. The pyloric sphincter opens, allowing the chyme to empty into the duodenum for further digestion.

Gastric retention occurs when food does not move through the stomach owing to such diseases as peptic ulcer, carcinoma, and diabetic gastric atony and to drugs.

The patient complains of a feeling of fullness accompanied by anorexia and nausea. Abdominal distention results. The primary cause of the symptoms needs to be diagnosed through x-rays and laboratory tests and treated accordingly. When no cause is found, gastric retention is called idiopathic.

Peptic Ulcer

Peptic ulcer, a general term for ulcers resulting from the action of the acid and pepsin on the mucosa, is found in the esophagogastric or gastroduodenal junctions or the stomach. Therefore, gastric, duodenal, and esophageal ulcers are peptic ulcers if their cause is gastric acid or pepsin.

The difference between an acute and chronic ulcer is measured by the degree of damage to the tissue. For example, in the case of an acute ulcer, the gastric juice has eroded the wall of the esophagus, stomach, or duodenum; in the chronic ulcer, gastric juices penetrate into the deeper muscular layers of tissue.

Gastric Ulcer

A gastric ulcer is a peptic ulcer of the stomach. Symptoms of gastric ulcer include burning stomach pain when the stomach is empty; the pain is relieved by eating, drinking milk, or taking an antacid.

Upper GI x-ray series including fluoroscopy may be used to diagnose gastric ulcer. Analysis of gastric secretions may also be significant in diagnosis.

Gastric ulcer may be treated conservatively with dietary counseling and drugs. If massive hemorrhage occurs, blood transfusions and immediate surgery are required. A gastrectomy—total, subtotal, or hemigastrectomy—is performed for gastric ulcers or carcinoma. Figure 12–33 shows a total gastrectomy.

A Billroth I procedure (Figure 12–34) is a subtotal or partial resection of the stomach; an anastomosis is established between the stomach and duodenum.

Duodenal Ulcer

The cause of a duodenal peptic ulcer is gastric juice that penetrates the mucosal lining of the duodenum at the gastroduodenal junction. Duodenal ulcers occur predominantly in males, with a ratio of 4:1, males to females. The average age of people with duodenal ulcers is 33 years. A duodenal ulcer often occurs in a person who is under tension and stress.

The patient describes epigastric pain as aching, gnawing, burning, and cramping, which has a pattern of occurring at night or when the stomach is empty.

Laboratory blood analysis may reveal hypochromic anemia; examination of the stool may show the presence of occult blood. GI x-ray series may not always be diagnostic because of the deformity of the duodenal bulb, which may obscure the

Figure 12–33 Total Gastrectomy

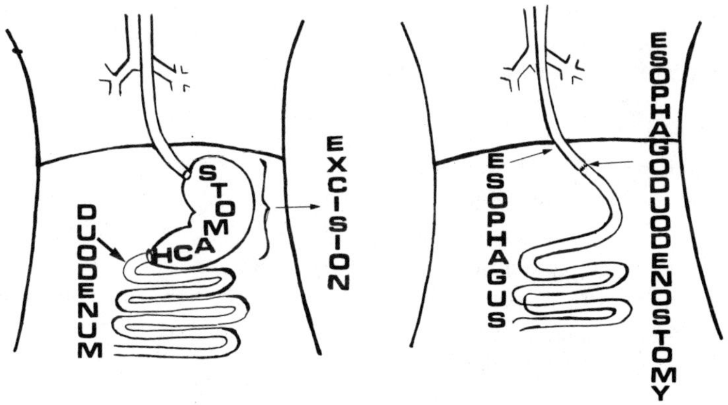

Figure 12–34 Billroth I Procedure

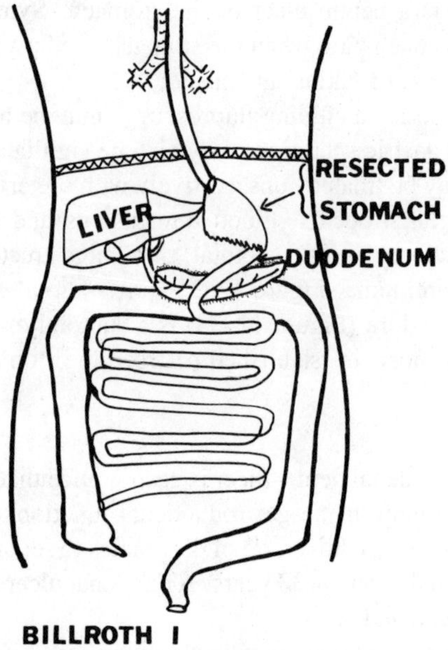

ulcer. Endoscopy may be valuable when radiology examination fails to diagnose the duodenal ulcer.

Conservative treatment may be indicated with dietary counseling or drugs. A patient with an acute duodenal ulcer and indications of hemorrhage may require surgery.

A Billroth II procedure (Figure 12–35) is the resection of the distal part of the stomach; an anastomosis is established between the stomach and jejunum.

Postgastrectomy Syndrome (Dumping Syndrome)

Under normal anatomical function the passage of food from the stomach to the duodenum is regulated. However, after a subtotal gastrectomy the control of food passing through the stomach to the duodenum is uncontrolled so that food passes too rapidly into the duodenum, causing the blood sugar to reach hyperglycemic levels owing to the rapid absorption of glucose.

Symptoms include weakness, nausea, pallor, palpitation, and, sometimes, hot flashes. These symptoms occur between 15 and 20 minutes after meals.[10]

Treatment includes low-carbohydrate and high-protein diet, frequent eating of small amounts, and rest after meals.

Figure 12–35 Billroth II Procedure

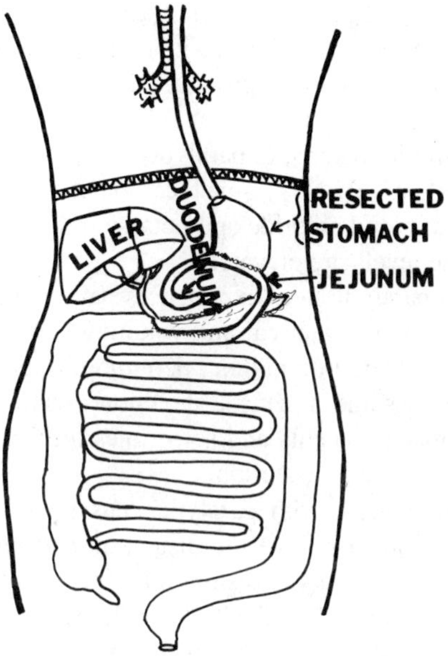

BILLROTH II

Ileus

Ileus is an intestinal obstruction. The two kinds of ileus are adynamic and dynamic.

Adynamic paralytic ileus is characterized by inhibition of bowel motility (peristalsis), which may be associated with serious diseases or injuries but most often occurs temporarily after anesthesia and abdominal surgery.

Dynamic mechanical ileus is an intestinal obstruction from blockage by organic or mechanical objects, such as a foreign body, worms, intussusception, and volvulus.

Differentiation between paralytic and mechanical ileus is important, since the patient with paralytic ileus is affected temporarily, whereas the patient with mechanical ileus generally requires emergency surgery.

In the early stages of paralytic ileus, bowel sounds are feeble; later there are no bowel sounds. However, in mechanical ileus, the bowel sounds are strong with a high pitch in the early stages of illness, gradually decreasing as the obstruction worsens.

X-rays are essential to confirm the diagnosis and distinguish between paralytic and mechanical ileus. Abdominal films taken in an upright position on a patient with paralytic ileus reveal gas–fluid levels; gaseous distention occurs uniformly in stomach, small bowel, and colon. In contrast, abdominal films on a patient with mechanical ileus reveal multiple gas–fluid levels; in an upright position, the distended bowel appears as a U on x-ray.

Comparing laboratory results, in paralytic ileus, blood chloride and potassium levels are decreased; pH, BUN, plasma bicarbonate, and hematocrit are elevated. In mechanical ileus, blood chloride and potassium levels are decreased; protein, amylase, and lipase levels are elevated.

The patient with paralytic ileus experiences pain in the upper abdomen that is mild, dull, but continuous; nausea; and vomiting. The patient with mechanical ileus experiences a sudden, intermittent, periumbilical pain. The peristaltic waves become strong and assume a reverse direction owing to the obstruction. The patient vomits stomach contents and sometimes fecal material and experiences constipation and abdominal distention.

Treatment of the patient with paralytic ileus is conservative, consisting of intubation with suction to relieve the distention and restriction of oral intake. Glucose is given intravenously to restore fluids and electrolytes. As bowel function returns, diet is increased gradually from fluids to solids. Generally, conservative treatment restores the patient to well-being.

Treatment of the patient with mechanical ileus is supportive, consisting of intubation with suction to relieve the distention, relief of vomiting, and prevention of aspiration. Small-bowel obstruction may be relieved in this manner. In addition, oral intake is restricted, with glucose administered intravenously to restore fluids and electrolytes. Antibiotic therapy (broad spectrum) should be given if strangulation of intestines is suspected. After supportive therapy, if fever and leukocytosis persist and blood is found in suctioned feces, emergency surgery is warranted. The procedure depends on the type of obstruction. An enteroenterostomy, the creation of a surgical communication between the intestines, may be performed to resolve a mechanical obstruction.

Intussusception and Volvulus

The prolapse of one part of the intestine into the lumen of the immediately adjoining part of the intestine is termed intussusception (Figure 12–36). *Ileocecal intussusception* occurs when the ileocecal valve prolapses into the cecum. *Ileocolic intussusception* occurs when the ileum prolapses through the ileocecal valve into the colon.

Volvulus is a twisting of a loop of the intestine, causing obstruction, infarction, and necrosis (Figure 12–37). Intestinal obstructions are often a predisposition to volvulus.

Figure 12–36 Intussusception

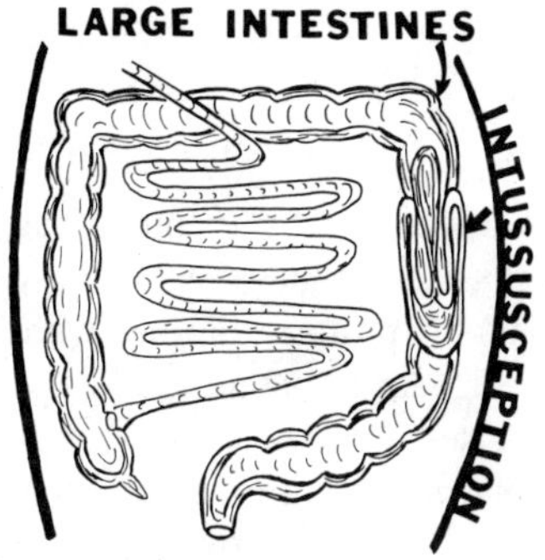

Figure 12–37 Volvulus

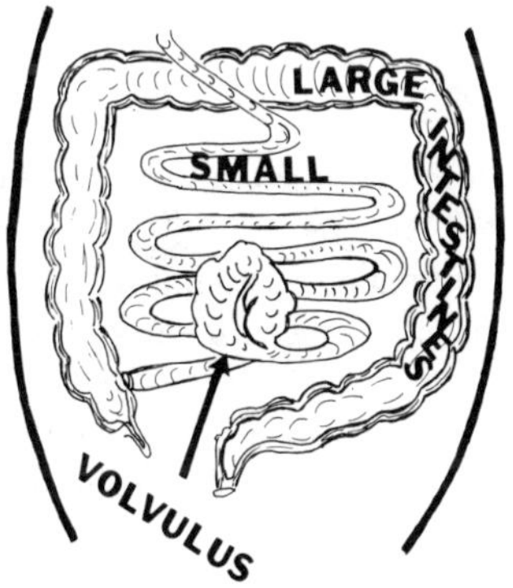

Intussusception and volvulus cause intestinal obstructions. Symptoms are similar to those of ileus and treatment follows the same pattern.

Mesenteric Vascular Occlusion

The mesentery is the membranous fold attaching organs to the body wall. Here, it specifically refers to the peritoneal fold attaching the small intestines to the dorsal body wall. An occlusion occurs when the blood supply has been reduced or cut off, so that the intestines do not receive an adequate supply of blood. Depending on the size of the vessels and the severity of the occlusion, infarction, followed by necrosis, may ensue or collateral circulation may take place.

Mesenteric vascular occlusion, depending on its extent and severity, may lead to intestinal angina or mesenteric infarction.

Intestinal/Abdominal Angina

Intestinal angina is characterized by crampy, postprandial pain caused by ischemia of the smooth muscles of intestines with mesenteric vascular insufficiency. The patient complains of postprandial pain with intensity related to the size of the meal; relationship of pain to eating gradually reduces food intake and, consequently, the patient loses weight.

Visceral angiograms confirm the narrowing of the mesenteric artery. Laboratory tests may show evidence of malabsorption.

Treatment consists of regulating food intake with small, frequent meals to help alleviate pain. If pain persists and the patient's physical condition permits, surgical revascularization of the bowel is the treatment of choice.

Mesenteric Infarction

Mesenteric infarction begins with an embolism that shuts off the blood supply through the mesentery to the intestines.

Symptoms are severe abdominal pain, vomiting, rectal bleeding, and, rarely, hematemesis. Abdominal distention occurs early, and bowel sounds may be absent.

Abdominal x-ray findings reveal gaseous distention of the intestines and evidence of peritoneal fluid. Laboratory findings reveal leukocytosis above 15,000 cubic millimeters.

Treatment consists of supportive therapy necessary to restore fluid and electrolyte balances, gastric intubation, and antimicrobial drugs. Surgery should be performed as soon as the patient's condition permits.

Irritable Colon Syndrome

Irritable colon syndrome is a functional disease characterized by a set of symptoms, including abdominal pain, nausea, vomiting, irregular bowel function of either constipation or diarrhea, hypersecretion of colonic mucus, anorexia, anxiety, and depression.

Physical examination reveals general abdominal tenderness. Sigmoidoscopy reveals spasm and mucus of the colon. Stool examination is necessary for occult blood and parasites and to rule out ulcerative colitis. GI x-ray series is without abnormalities.

Patient should be referred to a social agency for counseling and therapy for chronic anxiety and depression. The patient needs to be reassured that the symptoms are not caused by any organic disease.

Antispasmodic medication and sedative may be helpful. Regular meals and adequate sleep should be stressed. Alcohol and tobacco may be restricted. Metamucil may help to control diarrhea.

Ulcerative Colitis

Ulcerative colitis is recurrent ulceration of the mucosa and submucosa of the bowel to the extent that the colon cannot carry out its function of absorption. There are many types of ulcerative colitis, with such causes as anxiety, drug reactions, allergy, and bacterial infection.

Symptoms include lower abdominal pain and diarrhea streaked with bright red blood. There may be as many as 15 bowel movements per day, resulting in a serious reduction in body fluids and electrolytes. High fever may accompany severe diarrhea.

Diagnosis of the specific type of ulcerative colitis depends on the patient's historical data, stool examination, sigmoidoscopy, and lower GI x-ray series, including fluoroscopy.

Treatment is concerned with eliminating the underlying cause, resting the inflamed bowel, and restoring fluid and electrolyte balances. In severe cases, a temporary colostomy may be necessary to rest the bowel.

People with ulcerative colitis may have complications of arthritis, rheumatoid spondylitis, iritis, conjunctivitis, hepatitis, biliary cirrhosis, and carcinoma. Hard tubercles are often found on biopsy of the colon, along with scarring and strictures.

Cirrhosis

Cirrhosis is an inflammatory disease of the liver associated with the replacement of liver cells by fibrotic tissue and, finally, atrophy. Cirrhosis may be caused by viral infection, hepatitis, ingestion of drugs or alcohol, and obstructive liver disease.[11]

Laennec's cirrhosis is associated with alcohol ingestion and dietary deficiency. Symptoms are history of excessive alcoholic intake during which time the patient neglects to eat a nutritious diet. This pattern of alcoholic intake coupled with lack of eating over a period of time results in liver damage. Next, there is loss of weight and appetite, nausea, vomiting, distention of the abdomen with pains and hematemesis. In the advanced stage, fluid accumulates in the abdominal (ascites) and thoracic cavities, with jaundice of the skin and eyes owing to bile pigment in the blood. The liver and spleen gradually enlarge. Vascular spiders, or tiny bright-red formations of radiating arterial branches, may be present on the upper part of the body.

Biliary cirrhosis may be primary or secondary. Primary biliary cirrhosis is an inflammatory condition that causes obstruction of bile through the ductiles within the liver. Secondary biliary cirrhosis results from chronic obstruction of the bile ducts by calculus, stricture, or biliary atresia; any one of these conditions inhibits the flow of bile. Infection is often a complication.

Most people feel well during the early stages of primary biliary cirrhosis, complaining only of slight jaundice and pruritus. Later complications include bone pain; pathologic fractures may occur owing to osteomalacia and the lack of vitamin D; hyperpigmentation is evident. It is important to differentiate between primary and secondary biliary cirrhosis using laboratory and x-ray cholangiography.

There is no cure for primary biliary cirrhosis; treatment consists of calcium supplementation for osteomalacia; vitamins A, K, and D for steatorrhea; and cholestyramine for pruritus.

Symptoms of secondary biliary cirrhosis are jaundice, abdominal pain, hepatomegaly, and splenomegaly. The usual findings are choledocholithiasis (common bile duct stones), carcinoma of the bile ducts, or a bile duct stricture owing to the late effect of surgery.

Serologic tests of elevated alkaline phosphatase and 5′-nucleotidase indicate an interruption in the flow of bile from the liver to the duodenum. Cholangiography or computed tomography may demonstrate the obstruction. Relative to findings, surgery may be indicated.

Terminal neurologic events in cirrhosis of the liver are (a) slowness of mental ability and untidiness; (b) impending coma, including confusion, euphoria, drowsiness, and inappropriate behavior; (c) partial stupor, nearing complete unconsciousness; and (d) coma or unconsciousness.

Cholecystitis

Cholecystitis is inflammation of the gallbladder, generally precipitated by stones.[12]

Symptoms include indigestion with tenderness in the right upper quadrant of the abdomen, sometimes aggravated by taking a deep breath. There may also be a feeling of bloating, nausea, and vomiting after eating.

Diagnosis is generally accomplished by cholecystography. Conservative treatment is through low-fat dietary intervention. Treatment depends on the cause of cholecystitis.

Cholelithiasis

Cholelithiasis is the presence of stones, or calculi, in the gallbladder. When the rate at which the gallbladder empties is relatively slow, bile concentration increases. Stones are formed from the bile concentration in the gallbladder (Figure 12–38).

The results of chemical analysis of gallbladder stones have categorized them into (a) cholesterol and (b) pigment gallstones. Cholesterol gallstones form when the concentration of acid falls below a critical level. Analysis of pigment gallstones reveals that they are composed of bilirubin and calcium; the concentration of cholesterol has nothing to do with pigment gallstones. However, the majority of gallstones are composed mainly of cholesterol.

Symptoms are a vague sensation of fullness, dull distress in the right upper quadrant after eating, sour eructation, and flatulence.

Diagnosis is made through gallbladder visualization and laboratory blood chemistry for cholesterol level. Hypercholesterolemia has been associated with increased cholesterol in the bile.

The traditional method of treatment is cholecystectomy. However, in patients with cardiovascular or other diseases, symptoms can be relieved by low-fat diet, weight reduction, and drugs, such as anticholinergics, antacids, and sedation. Another alternative to surgery is the use of oral chenodeoxycholic (chenic) acid to dissolve cholesterol gallstones. The daily intake of chenic acid over a period of two years reveals an increased concentration of chenic acid in the bile, which chemically dissolves the precipitated cholesterol. The stones slowly disappear. Other drugs are also being tried.

Figure 12–38 Gallstones

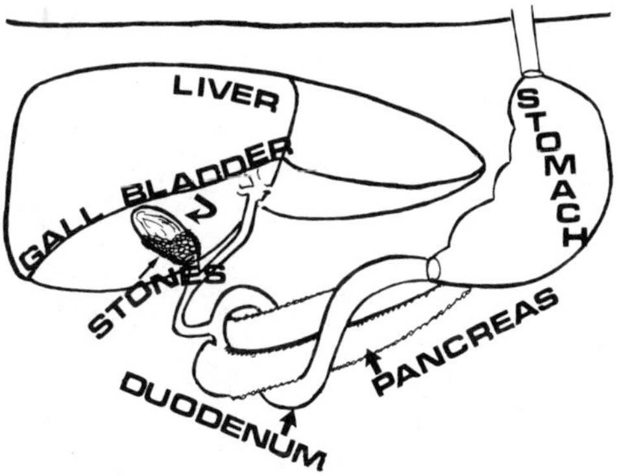

Choledocholithiasis

Although gallstones may form in the biliary ducts, generally they filter into the ducts from the gallbladder. They may not cause any discomfort, but they obstruct the flow of bile. Over a long period this can cause liver damage.

The patient complains of a sudden, severe right upper epigastric colic radiating to the right shoulder, accompanied by fever, nausea, and vomiting.

Physical examination reveals a jaundice patient with tenderness and rigidity in the epigastrium. The gallbladder is not palpable. Laboratory findings consistent with common duct obstruction reveal bilirubinuria and elevation of serum bilirubin and alkaline phosphatase levels. Computerized tomography and ultrasonography may assist in diagnosing the obstruction.

Traditional treatment is choledocholithotomy. However, it has recently become possible to remove common bile duct stones by passing an endoscope through the patient's mouth and stomach and into the upper small intestine. This enables the operator to identify the entrance of the common bile duct into the duodenum.

A small wire-like knife from the endoscope is used to cut the opening of the common bile duct, to widen it so the stone can pass through the duct into the intestines. This procedure often eliminates the need for surgery. Figure 12–39 traces a stone from the gallbladder through the cystic and common bile ducts to the Ampulla of Vater.

Pancreatic Disorders

The diseases of the pancreas are discussed in Chapter 8, The Endocrine System.

Figure 12–39 Progress of a Gall Stone

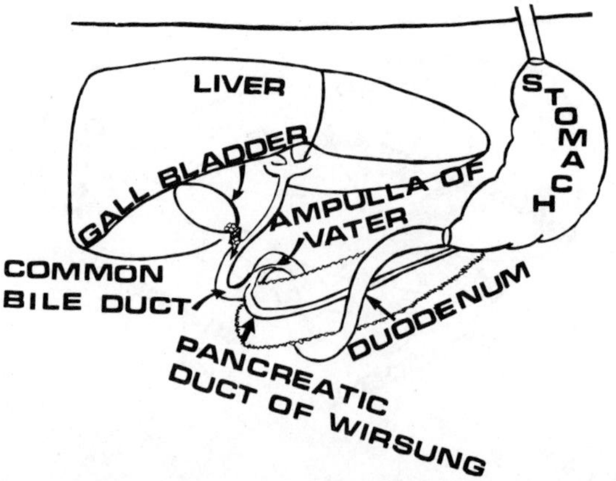

NOTES

1. Henry Gray, *Anatomy, Descriptive and Surgical,* 15th ed. (New York: Bounty Books, 1977), 908–909.

2. Ibid., 911.

3. Ibid., 921.

4. Robert Berkow, ed., *The Merck Manual of Diagnosis and Therapy,* 14th ed. (Rahway, N.J.: Merck Sharp & Dohme Research Laboratories, 1982), 1817.

5. Thomas M. Holder and Lucian L. Leape, ''Pediatric Surgery.'' In *Textbook of Surgery,* 11th ed., ed. David C. Sabiston, Jr. (Philadelphia: W.B. Saunders Co., 1977), 1378–1388.

6. Ibid., 1383–1384.

7. Ward O. Griffen, ''Meckel's Diverticulum,'' *Textbook of Surgery,* 1042–1044.

8. Holder and Leape, ''Pediatric Surgery,'' 1371–1373.

9. Willis C. Maddrey, ''Management of Esophageal Varices.'' In *The Principles and Practice of Medicine,* 11th ed., ed. A McGehee Harvey (New York: Appleton-Century-Crofts, 1980), 719–720.

10. Thomas R. Hendrix, ''Peptic Ulcer and Dyspepsia,'' *Principles and Practice,* 659–660.

11. Willis C. Maddrey, ''Chronic Diffuse Liver Disease: Cirrhosis,'' *Principles and Practice,* 735–745.

12. Thomas R. Hendrix and John L. Cameron, ''Abdominal Pain,'' *Principles and Practice,* 643–644.

Chapter 13

The Genitourinary System

Objectives

- Name the structures of the urinary and male reproductive systems.
- Explain the functions of the urinary system.
- Explain the functions of the male reproductive system.
- Contrast the symptoms of polycystic kidney disease and hydronephrosis.
- Compare nephrolithiasis and cholelithiasis.
- Compare a renal artery occlusion with a coronary occlusion.
- Contrast hyperplasia and hypertrophy.
- Explain the differences among perineal, retropubic, suprapubic, and transurethral prostatectomy.

Because the urinary system and the male reproductive system share common structures, they are combined in this chapter.

FUNCTION AND STRUCTURE OF THE URINARY SYSTEM

The urinary system includes the kidneys, the ureters, the bladder, and the urethra (Figure 13–1). It functions by:

- filtering impurities from the blood
- providing a system for these impurities to leave the body
- regulating the acid-base balance of body fluids
- maintaining the normal concentration of electrolytes in the body.

KIDNEYS

The kidneys, two bean-shaped organs, are located behind the abdominal cavity, one on either side of the vertebral column in the lumbar region of the spine. Surrounded by an outer covering called the renal cortex, the kidney is divided into

---

Figure 13–1 The Kidneys, Ureters, Bladder, and Urethra

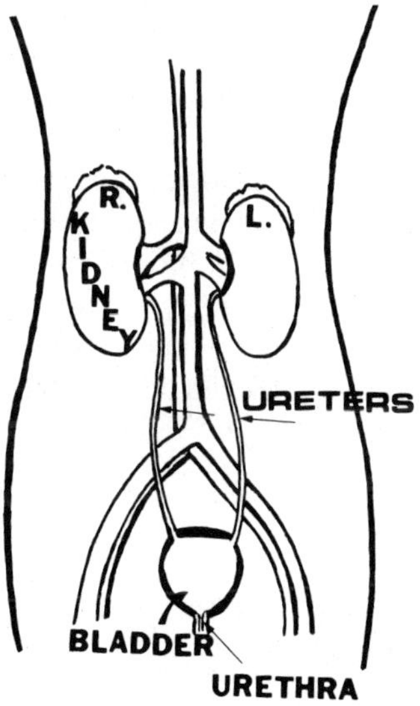

two parts: (1) the renal cortex, or outer shell, and (2) the renal medulla, or inner division. The renal cortex is composed mainly of glomeruli and convoluted tubules, which extend between the pyramids of the medulla. The renal medulla comprises an extension of the kidney pelvis, called pyramids, and renal tubules. The kidney pelvis, blood vessels, and nerves enter the kidney through the hilum, a depression on the medial border of the kidney that gives the kidney the appearance of a bean.

Nephron

Each kidney has approximately one million microscopic nephrons formed from the kidney cells and capillaries. The three main parts of the nephron are (1) the renal tubule, the stem of the nephron; (2) Bowman's capsule, which tops the nephron; and (3) the glomeruli, the network of capillaries stored in the top of the nephron (Figure 13–2).

Renal Tubule

The renal tubule, or proximal convoluted (twisted) tubule, is also the descending and ascending limb of the loop of Henle. The ascending limb terminates in a straight, or collecting, tubule that opens into the renal pelvis.

The renal artery entering the kidney at the renal pelvis progressively breaks up into smaller blood vessels until reaching the afferent arterioles of the glomerulus. The glomerulus is composed of small microscopic clusters of capillary loops, afferent arterioles, and is situated in the upper end of Bowman's capsule. As blood passes through the loops, a solution of water and solids diffuses into the space around the capillaries and passes down the convoluted tubule, where reabsorption of protein and electrolytes occurs. The urine then passes into the collecting tubules, where it becomes concentrated as water is absorbed. Next, it passes into the kidney pelvis. The amount of filtration and secretion of urine depends on the pressure under which the blood is forced through the glomerular capillaries. For example, if blood pressure greatly decreases, the production of urine diminishes and may cease altogether. From the foregoing one can see that two opposite functions are at work: glomerular filtration and tubular absorption.

URETERS

Two ureters, one for each kidney, carry the urine from the kidney by way of the kidney pelvis to the bladder.

Figure 13–2 The Nephron

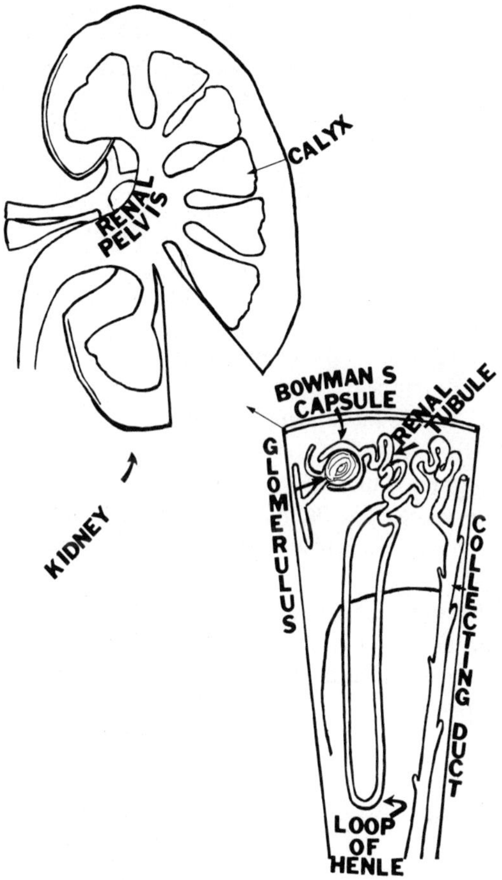

BLADDER

The bladder, a hollow membranous sac with muscular walls located in the anterior pelvic cavity, is joined to the kidneys by the ureters and to the body by the urethra. The function of the bladder is to store urine from the kidneys.

URETHRA

The urethra carries urine from the bladder to the exterior.

FUNCTION AND STRUCTURE OF THE MALE REPRODUCTIVE SYSTEM

Besides being the conveyor of urine from the bladder, the urethra is a passageway for seminal fluid in the male. The male reproductive system also consists of two testes, two epididymides, vas deferens, ejaculatory ducts, seminal vesicles, bulbourethral glands (Cowper's glands), and a prostate gland. The external genitals are the scrotum and the penis.

TESTES

The testes, consisting of several lobules, are located in a saclike organ covered with skin, called the scrotum. Each lobule of the testes has several long, coiled, seminiferous tubules for the manufacture of spermatozoa (sperm), a process that begins at puberty. The second function of the testes is to secrete testosterone, the male hormone that (a) masculinizes the body, (b) maintains the development of the male sex organs, and (c) aids in muscular development.

The production of testosterone in the testes depends on the luteinizing hormone (LH); the follicle-stimulating hormone (FSH) stimulates spermatogenesis. Contrasting this with the female, FSH stimulates follicular development to produce estrogen; LH stimulates the corpus luteum to produce progesterone.[1] (It would be well to review the material on anterior pituitary secretions in Chapter 8, The Endocrine System.)

EPIDIDYMIS, VAS DEFERENS, EJACULATORY DUCT, AND URETHRA

Sperm are formed by the millions in the seminiferous tubules, from which they flow into the coiled duct called epididymis. Through the epididymis duct, sperm continue the journey to the vas deferens, then into the ejaculatory duct, and, finally, into the urethra, where sperm travel to the exterior of the body. Figure 13–3 traces sperm from the seminiferous tubules to the urethra.

ACCESSORY MALE GLANDS

The accessory male glands—the seminal vesicles, prostate gland, and Cowper's glands—produce alkaline secretions that make up the gelatinous fluid of the semen. Alkali in the semen assures sperm survival and fertility.

Figure 13–3 The Tracing of Sperm from the Seminiferous Tubules to the Urethra

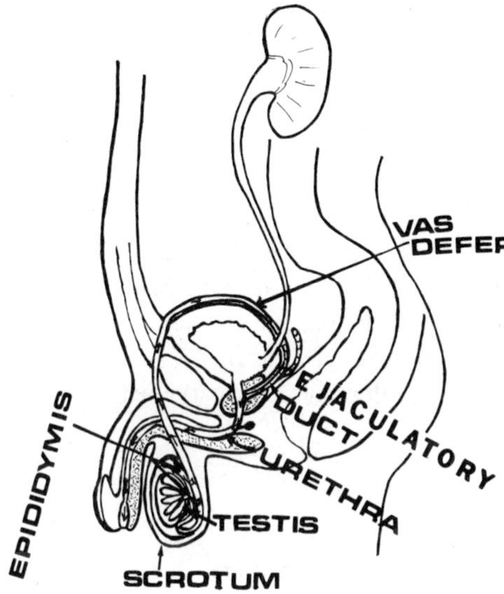

SCROTUM AND PENIS

The external male reproductive system is made up of the scrotum and the penis. The scrotum is the pouch that contains the testes and their accessory organs.

The penis, the organ of reproduction and urinary excretion, is attached to the lower portion of the pubic bone. The body of the penis is composed of two cylindrical bodies of erectile tissue. A third layer of tissue containing the urethra is found behind the head of the penis. The glans penis is the end of the penis; it contains the opening of the urethra.

The loose skin that covers the penis, the prepuce, allows the penis to become erect during sexual excitation. The inner surface of the foreskin contains glands that secrete a lubricating fluid that assists the penis to expand and retract past the foreskin.

CONGENITAL DEFECTS OF THE GENITOURINARY SYSTEM

Absence of Kidney

An infant may be born with only one kidney. In such a case, a kidney transplant must be performed; however, donor availability is generally a problem. Depending on the severity of the anomaly, plastic reconstruction of the urinary structures may also be necessary. Prognosis depends on the severity of the congenital defect and the availability of a kidney donor.

Exstrophy of the Bladder

Exstrophy of the bladder, occurring in embryonic development, is the absence of the lower abdominal and anterior vesical walls. Generally, there is also deformity of the urethra with separation of the pubes. There may be complete incontinence owing to the lack of a total bladder to store urine.

Treatment through plastic reconstruction of the bladder is in the experimental stage; urine is diverted surgically by placing the ureters in the large bowel, so that it can be excreted through an external orifice.

Patients with this defect are vulnerable to urinary tract infections and may die of an acute infection.

Phimosis

Phimosis is a congenital condition in which the prepuce is so tight that it prevents the retraction of foreskin over the glans. If not corrected, phimosis may result in inflammation of both the glans and the foreskin (balanoposthitis); urinary obstruction may also occur. Generally, prophylactic newborn circumcisions are performed.

Hypospadias

Hypospadias is a congenital defect in which the urethra is off center and opens on the underside of the penis or on the perineum. Depending on the severity of the anomaly, surgical correction is performed according to urologic and reproductive implications.

Multicystic Kidney

A multicystic kidney, usually found on autopsy of a stillborn infant, is the condition in which the kidneys resemble a cystic mass.

ACQUIRED DEFECTS AND DISEASES

Kidney diseases and defects may be acquired owing to inheritance, infection, trauma, and neoplasms (Chapter 15).

Polycystic Kidney

Polycystic kidney disease, an inherited disorder, appears shortly after birth, when the abdomen becomes enlarged and the infant shows signs of emaciation and dehydration. A cystic mass is palpable on the kidney.

The adult type of polycystic kidney disease makes its appearance in individuals between the ages 40 and 60, with onset of abdominal pain, polyuria, nausea, and vomiting. In the advanced stage, there is weight loss, hypertension, and uremia; the liver, spleen, and kidneys are all palpable.

Laboratory blood tests reveal anemia; urinalysis shows the presence of red blood cells, protein, and casts and a low specific gravity. A renal photoscan confirms cystic kidney.

In infants, prognosis is fatal; in adults, the disease shows slow progression.[2]

Hydronephrosis

Hydronephrosis is enlargement of the renal pelvis and the renal calices owing to urinary retention (retaining urine). This condition results from a urinary tract obstruction caused by tumors, adhesions, trauma, or congenital abnormality. The obstruction may represent a permanent condition owing to complete obstruction, or it may be a temporary condition, resulting from a partial obstruction of the ureter.

Symptoms accompanying a permanent obstruction are dull pain and an enlarged kidney; signs of a partial obstruction are oliguria with pain or polyuria with relief of pain.

Laboratory urine examination (catheterized specimen) reveals hematuria and low specific gravity. Pyelography reveals dilatation of the renal pelvis and calix. The usual course of the disease as observed in similar situations is serious.

Treatment consists of resolving the urinary tract infection if one exists. Catheter drainage may be satisfactory, but a severe obstruction may require a temporary nephrostomy for drainage until the obstruction can be removed.

Urinary Calculi

Urinary calculi is a general term used for a calculi (stone) anywhere in the urinary tract.

Nephrolithiasis is the presence of calculi in the renal pelvis that obstructs the flow of urine. Although the exact cause of renal calculi is unknown, predisposing factors include infection, dehydration, obstruction, and metabolic causes, such as gout. More common in males, nephrolithiasis appears in individuals between ages 30 and 40. Small calculi in the renal pelvis may pass out of the pelvis into the ureter and bladder, causing obstruction; they may also pass out of the urinary tract through the urine.

Symptoms are intermittent lumbar discomfort, dysuria, renal colic (sharp pain), nausea, and vomiting.[3]

Urinalysis reveals the presence of acid, urate crystals, red blood cells, and protein. Uric acid calculi is associated with gout.

The presence of calculi without infection may not require any treatment. When there is an infection, resolution of the infection is essential. Uric acid calculi alone may be resolved by prolonged urine alkalinization with drugs. Very small stones in the lower ureter may be removed by cystoscopic basket extraction. Large calculi in the ureter or renal pelvis are removed surgically.

Calculi obstructing the flow of urine out of the bladder may be removed through an endoscopic (through the urethra) technique called litholapaxy. In litholapaxy, the calculi in the bladder are crushed and the fragments immediately washed out of the bladder.

Urinary Tract Infection, Acute

A urinary tract infection is the invasion of bacteria in any part of the urinary tract. The microorganism may be found in the urine, or an organ, such as the testes or the prostate, may shows signs of infection.

Symptoms are burning pain on urination, chills, fever, and back pain. The urine generally smells strong and is dark in color.

Laboratory examination, culture, and sensitivity are indicated for isolation of microorganism and specific prescription for antibiotics.[4] White blood cell count reveals leukocytosis with shift to the left. In severe cases the blood culture may be positive.

Antibiotic treatment is begun on diagnosis and should continue for two weeks or until the infection is resolved.

Glomerulonephritis, Acute

Acute glomerulonephritis, inflammation of the capillary loops in the glomeruli of the kidney, may occur about two weeks after a beta-hemolytic streptococcal infection of the throat, ears, or sinuses. Glomerulonephritis is due to an immune response to streptococcus in the body.

Symptoms are malaise, headache, anorexia, fever, hematuria, and, possibly, tachycardia and hypertension. In severe cases, signs of cardiac failure may appear, resulting from sodium and water retention in the kidneys.

Laboratory analysis reveals blood and hemoglobin in the urine, with protein, hyaline, and granular casts. Blood urea nitrogen and serum creatinine levels are elevated; blood analysis reveals mild anemia.

There is no specific treatment for acute glomerulonephritis except for bed rest. The patient's condition is observed for clinical signs of cardiac failure characterized by hypertension and peripheral edema.

Pyelonephritis, Acute

Acute pyelonephritis results from bacterial infection of the kidneys. The most common causative organisms are *Escherichia coli, Pseudomonas, Klebsiella,* and *Staphylococcus aureus*.

Symptoms are back pain over the costovertebral region with frequency of urination, dysuria, nausea, vomiting, and chills.

Laboratory blood test reveals leukocytosis; urinalysis should be examined for microorganisms with culture and sensitivity. Pyelography may show enlargement of the kidney. The prediction of the probable outcome of the disease based on the condition of the patient is uncertain.

Antibiotic therapy should be initiated as soon as culture and sensitivity results are available and should continue for approximately two weeks or until repeated urine cultures are negative for infection.

Prostatitis

Infection may be carried to the prostate through the bloodstream or may be spread from another part of the urinary system.

Symptoms are acute perineal pain, fever, dysuria, and urethral discharge. The prostate may be enlarged and tender. If accompanied by urinary tract infection, there may also be pain in the lumbosacral area and frequent, painful urination.

Blood analysis reveals leukocytosis; culture and sensitivity of discharge from the prostate and urinalysis are necessary for isolation of the bacteria and prescription of proper antibiotic.

Treatment includes bed rest with adequate fluids, antibiotics, analgesics for pain, and warm sitz baths to reduce any swelling of the prostate.

Benign Prostatic Hyperplasia and Hypertrophy

In order to understand benign prostatic hyperplasia and hypertrophy, the reader should review the contrast between hyperplasia and hypertrophy given in Chapter 4.

The most common cause of bladder obstruction in men over age 50 is benign prostatic enlargement. This is hyperplasia of the lateral and subcervical lobes of the prostate with enlargement of the prostate, accompanied by urethral obstruction.

Although the phenomenon is not completely understood, it is recognized that androgen production diminishes after age 40, and enlargement of the prostate may occur with advancing years. As the prostate enlarges, the prostatic portion of the urethra is compressed, resulting in the restriction of urine flow and emptying of the urinary bladder.

Symptoms are enlargement of the prostate and bladder retention. Hematuria, uremia, and hydronephrosis may result from urinary retention.

Determination of blood urea nitrogen levels is diagnostic for the presence of benign prostatic hyperplasia.

Benign Prostatic Hypertrophy

Benign prostatic hypertrophy is the enlargement of the prostate with protrusion posteriorly into the anterior rectal wall, obstructing the bladder outlet. Examination reveals bladder retention. Cystourethroscopy confirms the presence of prostatic enlargement and the assessment of the bladder outlet obstruction.

Azotemia (an excess of urea or other nitrogen compounds in the blood) is diagnostic of bladder outlet obstruction. Phenolsulfonphthalein (PSP) test provides a basis for renal function and urinary retention.

Surgical intervention may be indicated after total assessment of benign prostatic hypertrophy. *Prostatectomy* is the removal of part or all of the prostate. There are several approaches: A *perineal prostatectomy* is the removal of the prostate through a perineal incision. A *retropubic prevesical prostatectomy* is the removal of the prostate through a suprapubic incision, without entering the urinary bladder. A *prostatectomy by transurethral resection* is an instrumental resection of the prostate through the urethra.

NOTES

1. Sylvia A. Price and Lorraine McC. Wilson, *Pathophysiology,* 2nd ed. (New York: McGraw-Hill Book Co., 1982), 738.
2. Ibid., 545–546.
3. John T. Grayhack, "The Urinary System." In *Davis-Christopher Textbook of Surgery,* Vol. 2, ed. David C. Sabiston, Jr., M.D. (Philadelphia: W.B. Saunders Co., 1977), 1727–1730.
4. Ibid.

Chapter 14

The Female Reproductive System

Objectives

- Name the structures of the female reproductive system.
- Compare the phases of the menstrual cycle.
- Explain the process of female reproduction.
- Contrast cystocele and rectocele and their repairs.
- Compare the symptoms of menorrhagia and metrorrhagia.
- Describe the three stages of labor.
- Differentiate among the uses of low, midforceps, and high forceps.
- Explain the types of infant presentation.
- Contrast the three types of ectopic pregnancies.
- Discuss the treatment of ectopic pregnancy.
- Compare therapeutic, habitual, and spontaneous abortions.
- Explain the difference between preeclampsia and eclampsia of pregnancy.
- Contrast low cervical and classic cesarean section.

FUNCTION AND STRUCTURE

Unlike the male reproductive system, the female system does not use urinary structures in the functions of reproduction. The female reproductive system includes the uterus, fallopian tubes, ovaries, vagina, Bartholin's glands, and vulva. (The breasts are discussed in Chapter 15, Neoplasms, since most breast diseases are neoplastic in origin.) Each of the foregoing female organs functions as an organ as well as within the system. This chapter includes gynecologic diseases and obstetric procedures. Obstetrics is the study of the normal process of birth and the procedures for delivery, complications of labor, delivery, puerperium, and postpartum. Figure 14–1 shows the female reproductive system.

UTERUS

The uterus, hollow and pear-shaped, is located in the lower part of the pelvis between the rectum and the bladder. It has an upper part, or fundus, that is broad and flat; a center, or corpus, that is pear-shaped; and a lower part, or cervix, that is narrow and elongated. The uterus has an outer muscular layer of tissue called myometrium; its hollow space is lined with mucous membrane called endometrium.

The function of the uterus is to provide shelter and nourishment for the developing embryo and fetus.

Figure 14–1 The Female Reproductive System

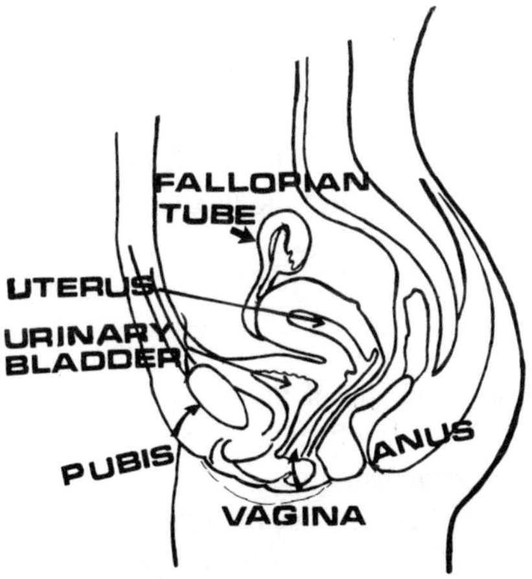

FALLOPIAN TUBES

The fallopian tubes, or uterine tubes, extend bilaterally from the fundus of the uterus. At the outermost end of the tubes are tentaclelike projections called fimbriae.

The function of the fimbriae is to grasp the mature ovum from the ovary and transport it into the fallopian tube. It is in the fallopian tube that the ovum becomes fertilized. After fertilization, the ovum moves to the uterine cavity, where it is implanted on the uterine wall.

OVARIES

The ovaries are two golf ball–sized organs located bilaterally at the fimbriated edge of the fallopian tubes. They are attached to the posterior wall of the uterus and the broad ligament.

The function of the ovaries is to release mature ova and steroid hormones of estrogen and progesterone.

VAGINA

The vagina, a tubular structure located at the distal end of the cervix, has an outermost layer of strong fibrous tissue, a middle layer of muscular tissue, and an inner layer of mucosa. The vagina at its upper end, at the lower end of the uterus, forms a cuff around the cervical uteri; at the lower end of the vagina are found the Bartholin's glands.

The function of the vagina is to provide (a) a passageway for menstrual flow, (b) a receptacle for sperm, and (c) a birth canal for the fetus.

BARTHOLIN'S GLANDS

The Bartholin's glands, located at the lower end of the vagina, provide lubricating secretion on the interior surface of the vagina.

VULVA

The vulva, the exterior genitalia of the female, has the clitoris on the upper center. The clitoris is composed of many nerve cells and a fold of skin called prepuce. It is the counterpart in the female for the glans penis in the male. The two folds of skin surrounding the clitoris are the labia majora and labia minora. Just inside the vaginal opening, between the opening and the labia minora, is an area called the vestibule. The functions of the vestibule are (a) to provide an opening for the urethra and (b) to house many glands. Figure 14–2 shows the exterior female genitalia.

MENSTRUAL CYCLE

The normal menstrual cycle of 28 days has three phases: (1) the follicular phase, (2) ovulation, and (3) the secretory phase.

Follicular Phase

The first phase, the follicular phase, is characterized by growth of the ovary initiated by the follicle-stimulating hormone (FSH) released by the anterior pituitary under the influence of the hypothalamus. The hypothalamus initiates the release of FSH when the level of estrogen in the blood is reduced. As they grow, the follicles manufacture estrogen. The endometrium, the inner lining of the uterus, responds to estrogen by (a) assisting the growth of epithelium, (b) restoring the connective tissue, and (c) maintaining the blood supply to the area. Even though many follicles commence growth under the influence of FSH, only one becomes fully mature.

Figure 14–2 The External Female Genitalia

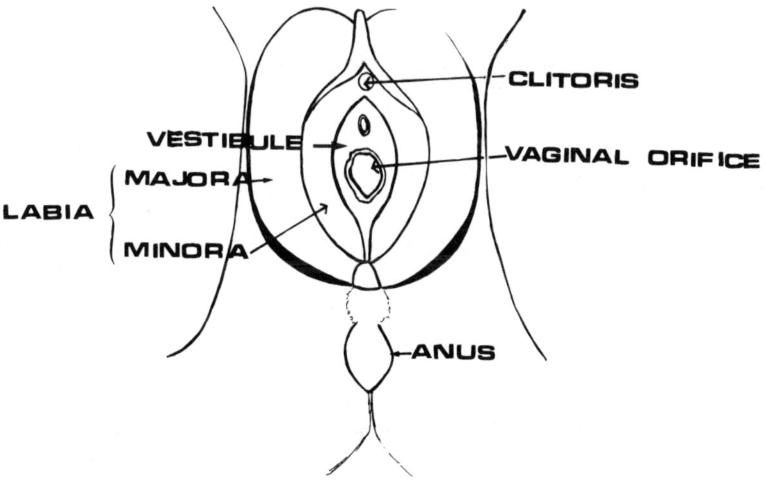

Ovulation Phase

In Chapter 13 a comparison was made between the action of FSH and luteinizing hormone (LH) in the male and female. The following discussion on the ovulation phase is a fuller explanation of the role of FSH and LH.[1]

Fourteen days after the beginning of the cycle, there is an increase of estrogen and FSH initiates the release of LH from the anterior pituitary. LH is responsible for the release of the mature ovum into the fallopian tube; this is called ovulation. The woman's body temperature rises. Under the action of LH, the follicle containing the mature ovum is transformed into a corpus luteum. Progesterone produced by the corpus luteum initiates the endometrium to pass into the secretory phase of the cycle.

Secretory Phase

Within 48 hours after its release from the ovary, the ovum should be fertilized.

A fertilized ovum takes approximately three days to travel through the tube as its cells divide. Reaching the endometrial cavity, it again divides for two to three days before attaching itself by implant into the endometrial wall of the uterus. The secretory glands of the endometrium provide nutrients for cell growth as the fertilized ovum divides itself into the embryo and the placenta (trophoblast cells). The trophoblast cells produce human chorionic gonadotropin (HCG), which maintains the production of progesterone in the corpus luteum. This prepares the uterus for the reception and development of the fertilized egg.

If the ovum is not fertilized, then the ovum and the corpus luteum disintegrate, hormone production wanes, the endometrium breaks down, and the debris appears externally as menstruation. The mentrual cycle is complete.

CONGENITAL DEFECTS OF THE FEMALE REPRODUCTIVE SYSTEM

Atresia of Vagina

Atresia of the vagina is the congenital closure of the vagina. The vagina is present, but there is no opening. This condition requires surgical opening.

Absence of Ovary

Congenital absence of both ovaries is rare, but absence of one ovary is not unusual. Replacement of estrogen is given to provide growth stimulus to the genital structures.

ACQUIRED DEFECTS AND DISEASES

The acquired defects and diseases of the female reproductive system may result from infection, static mechanical abnormality, metabolism, neoplasms, and uncertain cause.

Infection

Infection in the female reproductive system is often found to diffuse to the cervix uteri, fallopian tubes, and ovaries owing to the proximity of the organs. The same microorganisms are found to infect all female organs.

Cervicitis

Cervicitis is the inflammation of the cervix uteri owing to *Escherichia coli,* staphylococcus, streptococcus, and gonococcus. When only the mucosal layer of the cervical uterine is involved, the infection is called endocervicitis; inflammation of the entire cervix is called pancervicitis.

Symptoms are feeling of weight in the pelvis, dyspareunia, and dysmenorrhea. On examination the cervix is red, swollen, and bleeds easily when manipulated.

Chronic cervicitis reveals excessive vaginal discharge from a red, swollen cervix. There may be ulceration and erosion around the external os.

Diagnosis is made through smear with culture and sensitivity for micoorganism and cytology study of the tissue for malignancy involvement.

Colposcopy and colpomicroscopy are means of identifying any suspicious areas of the cervix, which should be treated before biopsy. Treatment is generally by electrodesiccation, by ultrarefrigeration (cryotherapy), or with silver nitrate. Cautery should include the involved exocervix and endocervical canal. Repeated cautery, surgical conization, and sometimes hysterectomy for women past childbearing years may be required for severe chronic cervicitis.

Pelvic Inflammatory Disease

Included under pelvic inflammatory disease are chronic salpingo-oophoritis, pyosalpinx, and hydrosalpinx. *Chronic salpingo-oophoritis* is a major complication of gonorrhea. It may be asymptomatic after the acute stage is resolved and the tube is agglutinized (fused together in the process of healing). *Pyosalpinx* (the tube filled with pus is dilated closed) may occur after gonorrhea. *Hydrosalpinx* (the tube filled with serous fluid) may follow pyosalpinx.

Chronic oophoritis may also result, since the ovary may become involved in an inflammatory disease of the tube. Pelvic adhesions (adhesions of pelvic viscera to bowel and omentum) sometimes occur.

Symptoms may be severe abdominal pain and menorrhagia, severe pain on manipulation of the cervix, adnexal mass, and fever.

Laboratory tests reveal elevated white blood count and erythrocyte sedimentation rate. Culture and sensitivity from smear should be completed for isolation of the microorganism and institution of antibiotic therapy.

Treatment of pelvic inflammatory disease may be either medical or surgical. Medical treatment involves bed rest; heat; antibiotic therapy with penicillin, ampicillin, or other antibiotics; and analgesics for pain. Surgical treatment of hysterectomy with salpingo-oophorectomy may be decided on after the acute infection is resolved. Bilateral oophorectomy requires estrogen replacement for younger women.

Static Mechanical Abnormality

Prolapse of the Uterus

The prolapse of the uterus is measured by the degree of downward displacement. The three degrees of uterine prolapse are characterized by (1) the displacement of the uterus in the vaginal orifice, (2) cervical uteri displaced outside the orifice, and (3) the entire uterus prolapsed outside the vaginal orifice. Prolapse of the uterus may occur after parturition, especially after a difficult delivery. This condition is less common today owing to good obstetric care. It is generally associated with cystocele and rectocele.

Symptoms are low backache, pressure sensation in the pelvis, frequent and painful urination, and leukorrhea.

Physical examination reveals a questionable mass in the lower vagina. Pelvic examination demonstrates prolapse of the uterus when the patient bears down or strains either in a standing or lying position.

Surgical intervention depends on the patient's age and physical condition. In the Manchester–Fothergill operation the cervix is amputated and the ligaments are attached to the anterior part of the uterus. Vaginal hysterectomy may also be performed. Vaginal pessary is an alternative to surgery.

Cystocele

A cystocele is the herniation of the urinary bladder into the vagina owing to the lacerations of the vagina in the delivery of a large baby or twins. It is often accompanied by urethral diverticulum in the vaginal canal.

This condition may be asymptomatic until menopausal age, when the patient complains of fullness in the vagina, urinary urgency and frequency, and dysuria.

Catheterization of the patient after voiding reveals approximately 60 ml of urine in the cystocele; it may also reveal urinary tract infection. Radiology with induction of contrast media into the bladder reveals the cystocele.

Surgical intervention with anterior vaginal colporrhaphy (plasty repair of the vagina) is the preferred treatment. A pessary may be an alternative to surgery.

Rectocele

A rectocele is the herniation of the rectum into the vagina owing to a tear in the fibrous connective tissue separating the rectum and vagina during rapid birth, delivery of a large baby, or forceps or breech delivery.

Symptoms are a sense of vaginal and rectal fullness with a continuous urge for defecation. Depending on the size of the defect, there may be constipation owing to the feces lodging in the defect. Cystocele and prolapsed uterus often accompany a rectocele.

Rectal examination is diagnostic. Radiologic lower gastrointestinal series outlines the rectocele.

Surgical intervention with colpoperineoplasty, vaginal and perineal repair, of the rectocele is the preferred treatment.

Menorrhagia and Metrorrhagia

Menorrhagia is excessive or prolonged menstrual bleeding during the regular menstrual cycle. This may be due to a uterine myoma, endometrial polyp, or salpingitis.

Metrorrhagia, bleeding that occurs between the menstrual cycle, may be an early sign of uterine malignancy.

Diagnosis of menorrhagia and metrorrhagia is accomplished through surgical cervical biopsy and diagnostic dilatation and curettage. Culture for microorganisms should also be carried out.

Intervention for acute blood loss is intravenous fluids and blood transfusions. The role and use of hormones to halt the bleeding should be considered.

OBSTETRICS

Obstetrics is a branch of medicine and surgery dealing with the management of pregnancy, labor, and puerperium. Pregnancy is not an illness, but a normal occurrence; however, sometimes complications make it life threatening.

Reproduction

Germ cells, oogenesis (female) and spermatogenesis (male), are the two types of reproductive cells found in the body. Mature germ cells contain chromosomes; chromosomes contain patterns of heredity in genes paired in 23 sets. Twenty-two pairs of chromosomes contain genes (autosomes) for determination of body characteristics. The one remaining pair contains sex genes.

Through sexual intercourse (copulation or coitus), reproduction takes place. This is accomplished by the ejaculation of the male germ cell into the woman. The male germ cell travels through the uterus to the fallopian tube to penetrate the ovum.

The ovary of the woman ejects ova, which are picked up by the tubal fimbriae and carried into the fallopian tube for possible penetration by the male germ cell. In the fallopian tube, fertilization of the ovum takes place. In fertilization, the nuclei of the two cells fuse; the one-cell zygote is now in the first phase of human development.

The zygote stage is characterized by cell division, and the zygote becomes surrounded by cells called trophoblasts. The trophoblasts aid in nourishment of the zygote and eventually evolve into the chorion. The cells and surrounding cavity (blastocyst) fill with fluid, and the cavity becomes the amniotic cavity. The blastocyst travels to the uterus, where attachment is made to the uterine wall. For the first two weeks of development the zygote continues cell division by layers: (1) ectoderm, (2) entoderm, and (3) mesoderm. These three layers of tissue ultimately begin the next phase, embryonic development.

By the third week, embryonic development begins and lasts for approximately six weeks. During embryonic development, rapid growth occurs. There is differentiation of the major organ systems and development of the main external features. Therefore, during this period, congenital anomalies occur.

The fetal stage begins at the end of the embryonic developmental stage, the seventh week of gestation, and continues until birth. The total period of 38 to 42 weeks is counted from the first day of the last menstrual period. Figure 14–3 outlines the stages of growth including the zygote, embryo, fetus, and newborn.

Pregnancy

A pregnant woman sometimes experiences pigmentary changes on her face (cholasma gravidarum), and a dark line (linea nigra) may appear on her abdomen. As the fetus grows, the abdomen enlarges; the stretching of the abdominal skin causes streaks called striae gravidarum. The mother feels the first movement of the fetus; this is called quickening. As the time for delivery grows close, the fetus drops into the lower position for birth; this is called lightening.

Presentation

The position in which the child drops into the lower cervix for birth is important. Presentation refers to the part of the infant's body that appears at the vulvar ring for delivery. The vertex presentation of the upper and back portion of the head is

Figure 14–3 Stages of Growth

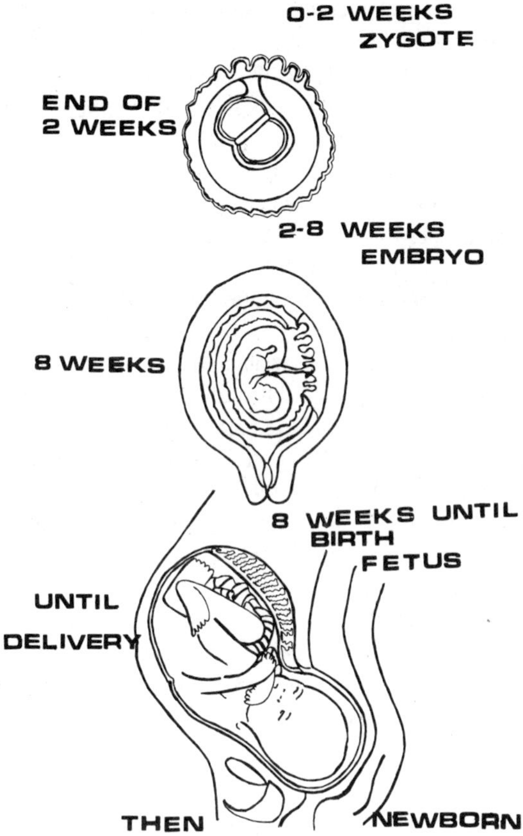

considered a normal presentation. The brow and fontanelle presentations are also considered head presentations. If other parts of the infant's body appear first for delivery, this is a breech presentation; it includes the buttock, footling, frank breech, and knee types. Deliveries of infants with breech presentations often require manipulation and skill. Sometimes a breech presentation requires delivery by cesarean section.

Stages of Labor

Childbirth begins with parturition, signalled by the discharge of a mucous plug from the cervix, called show. The first of the three stages of labor, from the commencement of labor to complete dilation of the cervix, is beginning. The cervix now begins to shorten and thin; this is effacement, as it becomes stretched beyond its normal limits. The opening enlarges; it dilates. The presentation of the infant's body appears at the external os of the cervix; this is the portion that will appear first. As the infant's body descends through the pelvic outlet, engagement occurs at this station. As the infant's body descends through the birth canal, it is eventually encircled by the vulvar ring.

The second stage of labor begins with the complete dilation of the cervix until birth. When the largest area of the infant's presenting part is encircled by the vulvar ring, the infant is crowning. The birth is completed; the infant is newborn.

The third stage of labor begins with the birth of the child and ends when the mother delivers the placenta. Within minutes after birth, the mother delivers the afterbirth, secundia, from the vagina.

Forceps can aid in delivery. The application of forceps are low, high, and midforceps. Low forceps are applied when the infant's head is on the perineum; high forceps are used before the head has passed the pelvic outlet; and midforceps are applied when the infant's head is at the ischial spine level.

An episiotomy, median or mediolateral, is performed to assist the delivery and prevent a perineal laceration. In a median episiotomy, the incision is made in the midline of the perineum; in the mediolateral episiotomy, the incision is made toward one side of the midline.

From the end of labor until the uterus returns to its normal size (involution), there is a period of about six weeks, called puerperium. A mother giving birth to her first child is a primipara and to successive children, a multipara.

Complications

Placenta Previa and Abruptio Placentae

The placenta is a highly vascular organ attached to the wall of the uterus through which the baby obtains oxygen, nutrients, and other substances in exchange for carbon dioxide and other wastes. The function of the placenta is interfered with when the placenta is abnormally implanted on the wall of the uterus.

Placenta previa occurs when the placenta is implanted very low, so that the external os is partially or completely covered.

Symptoms include bleeding, ranging from slight to hemorrhage, on dilation of the cervical os, when the placenta tends to break away from the uterine wall.

Diagnosis may be made by ultrasonography. Pelvic examination is contraindicated. Typing and cross matching of the patient's blood for transfusion is required. Cesarean section is preferred to stop the hemorrhage.

Abruptio placentae occurs when a normally positioned placenta breaks away from the uterine wall prematurely after the fetus is viable and before delivery. Generally, the hemorrhage brings immediate death to the fetus.

Symptoms are abdominal pain, uterine tenderness, and contractions. Shock and death may occur in minutes. Hemorrhage may or may not be visible. If hemorrhage is concealed, then blood trapped behind the placenta seeps into the myometrium and other female structures. Cesarean section is urgent.

Cesarean Section

A cesarean section is performed for dystocia, cervical stenosis, carcinoma of the cervix found during pregnancy, partial and complete placental previa, hemorrhage, and other reasons. A previous cesarean section is no longer a valid reason for performing another cesarean section.

A cesarean section is the removal of the fetus through incisions made into the abdomen and uterus. Types of cesarean sections are low cervical and classic. Essentially, in either type the abdomen is incised; the pelvis and uterus are entered; the infant's head is delivered; the infant's airways are cleared; the infant's body is delivered; the placenta is delivered; the uterus is closed; and the abdomen is closed.

Ectopic Pregnancy

An ectopic pregnancy is the implantation of the fertilized ovum outside the uterus. Types of ectopic pregnancies are abdominal, ovarian, and tubal pregnancies.

Abdominal pregnancy occurs when the ovum travels by error into the abdominal cavity and implantation of the conceptus is made in the abdominal cavity. This is rare, but it does occur. This type of pregnancy may be carried to full term with delivery of the baby by cesarean section.

An *ovarian pregnancy* occurs when implantation of the conceptus is made in the ovary. This rarely happens.

A *tubal pregnancy* occurs when implantation occurs in the fallopian tube. This type of ectopic pregnancy is common.

When the fetus that is lodged in the ovary or tube becomes too large for that area, the ovary or tube ruptures and hemorrhage takes place. The abdomen is entered with a lower midline incision; the blood is evacuated from the area; the ectopic pregnancy is identified; the fallopian tube or ovary (sometimes both) are mobilized and removed.

Abortion

An abortion is the termination of pregnancy by expelling the fetus before it is viable. Expulsion of the fetus after it is viable is called immature or premature delivery.

There are many causes for abortion; reasons may be maternal or fetal. Types of abortion are threatened, therapeutic, habitual, and spontaneous. An abortion is *threatened* when the cervix becomes soft and slightly dilated. Symptoms are backache, cramps, and spotting of blood. An abortion is *therapeutic* when medical or surgical intervention is necessary to terminate a pregnancy that might jeopardize the health or life of the patient. If a patient experiences three or more consecutive abortions, this constitutes *habitual abortion;* this condition is also referred to as *spontaneous abortion*. A *spontaneous abortion* occurs naturally without any warning.

Toxemia of Pregnancy

Toxemia of pregnancy on a continuum is preeclampsia on one end and eclampsia on the extreme other end. *Preeclampsia* is toxemia that occurs in the last three months of pregnancy. The patient progresses from preeclampsia to eclampsia. Symptoms are headache, dizziness, malaise, epigastric pain, nausea, and loss of vision. Physical examination reveals a rise in blood pressure and ankle edema.

Eclampsia, characterized by convulsions and coma, is associated with hypertension, edema, and proteinuria. The cause is unknown; however, the patient has predisposing factors that include renal and vascular diseases and sodium retention. Symptoms of preeclampsia develop into convulsions, coma, and hypertension.

Ophthalmoscopic examination reveals papilledema, retinal edema, or vascular spasms. Laboratory findings in eclampsia are greatly reduced blood carbon dioxide, increased serum uric acid, blood urea nitrogen, and nonprotein nitrogen.

The condition is serious for both mother and fetus. The patient with eclampsia or preeclampsia is given intravenous infusion of a balanced salt solution and 2 to 4 g of magnesium sulfate over four to six minutes to decrease the risk of convulsions. Blood pressure should lower with this treatment and stabilization should occur within four to six hours. The type of delivery depends on the condition of the patient. After delivery the patient's blood pressure needs to be monitored just as before delivery. In addition, repeat blood chemistry including complete blood count, urinalysis, blood urea nitrogen, and creatinine determinations must be obtained.

NOTE

1. Sylvia A. Price and Lorraine McC.Wilson, *Pathophysiology*, 2d ed. (New York: McGraw-Hill Book Co., 1982), 738.

Chapter 15

Neoplasms

Timothy E. Aldrich

Objectives

- Recognize and define specific terms from the vocabulary on neoplasms.
- Describe the general mechanism of carcinogenesis.
- List the major cancers in men and women.
- Discuss the diversity of neoplasms by anatomical site and cell type.
- Discuss the therapeutic approaches used for cancer management with specific examples for anatomical site.
- Describe the hospital- and population-based approaches for studying cancer.
- Discuss the epidemiologic descriptions (distribution, risk factors) for cancer in general and for selected anatomical sites.

Today the greatest medical concern facing Western society is cancer. As the nation's second leading cause of death (after heart disease), it is unchallenged in its capacity to instill fear in people. No other major disease exacts such a dramatic toll in human anguish and suffering. Accompanying this emotional tragedy is, all too frequently, a severe financial burden. Yet this is not the full story of cancer. In fact, there is much room for hope and optimism. This chapter presents some of the contemporary knowledge about this disease and its natural history.

Cancer is a cellular disease. As one studies it, this concept will reappear frequently. Cancer was first described clinically, the crablike appearance of the tumor being the basis for the Greek term—cancer. Today several terms are more frequently applied to the disease and in fact are more appropriate. A brief description of several key, cancer-related terms follows:

- *Neoplasm* Literally, new growth.
- *Carcinoma* A synonym for cancer; the most common cell type of the disease. The term applies to tumors arising from tissues of ectodermal (epithelial) origin.
- *Malignant* Implies proliferative growth, especially in a highly competitive and unrestrained manner. It is the attribute that distinguishes "cancer" from benign tumor.
- *Metastasis* The process of disease dissemination that results when single cells or groups of cells separate from the tumor and recolonize at remote body sites. This is a characteristic of cancer that is often substituted for the term malignancy.

These terms provide a basis for a superficial description of cancer. The disease begins on a cellular level. As the cell proliferates, a tumor is formed. Yet the behavior of this tumor, its malignancy, is what distinguishes cancer as the major health threat that it is today. As the malignant neoplasm grows, the cells comprising the neoplasm undergo a variety of changes; among these is metastasis and the appearance of remote foci of disease. As a consideration to the disease process, there is frequently a decline of body defenses.

The afflicted person often feels well for much of the early stages of disease. Since treatment is often aggressive, a misconception appears that the treatment is worse than the cancer. In advanced cancer, there is dramatic body wasting (cachexia). The lessened immune status of the patient often leads to severe infections, usually from casual pathogens. A frequent cause of death in cancer patients, then, is infection. It is fair to say that a person's body is simply overwhelmed by the growth of cancer. The process may continue for years, especially with heroic treatment. This leads to extended clinical courses and the lingering experience that is so frightening.

CANCER BIOLOGY

Let us look briefly at carcinogenesis. This is generally regarded as involving the steps of initiation and promotion.

Initiation

Initiation is the transformation of a normal cell into one that is (potentially) malignant. This step implies damage to the cell or its organizational units in such a way that the cell "looses its identity." Such a transformed cell will begin to behave differently from its neighboring cells and will begin to undergo changes in its metabolic processes. These changes may be gradual or delayed as the initiated cell lies "dormant."

Promotion

A second and separate step follows initiation to prompt the transformed cell(s) to grow. Often such growth will be more rapid than that of the surrounding tissue. The second event triggers the initiated cell to begin forming a neoplasm. Promotion may be removed in time from the initial event by years or even decades. The damaged cell line will begin to grow in an uncontrolled fashion and the process of carcinogenesis is complete.

As the tumor grows, the cells that constitute it compete with their neighbors. Such competition is often the basis for the weight loss and emaciation seen in cancer patients. Malignant tumors are characterized by necrotic centers, as their growth is too rapid to provide for adequate vascularization and thus nourishment. Therefore, the actively dividing cells are on the surface of the tumor, and as each new replication occurs, the cells change. The initally transformed cell retains characteristics of its original nature. Cancer cells go through generations of what might be termed "reverse evolution." That is, the cells become less and less differentiated. As the cells become more primitive, they exhibit less contact inhibition (adhesiveness) and, thus, are more likely to be swept away in blood or lymph. This is the process of metastasis. Furthermore, as the cells become less differentiated, they are more aggressive and will usually divide more rapidly.

Two points about the biology of cancer are often misunderstood by the lay public. First, as the cancer arises from once-normal cell lines, the body has an initial period of confusion in recognizing the change in the transformed cell. Too frequently, this failure on the part of the body's internal defenses leads to further failure later, when the differences in the cancerous cells become manifest. The body becomes reluctant to attack cells that it has difficulty distinguishing from "self," and in this weakened state, infections may flourish. Second, metastases are the most crucial aspect of cancer. The cells that spread to remote foci are, by selection, the most primitive and aggressive. Growth of these metastases is a frequent cause of cancer death, for vital organs, such as the liver, lungs, brain, and bone marrow, are predominantly affected.

THE CLINICAL COURSE

In many cancer diagnoses the finding is asymptomatic. The admonishment for annual examinations is valid. By the time cancer produces symptoms, the disease is often widespread and treatment efficacy is compromised. Several systematic elements of the clinical management of cancer are cited here briefly.

First, there is the concept of staging. Cancer begins at what is termed a primary site; this is the organ or tissue of origin. When the cancer is solid, as compared with fluid malignancies (i.e., leukemia, lymphomas), the identification of the primary site is often crucial. By identifying the originating cell line of the tumor, much information is garnered concerning its anticipated behavior. This deduction of cell type and the previously mentioned level of differentiation is the reason the pathological diagnosis of cancer is so vital. Elaborate coding schemes have been devised for identifying the anatomical site of cancer and the cell type. Also used for such data collection purposes is a graduated scale for the tumor grade, or level of differentiation, as shown in Table 15–1. These systems are included in the International Classification of Disease-Oncology; a subset of ICD-9-CM.

When a tumor is limited to its tissue or organ of origin, it is termed localized. Surgery is often successful for these circumscribed tumors, as they are removed en bloc. Cancer is a subtle illness, however, and owing to its cellular nature, the localized stage is rare for some body sites. As the cancer grows, it extends beyond the local tissues by the two mechanisms of (1) direct extension and (2) lymphatic drainage. This level of disease is termed regional and is generally treated by radiation therapy. Frequently, a course of radiation therapy may be prescribed as prophylaxis for occult regional spread in lesions not generally diagnosed at a localized stage (a good example of this is breast cancer).

When cancerous cells have extended beyond the directly contiguous tissues or the directly draining lymph nodes, this is termed distant disease. Chemotherapy is

Table 15–1 Grading Neoplasms

Grade	
I	Well differentiated
II	Moderately differentiated
III	Poorly differentiated
IV	Undifferentiated
V	Differentiation not determined

generally used to combat such multifocal lesions. Other systematic strategies may also be in order, such as hormonal manipulation and immunotherapy. Thus, staging has become an important aspect of clinical oncology (the study of tumors). The systems for quantifying the extent of disease involved with cancer are varied. The local, regional, distant descriptions are based on the American College of Surgeons' system. A more elaborate system is the TNM classification, which involves a site-specific quantification for the original tumor size (T), the number and size of lymph nodes involved with disease (N), and the presence or absence of distant metastases (M). Other site-specific systems are also commonly used, for example, the Dukes classification (colon cancer), Clark's levels (skin cancer), and the Lukes system and the Ann Arbor classification (both for lymphomas).

Second, there are the therapeutic strategies for cancer management. Surgery is a classic technique; the en bloc technique suggests that margins of normal tissue encompass the malignancy. When "clear" margins cannot be obtained, radiation therapy may be used to kill the faster-growing cancer cells. Here the rapid growth cycle of cancer cells increases their susceptibility to ionizing radiation, compared with healthy surrounding tissue. Radiation is given in cycles to permit recovery of the normal tissue, since this treatment can produce side effects. Likewise, chemotherapy can produce illness, especially in the debilitated patient. Chemicals intended to kill cancer cells necessarily will afflict normal cells as well. Great planning is needed for the administration of chemotherapeutic agents, strategy intended to maximize the drugs' effectiveness against the malignant cell lines.

Cancer cells have many attributes that can render them susceptible to chemical attack. They may have particular metabolic needs or growth characteristics that, if known, can be used against them. By using combinations of chemicals, lesser doses of any one chemical may be sufficient, yet cancer-cell killing may be maximized. Another systemic treatment for cancer cells is the manipulation of hormones. If the cancer arose from a cell line that is hormonally sensitive (e.g., breast tissue), then removal of that hormone or treatment with an antagonistic hormone may weaken the tumor. Removal of hormone-producing tissues may be part of cancer surgery; or a hormone may be included in a combination of chemotherapies. Another systemic treatment for cancer aims at reawakening the body's defenses to attack the cancer. These techniques of immunotherapy are still largely experimental, but such terms as interferon, monoclonal antibodies, and immune stimulation are becoming more common.

Another point on the clinical management of cancer is that each person's experience with this disease varies. Some general comments are offered, however. First, many cancers are slow growing (e.g., colon, breast). Even though the cancer cells are growing faster than the cells of their origin, this growth may still require several years or a decade to double the cancer cell population. Second, cancer is not inherited. However, some known familial syndromes do predispose to cancer; a family history of cancer is always a justification for careful medical follow-up. Third, most cancers arise from our environment. This includes the foods we eat, the things we drink (or inhale), as well as our work setting and place of habitation. These facts lead to an important point: Today more people die of cancers that can be cured than die of ones that cannot. Nearly one of every two cancer patients is clinically cured of their disease.

No discussion of the clinical aspects of cancer is complete without a mention of the many methods available for the early detection of the disease. When cancer is detected early, there is less cell volume to be combatted; the appearance of the more primitive, aggressive cells is lessened; and the therapeutic options are much greater. One of the best ways to detect cancer centers on the individual's initiative. Early recognition of some change in what is normal for one's self is a starting point, as shown in Exhibit 15–1. Cancer's warning signals are usually noticed by

Exhibit 15–1 Cancer Warning Signals

CANCER WARNING SIGNALS

CHANGE IN BOWEL OR BLADDER HABITS

A SORE THAT DOES NOT HEAL

UNUSUAL BLEEDING OR DISCHARGE

THICKENING OR LUMP IN BREAST OR ELSEWHERE

INDIGESTION OR DIFFICULTY IN SWALLOWING

OBVIOUS CHANGE IN WARTS OR MOLE

NAGGING COUGH OR HOARSENESS

IF YOU HAVE A WARNING SIGNAL, SEE YOUR DOCTOR.

the individual or an immediate family member. Additionally, a recognition of personal risk factors for cancer may lead one to be more cognizant of specific body systems and to any suspicious changes. There is no substitution for a regular medical examination. A fear of cancer should never immobilize one from a frequent check-up. ''Cancer phobia'' may generate its own justification by a reluctance to face up to one's own risks, thus leading to a dimmer prognosis if cancer is ever found. Many things may cause cancer death, but ignorance or fear should never be one of them.

GENERAL DESCRIPTION

Cancer is described as being more than 100 diseases. This means that there are some forty body sites at which cancer strikes, and with the combination of cell types at these sites, there are easily 100 separate pathologic entities. Oncology, the study of unusual growths in the human body, is beset by this diversity and the multitude of personal factors that influence clinical decisions. Yet there are characteristics that are known about the distribution of cancer, as well as about the determinants (risk factors) that are associated with these distributions.

OVERVIEW OF CONCEPTS

Consider these general patterns in the traditional epidemiologic triad of person, place, and time.

Person

Risk of cancer increases with age. Certain malignancies (e.g., the leukemias, some lymphomas) predominate in the first two decades of life. For most cancers, the age-specific incidence rates begin to incline most noticeably in the fourth decade and peak in the mid-to-late seventh decade. Men and women have different configurations of cancer, as shown in Table 15–2. Generally, women develop their cancers earlier in life than do men, yet men, overall, experience a higher rate of cancer. This information can be deceptive, as cancer occurrence should be considered on a site-specific basis.

Cancer varies by race. In the United States there are more white cancer cases than black ones, but this is due to the racial composition of the population. Blacks actually experience higher rates of several cancers than do whites (e.g., lung, esophageal, cervical). Generally, blacks tend to have higher cancer mortality than do whites. However, this has been associated with more advanced stages of disease at the time of diagnosis in blacks and lesser utilization of health care facilities.

Table 15–2 Estimates of Cancer Incidence by Site and Sex (1984)

	Male (%)	*Female (%)*
Skin	2	2
Oral	4	2
Lung	22	10
Colon and Rectum	14	15
Pancreas	3	3
Urinary	9	
Leukemia and Lymphomas	8	7
Prostate	18	
Ovary		4
Uterus		12
Breast		26
All Others	20	15

Cancer does not respect socioeconomic strata. All income groups and education levels are afflicted with cancer. Occupational risks for cancer are myriad, but these will not be elaborated on in this discussion. Some cancers are associated with affluent life styles; this is often a function of diet (e.g., colon cancer). Many cancers are associated with certain population groups; an example of this is the elevated risk of skin cancer in people with fair complexions and those with outdoor life styles. Certain religious groups (e.g., Mormons, Adventists) have characteristically lower rates of cancer; this is attributed to their vigorous life style. It is interesting to note that marital status (i.e., being married) is associated with earlier stages of diagnosis and better survival.

Place

The pattern of cancer occurrence is not static, either within the United States or internationally. Liver cancer is the leading cause of cancer death in the world, yet in the United States it is uncommon. Developing countries have higher rates of stomach cancer and cervical cancer than do the developed countries. As nations become more civilized or Westernized, their cancer patterns become similar to those seen in the United States. Lung cancer begins to predominate, with high rates of breast cancer, colorectal cancer, and the hormonally related tumors (e.g., uterine, prostate). A particularly interesting line of research has been the study of international migrants. As migrants tend to assume the cancer risks of their new home country, the large proportion of cancer risk that is environmental is evident.

Cancer patterns also vary within the United States, as shown in Figure 15–1. When one considers all sites combined, there are aggregations of high occurrence areas in the industrial Northeast and Midwest. As one inspects the site-specific maps, provocative patterns emerge that have given rise to several epidemiologic studies. The best example involves lung cancer investigations in Atlantic coastal counties. These studies identified asbestos exposure related to shipbuilding as the risk factor. The geographic patterns follow some known risk patterns, such as the north-to-south gradient in skin cancer rates; thus, the rate of sunlight exposure may be inferred. ''Place'' studies of cancer have been useful in identifying several rare relationships with cancer, such as the proximity to known emission sources and the risk of lung cancer.

Time

Cancer has been with us at least since the time of Hippocrates. Certainly, public emphasis and visibility of cancer have increased since the 1950s. Yet during that time most cancer rates have remained relatively constant. The most significant exceptions are lung cancer, stomach cancer, and uterine cancer. Lung cancer, especially in men and just recently in women, has shown a dramatic increase over time, which has been linked to a rise in cigarette smoking. Stomach cancer has declined since the 1930s; this trend is associated with more affluent, Westernized life styles. The decline in uterine cancer (specifically, mortality) is probably due to the advent of the Pap smear.

Figure 15–1 Estimated New Cancer Cases by State (1984)

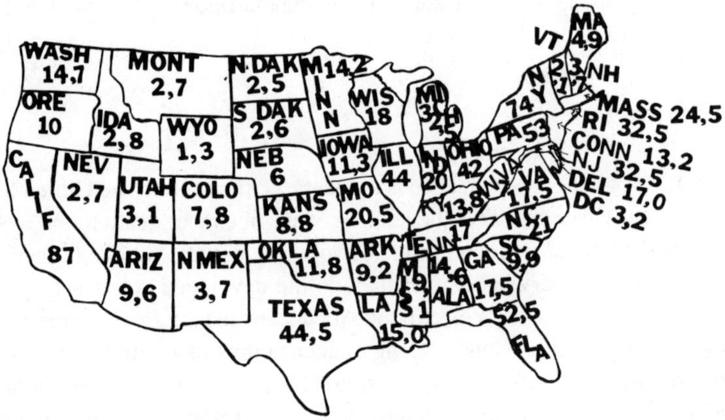

Source: Data based on rates from NCI Seer Program (1973–1979)
(Numbers × 1000; for example, Texas: 44.5 = 44,500)

This completes the survey of the board trends in cancer epidemiology. As a last point in this section, it is important to include a comment on major cancers and those for which the poorest survival is found. Lung cancer is the most common cancer in men; the fact that lung cancer is also a highly lethal disease leads to its domination of cancer statistics. As the male lung cancer epidemic approaches its apex, it is being followed by an incline in female lung cancer rates. As this severe cancer continues to lead the occurrence patterns in the United States, therapeutic advances made with other cancers have been overshadowed. Breast cancer is the leading cause of cancer death in women. However, recent advances in the detection and treatment of breast cancer have widened the gap between incidence and mortality.

The next most common cancer (in men and women) is cancer of the colon and rectum. This cancer is associated with dietary factors and is a disease of later life. Early detection is possible with several currently available, conventional techniques. Therapy can be successful with colon tumors diagnosed at an early stage. Sex-specific cancers are the next most frequently occurring cancers—prostate cancer in men and uterine cancer in women. Both types of malignancy are detectable at relatively early stages. These major cancers account for almost two-thirds of all cancers and well over half of all cancer deaths.

CANCER BY SYSTEMS

Circulatory System

The leading cancers of the circulatory system are the leukemias and the lymphomas. Leukemia is a disease of the blood-forming tissues (bone marrow). The two principal varieties are (1) myelocytic and (2) lymphocytic. Leukemia, by definition, is disseminated at diagnosis; there are, however, several successful combination chemotherapy regimens that are used for this illness. A distinctive attribute of leukemia is its bimodal age distribution; children (under age 15) and older adults (over age 60) are the main occurrence groups. Lymphomas strike young adults quite frequently but may occur at any age. There are myriad cell types of lymphomas, the most prominent being Hodgkin's disease. This lymphoma is characterized by Reed–Sternberg cells and has been treated successfully by radiation therapy and chemotherapy.

Respiratory System

Cancer of the nasal passages and pharynx (all subsites) is exceedingly rare. The general cell types are squamous-cell carcinomas. Therapy is almost exclusively a combination of surgery and radiation. Cancer of the larynx is common in smokers;

it is treated primarily by surgical removal of the larynx (laryngectomy). A form of esophageal speech can provide laryngectomy patients with a means of verbal communication after the loss of their voice boxes. Lung cancer is, of course, the most notable respiratory malignancy. Its association with cigarette smoking is a matter of sufficient fact that no elaboration is necessary. As mentioned earlier, lung cancer is not readily detectable and is a difficult malignancy to manage clinically. Survival with lung cancer is often expressed in months rather than years owing to its aggressive biology. This picture of lung cancer is not uniform; some types of lung tumors are more manageable than this gloomy depiction might suggest.

Squamous-cell carcinoma of the lung has the most dismal prognosis. This is the "smokers' cell type" and, unfortunately, is the most common. Adenocarcinoma (glandular cells) is the next most common variety of lung cancer, and some success has been found with chemotherapy against this cell type. Large-cell and small-cell (oat-cell) varieties, also common, are more successfully managed than the squamous-cell type. Surgery and radiation therapy can be used effectively against lung cancer when the lesions are diagnosed in a localized stage; unfortunately, this is an infrequent occurrence.

Several occupations are associated with cancers of the lung. Two of the most clearly linked are asbestos workers and uranium miners. Both these exposures provide an even higher risk of cancer when they are coupled with smoking.

Digestive System

Cancers of the oral cavity are predominantly squamous-cell types. Surgery and radiation therapy are the preferred methods of treatment, but some chemotherapy agents have been effective also (e.g., methotrexate). The association of these cancers with the combination of cigarette smoking and alcohol consumption is instructive for prevention. Local exposures, such as snuff dipping, tobacco chewing, and cigar smoking, are also risks for oral cancers. The highly vascularized tissues are a minus factor for advanced disease, yet diagnosis is often quite early and successful clinical courses are common. Significant strides have been made in the rehabilitation of these patients owing to use of individualized prostheses (artificial appliances, such as noses and cheeks). Cancer of the esophagus is essentially all squamous-cell type and the prognosis is bleak. This highly vascularized tissue is associated with rapidly fatal disease. The link to strong alcoholic beverages (as contrasted to wine or beer) is remarkable. Surgery is the principal therapy for esophageal cancers. Radiation therapy and chemotherapy are rarely used owing to the cachexic state experienced by such patients because of loss of nourishment. A supportive therapy, hyperalimentation, has been successful in sustaining these patients and others through a precarious nutritional state.

Cancer of the stomach is mostly adenocarcinoma cell type. The decline of this cancer in recent years is a distinctive attribute, since this pattern is so unusual. Consumption of smoked fish in Japan and a history of gastric ulcers are factors associated with this cancer. Like esophageal cancers, the lesions are primarily treated surgically. When advanced disease is forestalled, radiation therapy and, to a lesser extent, chemotherapy may be used. Stomach cancer is uncommon in the United States.

Several other rare digestive tumors are also noteworthy. Cancers of the liver are primarily hepatomas. Such cancers are so rapidly fatal that a heroic effort with chemotherapy is the main treatment. Cancer of the gallbladder or of the common hepatic ducts is likewise highly lethal and mercifully rare. Cancer of the pancreas has been termed ''epidemic'' by some researchers, yet even its increased occurrence ranks this cancer as extremely rare by comparison with the ''major'' cancers discussed in the preceding section (lung, breast, uterine, etc.). Cancer of the pancreas is usually of the islet-cell variety; the tumors are rapidly fatal and rarely diagnosed early. A distinctive surgical approach, Whipple's operation (pancreatoduodenectomy), and limited chemotherapeutic regimens are used to manage this cancer. Lastly, cancer of the small bowel is almost unheard of in the field of oncology. The rare occurrence is usually adenocarcinoma and surgical management is used most. The complete experience of digestive cancer above the ileocecal sphincter, however, is slight by comparison with the large bowel disease.

For years colon cancer was the second leading cancer killer in men and women; recently, lung cancer has eclipsed this distinction in women. Predominantly adenocarcinoma, this cancer site is readily studied by noninvasive imaging techniques (e.g., barium enema). Early detection of colon tumors is quite feasible, especially when screening is performed in high-risk audiences. People over age 40 should have regular bowel examinations; these may include the simple guaiac smear, a test that is designed to detect occult blood in the stool. Colon cancer occurs with disproportionate frequency in the descending portions of the tissue; this has the advantage of improving successful coloscoptic procedures for detection. Colonic polyps (especially familial) are associated with the disease, as is ulcerative colitis, diverticulitis, and chronic constipation. Slow bowel transit time has been deemed a major risk factor, thus the protective effects attributed to high-fiber diets and bulky stools.

The Dukes classification is the staging system used to define the extent of colon cancer. Colon cancers are managed mostly by surgical resection, often involving a temporary or permanent colostomy (a constructed, external orifice for fecal elimination). For nonlocal disease, radiation therapy has some utility and chemotherapy may hold promise. The potential for early detection of this slowly developing cancer is still one's greatest prognostic consideration. Rectal cancers, like most colon cancers, are readily accessible for early detection. They are also managed surgically and are generally included in descriptions of the risks linked to colon cancer. Rectal cancers are by no means rare, as mentioned for the upper digestive cancers; they simply represent an anatomical and systematic continuum with large bowel disease.

Musculoskeletal System

Sarcomas are the most common cell type for cancers of the musculoskeletal system. The prefix given to the sarcoma indicates the tissue of origin: osteo- (bone), myo- (muscle), leiomyo- (smooth muscle), rhabdomyo- (striated muscle). These cancers may occur at all body sites; pediatric lesions are relatively frequent. Lipomas (adipose tissue) and chondromas (cartilage) also occur, but rarely. These cancers are managed clinically by surgery and, to a much lesser extent, by radiation therapy and chemotherapy. An exception is pediatric osteogenic sarcoma (Ewing's sarcoma), which is often well managed by radiation and chemotherapy. Sarcomas are uncommon and detection usually follows a structural break (in bone), severe pain, or the detection of a mass (i.e., lipomas).

Nervous System

Nerve cell tumors occur at many sites, but cancers of the brain are the most prominent of the nervous system tumors. The various cell types include multiple types of gliomas, neuroblastomas, and astrocytomas. Benign tumors of the brain often prove fatal owing to the intracranial compression they can produce. Surgery is the foremost therapy for nervous system cancers, but radiation therapy and some chemotherapies have also been used.

Endocrine System

Cancers of the ductless glands are rare. Pituitary, adrenal, and thyroid cancers do occur, and the treatment of choice is surgery. Radioactive iodine has been used in the treatment of thyroid cancers and a freezing probe has been used experimentally with pituitary cancers. Owing to the vital function of the glands, these cancers are usually diagnosed secondary to metabolic disorders and are managed delicately. Benign tumors of these glands (e.g., thyroid adenomas) represent a serious health threat, although not as great perhaps as cancer. Mixed elements of benign and malignant are often found in tumor sections.

Genitourinary System

This complex grouping of body sites entails a diverse range of malignant tumors. Ovarian cancer is composed of a variety of germ-cell tumors, including a mixture of rare teratomas, sarcomas, and, notably, disgerminomas. Ovarian tumors are rapidly fatal and management is by surgery and radiation therapy. Cancer of the uterine fundus is associated with older women and a history of endometriosis. Surgery is generally the first desired course, followed by radiation therapy and, frequently, some form of hormonal manipulation. Often ovaries are removed (bilateral salpingo-oophorectomy) and additive hormones are given. Estrogen and progesterone receptor assays have enhanced hormonal therapy; these tests assist the clinician in anticipating which hormonal effects will affect the cancer's growth most adversely. Adenocarcinoma is the most common endometrial cancer cell type. Postmenopausal, additive estrogen therapy has been associated with this cancer, as has obesity, higher socioeconomic status, nulliparity, and anovulation syndromes.

Cancer of the uterine cervix is an important disease, not only because of its frequency, but because of its salutary place in early detection efforts. The advent of the Pap smear (named after Dr. George Papanicolaou) has led to a dramatic decline in the mortality of young women from this cancer. In situ carcinoma became a synonym for this squamous-cell lesion. This cancer is frequently diagnosed at the preclinical state. Surgical management of such tumors has become sophisticated, involving the use of lasers and freezing probes (colposcopy). Cervical cancer is aggressive when invasive (owing to the vascular tissue), yet this stage of disease is seen relatively less frequently today. This cancer is associated with a variety of venereal exposures, including herpes simplex virus type 2. Other tumors of the lower female genital system include cancers of the vagina and the vulva. The association of clear-cell carcinoma of the vagina with a history of in utero exposure to diethylstilbestrol is well known. Melanomas of the vulva are a common cell type.

Genital cancers in men are rare, as they are in females. Testicular cancers are mostly dysgerminomas or semiomas. Surgical resection (orchiectomy) is the most common first course; chemotherapy has recently been found to be a highly successful adjuvant (e.g., platinum). Cancer of the penis is exceedingly uncommon; surgery is again the choice for management. In males, the most common genitourinary cancer is of the prostate. This disease of older men (generally, age 60 and older) is almost entirely adenocarcinoma. It is often relatively indolent, one autopsy series reporting 10 percent of U.S. males having occult foci of cancer. Surgical resection is followed by radiation therapy and hormonal manipulation. Digital detection of this common cancer suggests the utility of screening, especially in high-risk populations.

Cancers of the bladder and kidney occur with about equal frequency in males and females. Kidney lesions are predominantly of the renal cell type, and the bladder ones are transitional cell. Surgery is the preferred course in these cancers, and an ileostomy (temporary or permanent) is not uncommon. Radiation therapy and chemotherapy are frequently adjuvant courses for advanced disease. These cancers are associated with cigarette smoking and some chemical exposures. Wilm's tumor, a pediatric kidney cancer, has a rare, genetic risk associated with it. Bladder and kidney cancers are not readily detected by any means useful for general screening, yet owing to their manifestation of urinary symptoms, early diagnosis is not infrequent.

Integumentary System

Skin cancer is essentially of three varieties: (1) squamous-cell carcinoma, (2) basal-cell carcinoma, and (3) malignant melanoma. Squamous-cell and basal-cell carcinomas are the "common" skin cancers owing to the expectation that almost half the population will develop one of these lesions during their lifetime. Fortunately, the success of surgical management for these cancers approaches 100 percent. These cancers are not even included in cancer statistics today, as they are so common and so curable. The third variety of skin cancer is a different entity. Malignant melanoma is characteristically a darkly pigmented lesion and most commonly occurs in sunlight-exposed areas and in the eye. The dermal variety is exceedingly aggressive if not detected early. Ocular melanoma is a rare and relatively indolent disease; it is associated with a long survival. Surgical resection is a successful approach for localized lesions, yet for disseminated disease, neither radiation therapy nor chemotherapy is effective. Exotic immunotherapies have been generally unsuccessful with dermal melanomas. Particular staging systems are used with melanomas, notably the Clark levels and the Breslow classification. These systems use depth of growth and surface area as indexes. Skin cancer is patently detectable, thus suggesting public screening of high-risk people. Included in this group are individuals of British or Scandinavian genetic stock, fair-complected people, those with a familial predisposition to moles or pigmented nevi, and, generally, anyone given to frequent sun exposure and an outdoor life style.

Breast cancer is included in this system rather than in the genitourinary, as the lesion is not directly related to the role of the tissue in pregnancy. Female breast cancer is the majority of the experience, yet men develop breast cancer too. Infiltrating ductal cell (adenocarcinoma) is the most common breast cancer for both sexes. Breast cancer is managed surgically, with recent innovations leading to less radical procedures. Radiation therapy and chemotherapy are highly effective with breast cancer. Hormonal manipulation is also a frequent adjuvant course, the strategy of additive or antagonistic hormones being based on tumor responsiveness. The estrogen receptor assay can aid oncologists in deciding whether estrogens will enhance the tumor's growth or whether androgens or progesterone may actually retard the cancer growth.

Breast cancer is associated with nulliparity, a positive family history, and life styles that lead to childbearing at later ages. Screening modalities for detecting breast lesions are led by mammography and its related forms (e.g., xeromammography). This low-level x-ray technique, coupled with palpation, can be an effective means of early detection, especially in high-risk people. The practice of regular breast self-examination has led to almost half of all breast cancers being self-detected. The increase in early detection and effective therapies has improved survival for this cancer. Effective rehabilitation programs and reconstruction techniques have improved the quality of life for mastectomy patients.

METASTATIC SITES

As mentioned earlier, the property of malignancy or the capacity for metastases is a distinctive characteristic of cancer. Not all cancers spread with the same degree of aggressiveness, however, nor with the same anatomical pattern. Breast and colon cancers, for example, generally spread initially by the lymphatic drainage systems. Lung cancer and melanoma spread most readily through the blood. The most common sites of metastases are the lungs, the liver, the brain, the lymph nodes, and bone marrow. Most solid cancers spread to one or more of these areas. As these tissues are patently vital, one sees how the actual cause of death frequently derives from the metastatic disease.

STUDYING CANCER

Cancer is a *chronic* disease; this adjective arises from the extended nature of the usual clinical course. Certainly, some tragically rapid deaths are involved in cancer, yet increasingly more patients are living longer with their disease and a larger portion of patients are being cured. These advances derive from the public's increased awareness of cancer, its response to early detection information, and knowledge of high-risk factors. Unfortunately, cancer's greater visibility leads many people to misconceptions about the disease, particularly the misunderstanding of its frequency and diversity. Cancer is a rare disease when studied on a population scale. Further, the disease is a mosaic of various body sites and specific cell types. The means by which cancer is studied or a population is studied are elaborated here.

Registries

Systematic identification and description of cancer patients has been the single greatest contribution to research in this field. Several types of registries exist and their nature and function will not be dealt with in detail here. Generally, the three types of registries are (1) hospital based, (2) population based, and (3) special group.

Hospital-based registries routinely review and prepare an abstract (record a condensed, specific data set) for all cancer patient records in their institutions. Case finding becomes an intricate process, and the data storage files are so elaborate as to have led to a proliferation of specialized computer applications. The cornerstone of hospital-based registries is the lifetime follow-up of all cancer patients. This ongoing appraisal of the patient's health has been the basis for much of the descriptive information on cancer today and has generated most of the major hypotheses related to advances in cancer (e.g., smoking and lung cancer).

Population-based registries are necessary for the study of cancer incidence, that is, the accurate reflection of the rate of new-case occurrence. Several states operate population-based registries, the oldest being in Connecticut. The U.S. government funds a set of SEER (surveillance, epidemiology, and end results) registries in strategic population centers. Population-based registries do not usually do follow-up because of the complexity and large numbers associated with such data systems.

Standard classification systems have been developed to facilitate the exchange of information between the population-based registries and the hospital-based registries. The TNM staging system discussed earlier is one such system; the International Classification of Diseases—Oncology (ICD-O) is another. The former is distributed by the American College of Surgeons and involves a site-specific measure of the clinical extent of disease. The latter is distributed by the World Health Organization and provides a numerical classification for both anatomical sites (topography) and the cell types (morphology).

Special registries have been created to follow groups who have specific characteristics related to cancer. Cancer patients receiving a particular therapy but who are not part of a clinical trial might be followed to form a case series. A special registry might be used to follow people who are of high risk of cancer owing to occupational or environmental exposures (e.g., Love Canal, Three-Mile Island). This procedure of lifetime follow-up is the critical specialty in registry science. As other diseases begin to practice the registry method of research, the need for this skill will increase.

One application of patient follow-up that is particularly germane to cancer is that associated with clinical trials. As registries have provided clues to the utility of certain therapeutic regimens, clinical trials have been performed to specify and quantify these advances. Clinical trials involve following similar groups of patients who are receiving different therapies to compare their responses. As previously mentioned, such follow-up often entails years of study. These expensive studies are not undertaken fully or done casually. Yet they are the basis for all therapeutic advances. Clinical trials represent a major aspect of the field of oncology.

CURRENT CONCEPTS

In concluding this chapter, some general comments are needed to address the most contemporary events related to cancer. These comments have been rather broadly grouped into the three topics: (1) risk factors, (2) genetic advances, and (3) prevention.

Risk Factors

An increasing focus is being given to the matter of chemical exposures in the environment. Certainly, the contamination of drinking water, soil, and air represent substantial issues. On the whole, however, exposures are at exceedingly small levels and the human body is amazingly resilient to such hazards. Attention is being given to the heavily exposed groups and to those who have an increased susceptibility to these exposures. Generally, the chemical environmental risks are associated with rare cancer (e.g., liver, brain, bladder). The major cancers continue to be associated with well-established risk factors: lung cancer (cigarettes), colon cancer (dietary factors), and breast cancer (parity and familial risks).

Genetic Advances

Cancer is a cellular disease. As the body of knowledge accumulates for the operation and mechanisms involved with cellular process, the secret to cancer draws closer. The discovery of latent genetic sequences that control cell proliferation and that may be triggered into action by environmental, viral, or even random events bodes great opportunity for the control of cancer. These so-called oncogenes may hold the secrets to why transformed cells become malignant and why some cancers grow much more aggressively than do others. Ultimately, a means for reversing or preventing these events may be found.

Prevention

Until such advances become a reality, however, the adages of public education and early detection pose the greatest opportunities to impact on cancer statistics. It is vital, therefore, to examine life styles and individual risk configurations in order to prevent cancer. Prevention is still the best strategy for dealing with this disease. Cancer control, like any other idea, only becomes possible when it is attempted.

REFERENCES

Philip Rubin, ed., *Clinical Oncology: A Multidisciplinary Approach,* 6th ed. (American Cancer Society, 1983), 1.

World Health Organization, *ICD-O: International Classification of Diseases for Oncology* (Geneva: World Health Organization, 1976).

Appendix A

The Practical Use of Diagnosis-Related Groups

On September 1, 1983, the *Federal Register* contained regulations on prospective payments for Medicare inpatient hospital services. Following these regulations, the examples in this appendix provide medical record abstracts in which the student may obtain practice in assigning one of the following for each case:

- Principal diagnosis/procedure
- ICD-9-CM codes
- Major Diagnostic Category (MDC)
- Diagnosis-Related Group (DRG)
- Diagnostic findings specific to the principal diagnosis

DEFINITION OF TERMS

Major Diagnostic Category (MDC). A major diagnostic category is a broad medical category based on the body system involvement and disease etiology. The categories were created by researchers at Yale University with a "sample of 400,000 medical records and classified into 23 major diagnostic categories."[1] For example, MDC 10 is endocrine, nutritional, and metabolic diseases.

Diagnosis-Related Group (DRG). Under major diagnostic categories (MDC) are related groups listed by diagnosis, age, and procedures. For example, listed under MDC 10 is DRG 285, amputations for endocrine, nutritional, and metabolic disorders. Figure A–1 shows MDC 10 and DRG 285.[2]

DRG Criteria. "The DRG criteria include the patient's age, sex, principal diagnosis, secondary diagnoses, procedures performed, and discharge status."[3]

Figure A–1 Endocrine Nutritional and Metabolic Diseases

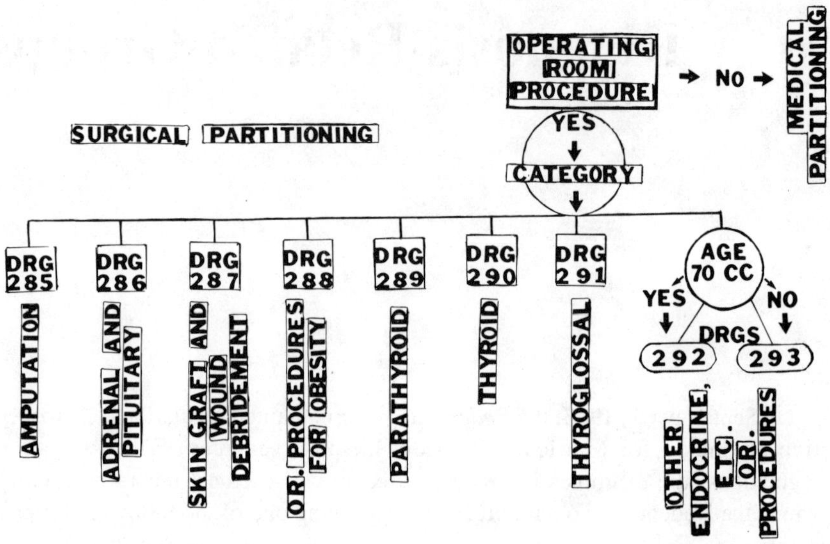

Principal Diagnosis. The principal diagnosis is the "diagnosis established after study to be chiefly responsible for occasioning the admission of the patient to the hospital for care."[4,5] Only one diagnosis can be listed as the principal diagnosis.

Secondary Diagnosis. Secondary diagnoses include comorbidities and complications. Secondary diagnoses should be listed according to resource consumption from highest to lowest. A *comorbidity* is a condition that existed before the patient's admission to the hospital and affects treatment received or length of stay.[6] A *complication* is a condition other than the principal diagnosis that occurred while the patient was in the hospital.[7]

Principal Procedure. A principal procedure is a definitive operation related to the principal diagnosis,[8] for example, an appendectomy performed on a patient admitted for acute appendicitis.

An operating room procedure unrelated to the principal diagnosis, but necessary to take care of a secondary diagnosis first in the order of resource consumption, and not performed for exploratory and/or diagnostic purposes, requires a special code 468, which appears later in this appendix.[9] For example, a patient may come into the hospital for pneumonia. However, during the stay an appendectomy is performed. The pathology report documents the secondary diagnosis, acute appendicitis. The resource consumption for the secondary diagnosis, acute appendicitis, is higher than the resource consumption in the primary diagnosis, pneumonia.

Resource Consumption. Resource consumption is the cost of services used by the patient owing to a specific diagnosis.[10]

Discharge Status. The discharge status of a patient may be leaving the hospital without the doctor's permission (AMA), being discharged to the home with the doctor's permission, expiring, or being transferred to another hospital or nursing facility.[11]

CASE STUDIES*

Case #1: Example

The patient is a 73-year-old white male who was admitted to the hospital after several episodes of weakness, numbness, and loss of sensation in his left arm and leg. His first experience of the foregoing symptoms lasted about 30 minutes and the last time, a day.

Significant findings on physical examination revealed diminished arterial pulsation and bruit.

Angiography revealed only minimal obstruction of the carotid arteries.

It was decided to try the patient on a trial of aspirin therapy before starting anticoagulants.

The patient was discharged after four days of hospitalization.

Final Diagnosis: Arteriosclerotic cerebrovascular disease
Cerebral ischemia
Principle Diagnosis: Cerebral ischemia
ICD-9-CM Code: 437.1
MDC: 01
DRG: 017

State the diagnostic findings that substantiate the principal diagnosis chosen. The diagnostic findings were periodic episodes of numbness, weakness, and loss of use of his limbs. The angiography revealed minimal obstruction of the carotid arteries.

Case #2

The patient is a 71-year-old obese white female admitted because of progressive anorexia, dehydration, lethargy, irritability, confusion, and muscle cramps.

---

*Answers to the case studies may be found at the end of Appendix A, preceding the Notes.

The patient is a known paraplegic after removal of a spinal cord tumor many years ago.

During the hospital course, it was found that the patient had an electrolyte imbalance, which was corrected. A CT scan of the brain was normal; there were no intracranial mass effect, hemorrhage, subdural collection, or hydrocephalus.

Clinical laboratory tests revealed dilution of serum Na concentration of 110 mEq/liter.

After seven days of hospitalization, the patient was transferred to a nursing home.

Final diagnosis: Electrolyte imbalance
Hyponatremia

Case #3

The patient is an 83-year-old black male admitted with diagnosis of status postcolostomy of the colon for carcinoma of the colon. Physical examination revealed a well-healed paramedian scar on the left side of his abdomen. He is admitted for a postoperative colonoscopy.

The patient underwent a colonoscopy with removal of multiple polyps in the area of the sigmoid colon. There was no evidence of the recurrence of carcinoma of the colon. The patient was discharged after two days of hospitalization.

Final diagnosis: Status postcarcinoma of the colon
Polyps of the colon
Procedure: Polypectomy
Colonoscopy

Case #4

The patient, a 66-year-old Latin female, was admitted to the hospital through the emergency room with the diagnosis of advanced metastatic carcinoma of the lung from previous carcinoma of the breast excised by mastectomy five years ago. Before this admission the patient received chemotherapy but failed to respond at this time. Chest x-ray reveals far advanced carcinoma of the lung. The patient continued to deteriorate and expired after the second day of hospitalization.

Final diagnosis: Metastatic carcinoma of the lung from previous carcinoma of the breast removed five years ago by mastectomy.

Case #5

This 77-year-old white male was admitted to the hospital with a diagnosis of abdominal pain with a history of inability to defecate for the past three days. The flat plate of the abdomen revealed evidence of fecal impaction but was otherwise within normal limits. Chest x-ray revealed arteriosclerotic plaques.

The patient was given an enema and discharged the next day.

Final diagnosis: Fecal impaction
Arteriosclerosis

Case #6

The patient, a 40-year-old white woman, was admitted to the hospital complaining of an abrupt onset of chills, fever, anorexia, malaise, arthralgia, and hematuria two days after a dental extraction.

Physical examination revealed petechiae of the skin, hemorrhages of the nail beds, Janeway lesions on the palms and soles, splenomegaly, and systolic murmur.

A clinical laboratory blood culture taken during chills revealed a staphylococcal infection sensitive to penicillin and streptomycin, which was given in massive doses.

The chills and fever abated after the third day of treatment. After a week the blood culture was negative for staphylococcal infection. The patient was discharged on the tenth day of hospitalization without fever and was instructed to continue antibiotic therapy for another week before returning to the doctor's office.

Final diagnosis: Bacterial endocarditis, staphylococcal
Post–dental extraction

Case #7

This 45-year-old black male with a blood pressure of 145/95 was admitted complaining of dizziness, weakness, nervousness, and palpitation. He stated that for about a week he had experienced a dull headache on awakening in the morning; the headache did, however, wear off during the day.

Physical examination revealed a five-foot, 160-pound obese black male. His blood pressure, taken on three occasions over two days by two nurses, was found to be 145/95. Ophthalmic examination revealed constriction of retinal arterioles. The lungs were clear to auscultation and percussion. The heart was found to be within normal limits in size.

Electrocardiography revealed P-wave abnormalities and a fourth heart sound. Chest x-ray revealed heart and lungs within the lower limits of normal. Blood and urine for sugar were normal.

The patient was placed on a low-salt, weight reduction diet to reduce blood pressure. During his week of hospitalization on a diet, his blood pressure dropped to 140/90. The patient was instructed by the dietician before leaving the hospital and he was told to return to the doctor's office the following Thursday.

Final diagnosis: Essential hypertension
Exogenous obesity

Case #8

This 50-year-old white male entered the hospital complaining of back pain in the costovertebral region, frequency of urination, dysuria, nausea, vomiting, and chills with fever of one-week duration.

Chemical laboratory culture of catheterized urine specimen revealed *Escherichia coli* sensitive to tetracycline. Urine also revealed red and white blood cells. Renal function studies were not significant.

Excretory urography revealed slight hydronephrosis and a small renal calculus of the right kidney.

The patient was placed on antibiotic regimen of tetracycline. Urine culture repeated within two days after therapy did not reveal bacteria.

The patient was discharged on antibiotic therapy after five days of hospitalization and was instructed to return to the physician's office in a week.

Final diagnosis: Pyelonephritis, *Escherichia coli*
Renal calculi

Case #9

This 33-year-old black female entered the hospital complaining of dull, aching pain and a bearing-down pressure in the lower abdomen and back area. The patient has a history of severe dysmenorrhea that began in her early 20s. She has also had problems with infertility; although she has been married for ten years, with frequent intercourse, she has never become pregnant.

The admission physical examination was entirely within normal limits. Routine blood chemistry and urinalysis were also within normal limits.

Diagnostic dilatation and curettage under general anesthesia revealed two small, superficial lesions on the cervix. Biopsy performed at the time of the examination revealed endometriosis.

The patient was placed on danazol 800 mg per day in an attempt to inhibit ovulation and suppress the endometriosis. The patient was discharged after three days.

Final diagnosis: Sterility
Endometriosis, cervix
Procedure: Diagnostic dilatation and curettage
Vaginal biopsy

Case #10

This 30-year-old Haitian male entered the hospital complaining of weight loss, weakness, irritability, and excessive thirst and urination.

The physical examination on admission was entirely within normal limits. X-rays and scans were reported to be within normal limits.

Admission blood chemistry revealed a fasting blood sugar of 140 and urinalysis was reported as 3+ for sugar. On the third day after admission, an oral glucose tolerance at the third hour returned a blood sugar of 200 and urinalysis was reported as 3+ for sugar.

The patient was regulated on a diabetic diet and 20 units of intermediate-acting insulin daily before breakfast. The patient was discharged after eight days of hospitalization with dietary and insulin administration instructions. He was to test his urine daily with the stick test and return to the doctor's office the following Wednesday.

Final diagnosis: Diabetes mellitus
Anxiety

Table A–1 Complication and Comorbidity (C.C.) Codes Pertaining to Case Studies

202.6-208.9,	276.1,	437.2,	592.1,
242,	276.9,	437.4-437.6,	593.5

Table A–2 Procedure Codes Pertaining to Case Studies

CODE	EXCLUDE (INVALID DRG CODES)
45	45.12-45.14, 45.19, 45.22-45.29
67	67.0
69	69.52-69.7, 69.91-69.94, 69.96

Exhibit A–1 Diagnosis Related Group Listings Pertaining to Case Studies

MDC 01 Nervous System

DRG 016 Nonspecific Cerebrovascular Disorders

All ages* with comorbidity or complication (C.C. see Figure 2) codes 348.3, 348.8, 348.9, 349.89, 349.9, 437.0, 437.1, 437.8, 437.9.

DRG 017 Nonspecific Cerebrovascular Disorders

All ages without C.C. codes 348.3, 348.8, 348.9, 349.89, 349.9, 437.0, 437.1, 437.8, 437.9.

MDC 04 Respiratory System

DRG 082 Respiratory Neoplasms

All ages codes 162–163, 164.2–164.9, 165.8–165.9, 195.1, 197.0–197.3, 212.2–212.5, 212.8–212.9, 213.3, 214.2, 231.1–231.9, 235.7–235.9, 239.1, 795.1.

MDC 05 Circulatory System

DRG 126 Acute and Subacute Endocarditis

All ages codes 036.42, 093.20, 098.84, 112.81, 115.04, 115.14, 115.94, 421.0–421.9.

DRG 134 Hypertension

All ages codes 401.0–401.9, 402.00, 402.10, 402.90, 404, 405.01, 405.09, 405.11, 405.19, 405.91, 405.99.

MDC 06 Digestive System

DRG 157 Anal Procedures

All cases ages 70 and over; ages 0–69 with C.C. codes (Figure 3 for invalid procedure codes). 45.33, 45.41, 46.4, 48.35, 48.73, 48.79–49.02, 49.04, 49.11, 49.12, 49.3, 49.44–49.46, 49.49–49.73, 49.79–49.99.

DRG 158 Anal Procedures

Ages 0–69 without C.C. codes 45.33, 45.41, 46.4, 48.35, 48.73, 48.79–49.02, 49.04, 49.11, 49.12, 49.3, 49.44–49.46, 49.49–49.73, 49.79–49.99.

*The term "ages" refers to the patient's age.

Exhibit A–1 continued

DRG 180 Gastrointestinal Obstruction (G.I.)

All cases ages 70 and over; ages 69 or under with C.C. code 560.

DRG 181 G.I. Obstruction

Ages 69 or under without C.C. code 560.

MDC 10 Endocrine System

DRG 294 Diabetes

All cases ages 36 and over codes 250.0–250.4, 250.6–250.9, 791.50.

DRG 295 Diabetes

Ages 35 and under codes 250.0–250.4, 250.6-250.9, 791.50.

DRG 296 Nutritional and Miscellaneous Metabolic Disorders

All cases ages 70 and over; ages 18–69 with C.C. codes 251.0, 251.2–269.9, 275.2, 275.4, 276–277.0, 278, 781–790, 791.6.

DRG 297 Nutritional and Miscellaneous Metabolic Disorders

Ages 18–69 without C.C. codes 251.0, 251.2–269.9, 275.2, 275.4, 276–277.0, 278, 781–790, 791.6.

DRG 298 Nutritional and Miscellaneous Metabolic Disorders

All cases ages 0–17 codes 251.0, 251.2–269.9, 275.2, 275.4, 276–277.0, 278, 781–790, 791.6.

MDC 11 Urinary System

DRG 323 Urinary Calculi

All cases ages 70 and over; ages 0–69 with C.C. codes 274.11, 591–592, 593.4–593.5, 594.1–594.9, 788.0.

DRG 324 Urinary Calculi

Ages 0–69 without C.C. codes 274.11, 591–592, 593.4-593.5, 594.1–594.9, 788.0.

MDC 13 Female Reproductive System

DRG 364 Dilitation and Curettage and Conization, Nonmalignant.

All ages codes 67.1–67.2, 68.21–68.22, 69.09, 92.27.

MDC 23 Factors Influencing Health Status

DRG 468 Unrelated Operating Room Procedure

ANSWERS TO CASE STUDIES

1. Cerebral ischemia: ICD-9-CM code 437.1, MDC 01, DRG 017, verified by historical data.
2. Hyponatremia: 276.1, 10, 298, laboratory reports.
3. Polypectomy, polyps of colon: 45.41, 211.3, 06, 157, pathology report.
4. Metastatic carcinoma, lung: 197.0, M8000/6, 04, 082 radiology report.
5. Fecal impaction: 560.39, 06, 180, radiology report.
6. Bacterial endocarditis, staphylococcal: 421.0 and 041.1, 05, 126, physical examination and blood culture results.
7. Essential hypertension: 401.9, 05, 134, blood pressure and electrocardiograph.
8. Pyelonephritis, escherichia coli and renal calculi: 592.0 and 041.4, 11, 324, radiology report and urine culture results.
9. Dilitation, curettage, and conization, cervical endometriosis: 67.2, 617.0, 13, 364, pathology report.
10. Diabetes mellitus: 250.01, 10, 295.

NOTES

1. Health Care Financing Administration (HCFA), ''Medicare Program; Prospective Payments for Medicare Inpatient Hospital Services; Interim Final Rule, with Comment Period,'' *Federal Register* 48 (September 1983):39760.

2. Ibid., 39882.

3. Ibid., 39761.

4. Ibid.

5. Report of the National Committee on Vital and Health Statistics, *Uniform Hospital Discharge Data: Minimum Data Set* (Hyattsville, Md.: National Center for Health Statistics, 1980), DHEW No. PHS 80–1157, 12.

6. Joan Loughran and Barbara Moore, ''Medical Record Association of New Jersey Technical Seminars on 1982 ICD-9-CM DRGs,'' November 1981.

7. Ibid.

8. Ibid.

9. HCFA, ''Medical Care Program,'' 37961.

10. This is my explanation from 14 years of work in the area of accounts receivable.

11. HCFA, ''Medical Care Program,'' 39759–39760.

Index

B

C

D

F

I

J

M

N

O

P

Q

R

S

T

About the Author

FLORENCE C. AMATO is an Associate Professor and Director of the Medical Record Administration Department at Florida International University in Miami, Florida. Before starting this program in 1977, for five years Florence Amato was the coordinator of a medical record technology program in Cincinnati, Ohio. Her affiliation with the health care industry spans 40 years and includes positions as hospital administrator, director of medical record departments, director of admissions and accounts receivable, transcriptionist, and nurse's aide. *Fundamentals of Medical Science for Medical Record Personnel* is the culmination of a lifetime of dedication and study and the desire to share her knowledge with others in her own profession.

Born in St. Louis, Missouri, Dr. Amato has also lived and worked in Tennessee, South Carolina, Ohio, Kansas, and Wisconsin. She currently resides with her husband, Paul, in North Miami Beach, Florida. In addition to a bachelors degree in Medical Record Administration, Dr. Amato holds two masters degrees, one in social work and the other in human relations research. Her doctorate is in the philosophy of education. In her next book, on research techniques for department administrators, she intends to use this extensive and versatile background to again write for medical record personnel.

About the Contributors

TIMOTHY E. ALDRICH is a faculty associate in the School of Public Health, University of Texas, Houston, Texas, and an adjunct faculty member of the Department of Epidemiology, University of Miami, Miami, Florida. He is currently working on a special project at the Oakridge National Laboratory, Health and Safety Research Division, Oakridge, Tennessee.

Born in Alabama, Dr. Aldrich's work and study have taken him all over the United States. At the University of Alabama, he earned a masters degree in public health with a major in cancer epidemiology. At the University of Texas he pursued his Ph.D. in epidemiology with minors in biostatistics and environmental health. This rich educational background is coupled with extensive research and work experience in cancer studies.

JUANITA S. PURSEL is an Assistant Professor in the Medical Record Administration Department at Florida International University, Miami, Florida. She holds a bachelor of science degree in medical record administration and a masters in social work. Ms. Pursel is currently pursuing her doctorate in public administration at Florida International University.

Born in Los Angeles, California, Juanita and her three children have lived in Miami Springs, Florida, since 1975. Although her specialization in teaching is administration, Ms. Pursel maintains her involvement with the medical science aspects of her field through study and research. Her current research involves medical records in a medical examiner's office.